The Neurodiversity Affirmative Child Autism Assessment Handbook

of related interest

The Adult Autism Assessment Handbook
A Neurodiversity Affirmative Approach
Davida Hartman, Tara O'Donnell-Killen, Jessica K Doyle, Dr Maeve
Kavanagh, Dr Anna Day and Dr Juliana Azevedo
ISBN 978 1 83997 166 2
eISBN 978 1 83997 167 9

The Little Book of Autism FAQs
How to Talk with Your Child about their Diagnosis and Other Conversations
Davida Hartman
Illustrated by Margaret Anne Suggs
ISBN 978 1 78592 449 1
eISBN 978 1 78450 824 1

A Therapist's Guide to Neurodiversity Affirming Practice with Children and Young People
Raelene Dundon
ISBN 978 1 83997 585 1
eISBN 978 1 83997 586 8

THE NEURODIVERSITY AFFIRMATIVE CHILD AUTISM ASSESSMENT HANDBOOK

Dr Maeve Kavanagh,
Dr Anna Day, Davida Hartman,
Tara O'Donnell-Killen, Jessica K Doyle

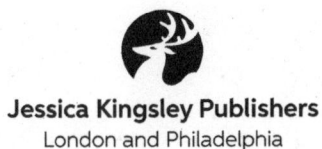

Jessica Kingsley Publishers
London and Philadelphia

First published in Great Britain in 2025 by Jessica Kingsley Publishers
An imprint of John Murray Press

2

A CIP catalogue record for this title is available from the British Library and the Library of Congress

ISBN 978 1 80501 165 1
eISBN 978 1 80501 168 2

Printed and bound in Great Britain by CPI Group

Jessica Kingsley Publishers' policy is to use papers that are natural, renewable and recyclable products and made from wood grown in sustainable forests. The logging and manufacturing processes are expected to conform to the environmental regulations of the country of origin.

Jessica Kingsley Publishers
Carmelite House
50 Victoria Embankment
London EC4Y 0DZ

www.jkp.com

John Murray Press
Part of Hodder & Stoughton Ltd
An Hachette Company

The authorised representative in the EEA is Hachette Ireland,
8 Castlecourt Centre, Dublin 15, D15 XTP3, Ireland (email: info@hbgi.ie)

CHILD'S VOICE

EDIE, AGE 7

I have situational mutism so when my Mummy and Daddy told me about my assessment I was happy and excited to find out what type of brain I have too. But I was really really scared to go to meet new adults. I sat on my Mummy's lap but the adults were kind and nice and I really wanted to play with some of their toys. They had fidgets I didn't try before and I really liked them and the noise they made and the adults were really funny. After a while I forgot that I was nervous and I was even able to talk. And I was laughing a lot. I liked lying on the floor and winning all the games. I didn't want to go home. It was my favourite best day because that was the day we figured out that I'm Autistic.

This book is dedicated to the Autistic young people we have been lucky enough to meet and know. We are grateful to them for trusting us with their stories and giving us the privilege of walking this part of their journey with them.

It is also dedicated to the wider Autistic community: those who share their stories and found connection on social media, the advocates who have borne the brunt of the prejudice against Autistic people as they push for basic human rights and demand that our voices are the ones leading the conversation about us, the Autistics who remain in institutions around the globe, punished by a world that seeks to extinguish that which it does not understand, Autistics who hold multiple marginalised identities and have exponentially greater barriers and prejudices to navigate, Autistic parents/caregivers who daily navigate outside pressure to force their children to conform to neurotypical societal norms and the Autistic clinicians, practitioners and researchers who work tirelessly and bare their soul daily, all for the greater good of protecting and promoting the rights and well-being of the Autistic community.

Contents

Acknowledgements.. 12

1. **Introduction** 15
   1.1 Who We Are and Why We Wrote This Book   15
   1.2 Introduction   16
   1.3 Making a Paradigm Shift: Reorientation   19

2. **Language Use** 21

3. **A Brief History of Autistic People and the Neurodiversity Movement**...... 35
   3.1 A Brief History of Autistic People and the Neurodiversity Movement   35
   3.2 Common Criticisms of the Neurodiversity Movement   52

4. **Learning from Lived Experience**...................................... 56
   4.1 Introduction   56
   4.2 Stories and How They Shape Us   56

5. **The Neurodiversity Paradigm and Neurodiversity Affirmative Practice**..... 68
   5.1 Introduction   68
   5.2 What Is the Neurodiversity Paradigm?   68
   5.3 What Is Neuro-Affirmative Practice: How to Work in This Way   73
   5.4 Conclusion   80

6. **Understanding Autistic Experience** 82
   6.1 Introduction   82
   6.2 Label vs. Identity   82
   6.3 Examining the Information We Hold   84
   6.4 Whose Voices Are Heard, and in Which Circumstances?   86
   6.5 The Notion of 'Normal'   87
   6.6 Construction of the 'Normal Child'   88
   6.7 What Is Being Autistic?   91
   6.8 Understanding Sensory Needs: A Brief Overview   106
   6.9 Executive Functioning   114
   6.10 Double Empathy   121
   6.11 Masking   125
   6.12 Monotropism   128
   6.13 Conclusion   130

7. **Autistic Developmental Trajectory** **131**
   7.1 Introduction   131
   7.2 Language Used in Developmental Descriptions   131
   7.3 Developmental Delay or Developmental Difference   133
   7.4 Autistic Developmental Trajectory   133
   7.5 Interest-Led Development and Monotropism   138
   7.6 Cognitive Development and How It Is Measured   139
   7.7 Conclusion   142

8. **Other Neurodivergencies** **144**
   8.1 Introduction   144
   8.2 ADHD   144
   8.3 Specific Learning Difficulties   150
   8.4 Intellectual Disability   153
   8.5 Giftedness   156
   8.6 Conclusion   159

9. **Mental Health, Trauma and How They Intersect with Autistic Identity** **160**
   9.1 Introduction   160
   9.2 Mental Health   161
   9.3 Trauma   163
   9.4 Conclusion   166

10. **Important Considerations** **167**
   10.1 Introduction   167
   10.2 Power and Process Issues within a Formal Autism Identification Process   167
   10.3 Working with Families with Previous Difficult Service Experiences   169
   10.4 Gender Variance and GSRD   171
   10.5 Intersectionality / Ethnic Minorities   173
   10.6 Autistic Neurology – Age for Identification   176
   10.7 Children in Care   176
   10.8 Self-Identification and the So-Called 'Widening' of Diagnostic Criteria   178
   10.9 Conclusion   179

11. **Conducting a Sensory Audit** **180**
   11.1 Introduction   180
   11.2 Sensory Audit Preparation and Key People   181
   11.3 Conducting Your Audit   183
   11.4 Assessment of Flexibility in Appointments and Space Settings   192
   11.5 Conclusion   194

12. **Making the Identification Process Accessible** **195**
   12.1 Introduction   195
   12.2 Barriers to Accessing Healthcare Settings   196
   12.3 Accessibility Considerations for Young People and Caregivers   202
   12.4 Conclusion   212

13. **Best Practice Guidelines** **213**
   13.1 Introduction   213
   13.2 Best Practice Guidelines   213

13.3 Evaluation of Current 'Diagnostic' Criteria – What Is Helpful and What Is Not   216
13.4 Conclusion   221

14. A Neurodiversity Affirmative Perspective on Autistic Neurology Assessment Tools   **222**
14.1 Introduction   222
14.2 Issues with Current Assessment Tools   223
14.3 Screening Tools   227
14.4 Assessment Tools   230
14.5 Helpful Questionnaires   235
14.6 The Pathway Forward   240
14.7 Conclusion   241

15. Conducting the Identification Process   **242**
15.1 Introduction   242
15.2 Preparing for the Process   242
15.3 Selecting Tests / Questionnaires and Working with Other Informants   246
15.4 Steps in a Neuro-Affirmative Process of Exploring Autistic Neurology with Children and Adolescents   249
15.5 Supporting Children and Young People Who Do Not Wish to Attend   275
15.6 Involvement of Multi-Disciplinary Team Professionals   276
15.7 Cognitive and Other Assessments   277
15.8 Reports and Other Documentation   279
15.9 Conclusion   284

16. Post-Identification Support Recommendations   **285**
16.1 Introduction   285
16.2 Within a Neuro-Affirming Framework, Is Support Needed?   286
16.3 Educational and School-Based Recommendations   289
16.4 Home-Based Support Recommendations   303
16.5 Pervasive Drive for Autonomy and Low-Demand Parenting   313
16.6 Clinical Recommendations   314
16.7 Conclusion   320

17. Conclusion   **321**

Appendices   324
Appendix 1: An Outline of Many Aspects of Current Criteria Re-Framed Within a Neuro-Affirmative Framework   324
Appendix 2: Sensory Audit Checklist   328
Appendix 3: Questions to Send to Young People in Advance of Their Session to Help Them Prepare and Provide Predictability   334
Appendix 4: Neuro-Affirmative Autistic Criteria – Mapping Document – Option 1   337
Appendix 5: Neuro-Affirmative Autistic Criteria – Mapping Document – Option 2   339

References   342

Subject Index   360

Author Index   372

Acknowledgements

Thank you to Helen Edgar, Katie Kerley and Elaine McGreevy for their invaluable input into this book.

Thank you to the amazing and dedicated teams of clinicians in Childversity, The Children's Clinic, The Adult Autism Practice and Thriving Autistic, who strive so hard for excellence in supporting Autistic young people and their families, and do it with such empathy and kindness.

Thank you to Philomena McCarthy for her invaluable input and thoughtful insights.

Thank you also to all the children and young people who contributed their own stories and experiences to the book.

Thank you to our families and those most precious to us:

Maeve would like to thank Barry, Maisie, Ben and Penny; Vera, Barry, Kieran and Elaine; Karen, Suzanne and Nem; and Jane for always listening.

Anna would like to thank Daisy for all her wisdomous wisdom, Flower, Peanut and Teddy (and Basil) for feline joy, and Nosh and Phil for their support. Thanks also go to Rebecca of Sussex Police (who made it safe to unmask), Julia (and Flora) for all their support which meant writing somehow continued. For Camelia, always remembered, always loved x

Davida would like to thank Max, Ely and Juno, William, Riona, Martina, Amy, Deirdre, Gloria, Ida and Roisin. I would especially like to thank my forever sister Annemarie and Márcio for their life saving support over the course of this book writing year.

Tara would like to thank her wonderful, funny, kind and inspiring children:

Lucas, Ray and Oisín. Gavin for his boundless encouragement and for never letting a day pass without sharing deep belly laughs, Sam for her unwavering faith and wise feedback. Jenny, Katherine and Fiona for the forever fun, and all the Autistic young people in her life who infuse it with such vibrancy and meaning.

Jessica K would like to thank Owli and Astro for their company, cuddles, mayhem and mouse adventures. Fred for being the best critic; Penelope and Cat for their hugs, body doubling and tea; Ruth and Oana for their support, friendship and wisdom; Mum for providing a space for our deep reflective talks even when I haven't talked to her in weeks; and Dad for all his reminders and nagging me to do all the things I always forget to keep me healthy and alive.

And finally, thank you to our editor Amy Lankester-Owen for all her ongoing support and enthusiasm and the entire publishing team at Jessica Kingsley.

Multi-Disciplinary Contributions

Occupational Therapy contributions for this book were provided by Katie Kerley, Autistic Clinical Specialist Occupational Therapist, Clinical Director of Horizons Therapy Services.

Speech and Language contributions for this book were provided by Elaine McGreevy, neurodivergent Speech and Language Therapist, Access Communication Ltd and Co-Founder of Divergent Perspectives.

Teaching and Education contributions for this book were provided by Helen Edgar, Autistic Teacher (Early Years / Primary, Special Educational Needs), Founder of Autistic Realms and Neuro-Affirmative Family Support Specialist with Thriving Autistic.

Childversity, The Children's Clinic and Thriving Autistic

Childversity was established in 2021 and is based in Kildare, Ireland. The team is a mixed neurotype, multi-disciplinary team specialising in neurodiversity affirmative exploration of Autistic identity with children and adolescents up to the age of 18 years. The importance of working closely with the Autistic community and of being informed by the preferences and needs of the community is at the heart of Childversity.

The Children's Clinic is a mixed neurotype, multi-disciplinary team of clinicians based in Dublin, Ireland which was founded in 2017. The clinic specialises in neurodiversity affirmative support for Autistic and otherwise neurodivergent young people aged 0–18 and their families, with an emphasis on neurodiversity affirmative Autistic identification exploration. It has a strong reputation for clinical excellence in the field.

Thriving Autistic is a non-profit dedicated to promoting the human rights of neurodivergent people. Founded in 2020, Thriving Autistic provides an online platform for Autistic and otherwise neurodivergent psychologists, therapists and allied health practitioners to promote their services. The team at Thriving Autistic partner with several neurodiversity affirmative clinics to offer post-identification support services for families.

As authors, we are mindful of the privilege, power and platform that we have in writing about Autistic experience, one that is not available to many Autistic people. In this book, we therefore seek at all times to honour our privilege and use it with great care and respect whilst we acknowledge that we do not and cannot speak for all Autistic experience. For example, those of us in the author team who are Autistic are mindful that we have educational privilege in being able to write about Autistic experience, and that our personal experiences of being Autistic will be very different from others' given the diversity of Autistic experience (e.g., we need to consider multiple marginalisations, intersectionality, co-occurring learning disabilities etc.).

CHAPTER 1

Introduction

Everything I say makes sense, it just depends who's listening.

DAISY (2023, AGE 13)

1.1 Who We Are and Why We Wrote This Book

We are a mixed team of neurodivergent and neurotypical colleagues. We are one of the only groups of psychologists worldwide providing neurodiversity affirmative autism assessments for children and adults across different settings in a progressive, neurodiversity affirmative framework (while still operating within the current best practice diagnostic frameworks). We are an adjunct professor, educational, clinical and coaching psychologists, an assistant psychologist/Autistic researcher, friends and colleagues who have come together with the shared purpose of, and passion for, supporting Autistic children and adults to live their best lives, in the recognition that for this to be within access of every Autistic person, there are significant societal changes (see Chapman, 2023) that need to be made in relation to how we understand and assess Autistic neurology.

This book approaches the collaborative assessment of Autistic identity ('diagnosis') from a neurodiversity affirmative standpoint that is rooted in the authors' allyship with and membership of the Autistic community. From this perspective, being an Autistic child is conceptualised as being as a valid a way to be in this world as the perceived neuro-majority, rather than considering being Autistic as reflecting 'deficits' in social communication etc. We have all seen first-hand in our work and private lives the enormous positive benefits that correct identification of being Autistic brings to children. We have seen how it can change the trajectory of a child and their wider family's life significantly to not only have been correctly identified as Autistic, but also to have been assessed through a neurodiversity affirmative framework. We have also unfortunately seen the real damage done when a child is not correctly identified as Autistic, or an assessment is carried out in way that it causes trauma and long-lasting harm.

Some of the authors of this book are parents/caregivers as well as professionals and have lived experience of wrestling with systems which do not mirror our neurodiversity affirmative approach to our young people's neurology, or our professional practice. As professionals we passionately advocate for neuro-affirmative practice, both for our own young people and those with whom we work, in the knowledge that we might not always 'get somewhere' but what matters is we worked towards change (Ahmed, 2021).

1.2 Introduction

Whilst there are many books published on how to undertake child autism assessments (typically these draw from a medical model with a deficit-based framing of Autistic experience), this book is the first published on how to undertake child autism assessments using a neurodiversity affirmative approach. It is our intention with this book, therefore, to support professionals already assessing and working with Autistic children to make a shift in practice to neurodiversity affirmative child autism assessments. The book is not intended to provide a complete training for professionals with no experience of autism assessments.

We hope that through changing your practices to be more neurodiversity affirmative, you too will experience the rich, genuine and moving connections that we have daily with the children that allow us the privilege of taking this part of their journey with them. These have been some of the most profound connections of our clinical experience, reflected in the beautiful words that many Autistic children have shared with us about their experience. This way of working is life-affirming and joyous.

We aim in this book to provide as much practical, 'how to' information as possible, whilst also covering the vital background information and up-to-date research that professionals need to know before starting, as it is the shift in thinking and perspective from a medical model to a neurodiversity affirmative model that will be the most vital learning for assessing clinicians.

Whilst we have sought to present practical and accessible material, readers will also note that we present a considerable amount of academic discussion and cite a significant amount of research. This was a deliberate decision because there is so much guidance about and research underpinning deficit-based assessments to counterbalance. We seek both to provide practical guidance for conducting a neurodiversity affirmative identification piece as well as discuss the underlying research/knowledge base.

Undertaking neurodiversity affirmative assessments is a new and emerging area which many professionals feel ill-equipped to work within because of a lack of knowledge, or they can often feel hindered in adopting this approach by the current systems in which they work. Whilst we know many healthcare teams that have already adopted this neurodiversity affirmative approach with enthusiasm, we are aware that worldwide the vast majority of teams and individuals undertaking this work are coming from a medical model. It can be hard therefore for individual, progressive clinicians to make changes in the teams they are working in. Our book seeks to empower clinicians to make this paradigm shift whilst acknowledging the challenges of working within a system that is inherently deficit-based, providing practice points and clinical reflections on how to embed neurodiversity affirmative principles in their individual practice.

We discuss this also in our book *The Adult Autism Assessment Handbook* (Hartman et al., 2023), which provided a detailed account of working within a neurodiversity affirmative approach during the collaborative identification process, in that case with Autistic adults. In this book for working with children, we will address many of the same areas we covered in the adult book, as they are highly relevant here also, and derive from the shared principles that underpin neurodiversity affirming assessment approaches.

We include here tips and methods that we have found helpful during the assessment process (e.g., preparing children, teenagers and their parents/caregivers for the process such as giving advance notice of questions, providing video clips of the assessing professionals, and reducing language load through methods like the chat function on Zoom, and adapting the clinical space to meet sensory needs within the constraints of the setting). We also provide guidance in how to undertake a collaborative identification piece that is both best practice and meets current traditional diagnostic (medical model) criteria while at the same time considering newer, more respectful ways of understanding Autistic identity. We include first-person accounts from Autistic professionals, parents and children who have been through an assessment process. We include reflective practice examples to help professionals with adapting their approach. Information about post-identification support and recommendations for parents/caregivers and young people are also detailed.

Finally, we explore the wider systems in which the identification process is located (e.g., school, health, social care) and make practice recommendations for working within these (often deficit-driven) systems whilst adopting a neuro-affirmative approach. We explore ideas underlying the importance of making a paradigm shift, critically examining the underlying knowledge base, such as considering how diagnostic criteria can be re-used (mindful that longer term, we would seek to advocate for a wider conceptualisation of Autistic experience that does not involve being designated as disordered).

Put simply, we will guide clinicians into framing an understanding of Autistic experience as a natural part of diversity and difference and how to adapt current child assessment approaches to become neurodiversity affirmative.

SOME NOTES ON LANGUAGE AND RESEARCH CITATIONS IN THIS BOOK

1. As you move through the book, you will notice that we choose to capitalise Autistic. We do so intentionally to reflect that being Autistic is both a neurology and an identity.

2. We make no assumption in this book that any reader is neurotypical and intentionally challenge neuro-normative assumptions. We therefore deliberately alternate between writing about Autistic people and using 'we' when describing Autistic experience as we also invite the reader to join us in not perpetuating 'us' and 'them' perspectives in writing about our community.

3. We have chosen not to repeat the rhetoric of deficit in relation to the Autistic experience, or to cite directly researchers whose work is both rejected by and has caused harm to the Autistic community. Whilst doing so, we hold in tension the need to follow best practice research whilst evaluating that research critically and

through a neuro-affirmative lens. Throughout the book, to echo our position that as clinicians we should always question the authority of knowledge sources, by whom it was produced and whose position was privileged, we deliberatively reference Autistic writers, researchers and bloggers where possible, recognising that all sources of knowledge are valid but some people do not have the privilege of sharing that knowledge widely (Gray-Hammond, 2022).

1.3 Making a Paradigm Shift: Reorientation

Each of us has travelled different journeys in making our shift to neurodiversity affirmative practice and come to different understandings of why we have done so. Our paths unify in passionate commitment to advocating for change. Wherever you are starting from in your work with Autistic children, the beginning is learning about the Neurodiversity Paradigm. However, making a shift in our clinical practice requires engaging not just intellectually but emotionally. Making this shift in practice seems like a huge undertaking. It requires reading work by Autistic researchers, writers, bloggers etc. and being aware of epistemic violence, which is the harm done in the process of knowledge production, e.g., by not including Autistic people in producing research about their own experiences; or non-autistic researchers dominating research about Autistic experience (see Fricker, 2007). And yet paradoxically, it is also not a huge undertaking. The biggest piece is wanting to learn, develop, do things differently with the children and families you work with.

We offer you in this book some reasons to make a shift in practice, including highlighting the injustices surrounding the construction of past and current knowledge around the Autistic experience, exploring current conceptualisations of being an Autistic child and adult, and an overview of the Neurodiversity Paradigm. We also invite reflection on the context in which diagnostic criteria were developed (e.g., whose voices were included in the research driving those criteria, were they developed by neurotypical clinicians privileging neuro-normative communication?). Exploring the 'ethics of autism', Hens (2021) reminds us to question the idea of 'dysfunctioning' and who gets to decide what this even is. We aim to support you to locate your personal reasons for making a paradigm shift, but there is no right reason. The most important part is seeking to make a change, whatever route you have come by to read this book and whatever reason you find to motivate a shift in practice. We welcome you.

IMPORTANT NOTE ON THE LANGUAGE OF 'ASSESSMENT'

Although we have used the word 'assessment' here and in the title of our book, as neurodiversity affirmative clinicians, we prefer to call this work 'collaborative Autistic identification' as the word 'assessment' is steeped in the medical model and has the connotation of something being 'done' to someone by someone else with power. In contrast, what we do is support children and their parents/caregivers collaboratively to discover their neurology, which is going to be their neurology whether they meet with us or not. Therefore, throughout this book you will mostly see the use of the term 'collaborative identification', or similar, instead of assessment. Where we do use the word assessment, we use it for ease of reading and so people will understand what we are referring to. However, we continue to advocate for changes so that in the future the terminology of 'collaborative identification' will be used instead.

Language Use

This chapter summarises key issues around language use when discussing difference and disability, and the preferred terminology of the Autistic community. The content is adapted from our adult book (Hartman et al., 2023, Chapter 2, pp. 16–27). It is so important to use language respectfully and aligned to the community it describes that we choose to reproduce key points here for readers not familiar with our previous text.

When embarking on an exploratory piece in relation to Autistic identity with a young person and their family, it is essential for clinicians and professionals to be aware of and up to date in terms of current language and terminology. When working with young people, clinicians are working with a wide variety of adults in the young person's life. The language used in relation to a young person has a significant impact on perceptions about them, and the language used by clinicians during the process of exploring Autistic identity is extremely important in terms of their sense of identity.

Many parents, families and caregivers begin the process having heard much alarming language in relation to their child, usually during the referral stage of the process. 'Concerns', 'red flags', 'delays' etc. are just a few examples of the type of language that is attached to any difference in development, and this type of language communicates to parents and caregivers that being Autistic is something negative that they should be worried about in relation to their child. Meeting with parents and caregivers at the initial stages of the process provides an opportunity to introduce affirmative language to the process, if it isn't already there. This is hugely important in terms of cultivating a positive Autistic identity, should their young person be identified as Autistic.

Honouring the language preference of any disability group is a sign of both professional awareness and respect, as well as a way of offering solidarity (American Psychological Association, www.apastyle.apa.org/style-grammar-guidelines/bias-free-language/disability). By using a community's language of choice, and avoiding ableist and damaging language, we can help build more accommodating and understanding societies for Autistic (and otherwise neurodivergent) people to thrive in. Changing our language is, of course, not easy and is a constant process of attention to, and reflection about, the words we use. It also means staying up to date with a community's preferences as language choices evolve over time. We need to focus deliberately on moving away from our bias for familiarity and challenge ourselves to change the language we are used to using. You may feel uncomfortable changing your language or have your own preferences but unless you are part of the community being described, set aside your preference and respect those of the community. It is part of our role as health and caring professionals to keep up to date with respectful language use for a community or population of people. Using outdated, harmful or incorrect terminology is a sign to Autistic people that you do not care about their voice, that you do not know or listen to any Autistic people and ultimately it damages your professional reputation with them. Using the language choices of a community shows that you are a professional who is respectful, sensitive and inclusive.

As professionals working with Autistic children, it is not only our responsibility to identify or provide therapeutic support to the best of our ability and knowledge, but also our responsibility to more broadly support and advocate for the community we serve. This, of course, includes listening to the communities with which we work who have a right to decide for themselves how they choose to be spoken about.

> Language continually evolves over time, and will no doubt continue to change for the Autistic community also. This means that the language recommended in this book may not always be correct in the future. If you are unsure of the language to use, seek guidance from self-advocacy groups, such as groups that are led by Autistic people,

> Sometimes the language individual people use to describe themselves will differ with wider community preferences. When working with individual people, always use the language they choose to use to describe themselves.

WHAT IS 'NEUROTYPICAL'?

Neurotypical is a descriptive term that refers to having qualities related to one's neurotype that are compatible with the design of the dominant systems (i.e., not 'neurodivergent' as defined by being Autistic, being an ADHDer, having obsessive-compulsive disorder (OCD) etc.). For more on this, see: www.verywellhealth.com/what-does-it-mean-to-be-neurotypical-260047.

According to Walker (2021), being neurotypical is a term for those who align their thoughts, feelings, behaviours, self-expression etc. with societal norms for neurotypicality. Walker suggests that neurotypicality is not a fixed entity and that anyone can harness their 'weird potentials' to become neurodivergent. We use neurodivergent in its broadest sense (including autism, dyspraxia, dyslexia, ADHD, acquired brain injury, post-traumatic stress disorder (PTSD), depression, Tourette's, OCD etc.).

We acknowledge that the terms neurodiversity and neurodivergent are framed in ways that hold both similarities and differences between different epistemologies (e.g., disability studies, critical autism studies, Neuroqueer Theory) and allow space for understandings that differ from our own.

The following are the current language preferences for the majority of the Autistic community.

Use 'Autistic person', not 'person with autism'

The majority of the Autistic community and Autistic-led Autistic organisations prefer the use of identity-first language (i.e., Autistic person) over person-first language (i.e., person with autism). This is well-established by countless research, blogs and opinion polls conducted with and by Autistic people. Person-first language is typically experienced by Autistic people as offensive and disrespectful to their neurotype. It is disrespectful for professionals to continue using identity-first language rather than following the preferences of the Autistic community.

There are many different perspectives amongst parents, caregivers, teachers and professionals on whether person-first language (i.e., 'I am a person with autism') or identity-first language (i.e., 'I am an Autistic person') should be used when referring to Autistic people. However, research has consistently shown that the Autistic community in English-speaking countries themselves have indicated that they wish to use identity-first language and do not wish to use person-first language (Botha et al., 2023). Some arguments in favour of the use of identity-first language relate to the intrinsic nature of Autistic identity (i.e., it is not something an Autistic person can 'remove' or change about themselves), and how with person-first language, the 'person with...' is usually followed by something negative. For example, we don't say 'I am a person with talent', we say 'I am a talented person'. Conversely, we don't say 'I am a cancer person', we say 'I am a person with cancer'. The use of person-first language in relation to Autistic people has been shown to have material risks for the Autistic community as language shapes understanding, concepts and perception, and may accentuate stigma (Gernsbacher, 2017). These material risks include an increased risk of mental health challenges and also interpersonal victimisation, especially for those who are non-speaking (Botha et al., 2023).

Language preferences may differ within Autistic communities across different countries and languages. A number of studies have demonstrated a preference among the Autistic community within Dutch-speaking countries for person-first language (Buijsman et al., 2023; De Laet et al., 2023), with the authors concluding that Dutch language and culture play a role in word preference. Little research has been carried out in other non-English-speaking countries as to terminology preferences, and factors such as less knowledge and/or more stigma in relation to being Autistic may be influential in terms of language connotations (Bosman & Thijs, 2023).

Many professionals will have attended a multitude of training courses which frame the Autistic neurotype as an overwhelmingly negative experience and a disorder, and suggest that all co-occurring conditions (e.g., epilepsy, intellectual disabilities and OCD) and responses to environment (e.g., mental health issues and anxiety) are a direct consequence of being Autistic. It is likely that within these courses person-first language was used and recommended, either explicitly or implicitly. Unless you are Autistic yourself, outside of your professional life, in the media and in non-autistic-led community groups, person-first language has also likely been the dominant framing.

Jim Sinclair (an Autistic activist who wrote some of the formative Autistic rights essays, including 'Why I dislike person first language' in 1999) pointed out that the only time we separate a person from their condition is when we see that condition in negative terms or believe it is incompatible with their human side.

Whilst we would hope that in the present day, most professionals working with Autistic children and adults would know that identity-first language is the community's preference, you will probably continue to encounter professionals incorrectly using person-first terminology. Adapting to a new understanding and new language use is challenging and requires conscious and consistent effort, and begins with making the choice to do so. For those who take the steps to reflect and examine thoughtfully, the feelings that identity-first language bring up in us can reveal a lot, highlighting our ableism, bias for familiarity and unconscious negative attitudes towards Autistic people. It shows just how much being Autistic is categorised in our heads alongside burdens and life-limiting medical conditions.

If you are new to using identity-first language, for all the reasons outlined here it can feel uncomfortable for a while. It was for the neurotypical authors of this book, who were using identity-first language for months before it felt natural.

Respecting individual preferences when working with people is important. But for books, reports, research papers, policy documents and people for whom you do not yet know their preference it is vital to choose identity-first language.

Interestingly, it would appear that most Autistic people who prefer person-first language have spoken mostly to professionals (who used outdated language) only and have not yet linked in with the Autistic community or are aware of the Neurodiversity Paradigm or Movement. The first professional to talk to a person about being Autistic will have a lasting impact on their language use going forward.

Many professionals worry that by using identity-first language they will upset or alienate clients or their families (or indeed other professionals). Of course, as clinicians we want to be seen as caring and respectful, and it is true that some people around you may not be up to date with respectful language choices and may query your choice of words. But if this is the case, be a force for change. Explain to people why you are using identity-first language. Use these situations as a learning opportunity to teach people about the Autistic community, and the importance of listening to them. It may be one of the most valuable lessons you impart.

Use 'disabled person', not 'person with a disability'

In modern discourse, many disability groups choose identity-first language as a preference ('disabled person' as opposed to 'person with a disability').

Disability groups who embrace being disabled as part of their cultural and/ or personal identity are more likely to prefer identity-first language. For them, the use of identity-first language is an expression of cultural pride and a reclamation of a disability that once conferred a negative identity.

This has not always been the case, as previously person-first language (i.e., a 'person with a disability') was how the majority of disabilities were framed and spoken about in the media and research journals. This changed over time as disability activists fought hard for the use of person-first language to combat how they had been dehumanised and abused historically. They sought to be treated and spoken about with the same respect and dignity as those who weren't disabled. Now, paradoxically, it is mostly non-disabled people who advocate for the retention of person-first language.

Again, the common argument used to promote person-first language in relation to being disabled in general was that it helped the person using that language to remember that the person is a 'person first' and not just 'their disability'. This highlights a misunderstanding of why identity-first language is preferred. Today, it is recognised and understood that identity-first language (i.e., disabled person) is preferred because it acknowledges that it is not that the person 'has' disabilities, but that they are a 'disabled person' because they are disabled by society and how it is not designed for, or indeed by them. Identity-first language acknowledges the role of the environment and the external factors that disable the person. A disabled person is disabled because they are actively disabled by the environment (an external force), rather than focusing on a person 'having' a disability which incorrectly suggests the disability as being within the person, belonging to the person, an issue with the person or something that is the sole responsibility of the person to change or live with.

There are some disability groups who prefer person-first language. In addition, there are some disability groups who, while being similarly disabled, live in different countries or regions and disagree with each other on how they would like to be referred to. Where it is unclear, you should research preferred language choices by contacting advocacy groups and organisations in the country you are working in. Again, make sure that the organisation is led, or at least heavily influenced by (e.g., having a high percentage of disabled people on the board of a charity), the community you are investigating.

Most important in our minds should be the Autistic children we are supporting, and the effect on them of growing up feeling that 'autism' is something that is a small and detachable part of them, that could or should be removed.

There is a need at times to gently introduce these concepts because many parents (who remember have quite a high likelihood of being Autistic themselves) and caregivers also grew up in a world with negative messaging about Autistic people and being taught to 'see the person first' which is shorthand for 'see the neurotypical person first'. If you are identifying Autistic children, you will of course meet many parents/caregivers with a strong preference for their child to be spoken about using person-first language, and this needs to be explored in more depth with them in relation to the foundations of where this comes from (as outlined in this book).

The neuro-affirmative concepts described within this book need to be introduced with compassion. It is also our job as clinicians to educate and support parents/caregivers to understand that language is powerful, and how parents/caregivers conceptualise the Autistic experience (and neurodiversity in general) now will have an impact on how their children understand themselves and their community in the future. Educating families helps break ongoing stigma and ultimately links parents/caregivers in with an important community that their child (and likely at least one of the parents) belongs to. This is a community of people who care about their child, and the future of their shared community. The way you as a professional frame being Autistic to these families will affect how these children come to understand themselves, how they value themselves and being Autistic, and how others see them and value them and their integral Autistic neurology.

Parental priorities are heavily influenced by the professionals they first meet as well as the resources and books they are then provided with post-diagnosis. Remember that many parents/caregivers you meet may actually have already discovered they are Autistic (and have chosen not to disclose to you) and so when talking about their child being Autistic, you are also talking about them. Respecting the place that parents/caregivers are at in their journey is vital for trust, but continuing to educate and gently point them towards information that is up to date and respectful is also vital and will benefit the family as a whole in the long term.

Talk about Autistic neurology, Autistic experience and Autistic people. Do NOT use autism spectrum disorder, ASD, autism spectrum condition or ASC

Using the words disorder or condition (which is inherent in ASD and ASC) is not neurodiversity affirmative and fully rejected by the Autistic community. More and more, these authors also have been avoiding using the word 'autism' by itself, instead using terms such as 'Autistic experience' or 'Autistic people'. This is because 'autism' itself is an abstract construct created within a specific societal context. What do exist are Autistic people, Autistic experience and Autistic neurology.

Talk about high or low support needs in specific areas. Do not use high functioning / low functioning

Two other terms that are frequently used are 'high functioning' and 'low functioning'. These are misleading and harmful. 'High functioning' is often attached to Autistic people who speak, are not intellectually disabled and who are likely to attend mainstream school. Low functioning is usually attached to those who are less likely to use spoken language, who are intellectually disabled, and who likely attend specialist school settings. The implication is often that those who are 'high functioning' are 'mildly Autistic', while those who are 'low functioning' are more 'severe'. Despite much research to the contrary, the term 'high functioning' has become synonymous with expectations of strengths in language, higher IQ, lower support needs, and better long-term outcomes (Fein et al., 2013; Howlin et al., 2014).

This conceptualisation of there being 'high' or 'low' functioning is incorrect and damaging. Conceptualising Autistic people as 'high functioning' implies that they need lower levels of support, which is often not the case. Conversely, conceptualising people as 'low functioning' implies that they need higher levels of support, which is also often not the case. All Autistic people (whether they speak, are intellectually disabled or regardless of the school setting they attend) have support needs that fluctuate. Support needs depend on the environment a person is in, their level of stress, their access to regulation and their mental health. A person who uses spoken communication and who has average intelligence may have very high support needs (and be 'low functioning') if they are in an environment that is over-stimulating and overwhelming. Similarly, a person who does not use spoken communication and who is intellectually disabled may have access to environments that are low stimulation and that promote regulation, and their support needs may be relatively low. Level of intelligence has been shown to be a poor predictor of functional capacity amongst Autistic people, particularly for those who are not intellectually disabled (Alvares et al., 2020) and the term 'high functioning autism' has been identified as an inaccurate clinical descriptor (Alvares et al., 2020).

Using high and low functioning is an outdated and disrespectful way to talk about people. Instead talk about a person's individual support needs and be specific about the areas you are talking about. Here is an example: 'Zavier currently has high support needs in relation to mobility in busy places and currently needs and wants a person to accompany him when out in the community. Zavier has low support needs in relation to advocating for his own needs. He prefers to communicate by text or email and has good IT skills.'

When someone is labelled 'low functioning', what naturally follows are low expectations and segregation. Yet when someone is labelled 'high functioning', what naturally follows is people not believing how high some of this person's support needs may be, for example not believing or understanding that this person may experience burnout, shutdown or be unable to speak at times. Thus, they are expected to struggle through difficult situations often to the detriment of their mental health. There is also ableism inherent in these terms, how they imply that to be Autistic and to openly show Autistic traits (e.g., stimming) is wrong in itself and means someone is lesser than another. An often-quoted phrase in the Autistic community is 'High functioning doesn't have to do with how disabled someone is. It is to do with how well they pass as neurotypical.'

The experience of being Autistic in a world not designed for you can bring to light different strengths and throw up challenges that are individual to the person within different environments. These challenges and strengths are not static and are dependent on context. They change depending on environment, internal states, external influences, energy levels, life events and seasons, moment by moment. There are so many different ways of being Autistic that using terms such as high or low functioning is nonsensical and unhelpful. Within the Autistic population there is the same amount of diversity that exists in the neurotypical population. Across both populations there are children and young people with, for example, different skills, preferences, abilities, types of intelligence, sensory systems, values, levels of support required, ways of being independent, things that are considered important to them. Using high and low functioning is like using a blunt axe to pick apart and describe the multitude of layers and depths that make up each individual child. Time and context add even more layers to be considered, as all people change, grow and fluctuate in the levels of support they need depending on their age, health, life stage, environment and personal circumstances.

That is why the concept of a spectrum is so helpful when understanding Autistic children and young people (although please do not use 'on the spectrum' as it implies again that someone is separate and 'on top' of something rather than it being part of their being). The spectrum concept allows children and young people to be individuals, who will need support at different times of their lives, individual to them.

Lived experience: Voice of a parent in response to medical model, non-neurodiversity affirmative language used in documentation.

Dear Clinician,

Thank you for your letter which arrived today. Please can you amend and reissue to correct some inaccuracies.

Please use Autistic, not Autistic spectrum disorder, in line with the preference with the Autistic community. Being Autistic is our neurology, not a deficit, as outlined by the Neurodiversity Paradigm. Please do not refer to X having a diagnosis. This is not neurodiversity affirmative language and is not the language I use professionally, and nor does X. Please state simply X is Autistic or has been formally identified as Autistic.

Please remove 'due to X's diagnosis' and replace with 'Consistent with Autistic experience, X can become overwhelmed...'

Other ableist language to avoid:

- Talk about 'passions'; avoid the use of the term 'special interests' which is deemed as patronising.

- Avoid referring to neurotypical milestones. For example, instead of saying 'Mary was delayed in reaching her milestones', use phrases like 'increased likelihood of being Autistic'. Do not use 'at risk for autism' or 'red flags for autism' (both of which are medicalised and deficit-based).

- Talk about the Autistic developmental trajectory instead of developmental issues or delay. If you are going to refer to 'developmental milestones', it could be stated that 'Mary began using words to communicate at 3 years old, which does not align with neurotypical developmental milestones, but may be more in keeping with an Autistic developmental trajectory' (see Leadbitter et al., 2021).

- Avoid talking about 'concerns' in relation specifically to Autistic traits or characteristics, as this implies that these are inherently negative, or even dangerous. This does not mean that you cannot highlight concerns about areas that are causing distress, e.g., self-harm, intense pain from sensory experiences, loneliness or mental health issues.

- Talk about Autistic 'characteristics' or 'features' instead of 'symptoms' or 'impairments'.

- Talk about Autistic communication styles or Autistic communication preferences instead of 'social impairment' or 'lacks social skills' (see information about the double empathy problem in Section 6.10).

- Talk about providing 'supports' or 'adaptations' instead of 'treatment' or 'treating'.

- Talk about the co-occurring needs and challenges instead of attributing all difficulties to being Autistic.

See the box below for a speech and language therapist's view on neurodiversity affirmative language and terminology.

PERSPECTIVES OF AN SLT: NEURODIVERSITY AFFIRMATIVE LANGUAGE AND TERMINOLOGY

ELAINE MCGREEVY

To disrupt and dismantle the medical model pathology approach to the Autistic experience, speech and language therapists (SLTs) should address the language of deficit and of subjective value judgements. CommunicationFIRST is a civil rights organisation led by and focused on the estimated five million people in the United States with speech-related communication disabilities. To reflect the diverse experiences and preferences of those with communication disabilities, they produced a language guide in 2023. They propose using the phrase, 'people who cannot rely on speech alone to be heard and understood', as an inclusive term referring to people who cannot speak at all, as well as people who may be able to use speech some of the time to communicate their thoughts effectively and be understood by others. Zisk et al. (2023) identified terms that were more and less preferred in a survey of 556 people with a variety of relationships to augmentative and alternative communication (AAC) on behalf of AAC app developers, Assistiveware. Drawing on this guidance, the following preferred terms are proposed for use in clinical practice:

- 'AAC users' or 'people who use AAC' are preferred over terms such as 'people who rely on AAC'. Information about working with children and young people who use AAC is provided on page 204.

- 'AAC supports' and 'communication supports' are preferred over terms such as 'AAC strategies'.

- 'Speech generating device' is a less preferred term.

- 'AAC device' is preferred over infantilising terms such as 'talker'.

- 'Non-speaking' is a commonly used and preferred term to describe a person who does not use spoken language. The term 'non-verbal' is least preferred, especially within the Autistic community. The term verbal refers to language, a cognitive skill. Language is produced by a motor action, such as speaking, signing, using gestures or typing. Use of the term non-verbal may lead to incorrect and potentially dangerous assumptions that a person does not have language or does not think. Use of non-speaking reminds the observer or supporter to avoid falling into the trap of making false assumptions about a person's capabilities based on their ability to use mouth words.

- Terms such as 'beginning', 'emerging' or 'emergent' communicator disregard and devalue the person's already established forms of communication. Similarly, the terms, 'preverbal' and 'pre-intentional' are used to describe a person's language based on neuro-normative assumptions about communication. 'The inability to demonstrate language by using speech or sign or gesture is not evidence of its absence' (CommunicationFIRST, 2023).

- Avoid the term 'non-communicative'. It is not possible for an observer to accurately determine the intentions behind someone's body language, movements or vocal sounds.

- 'Mouth words' is a community-specific term preferred by neurodivergent AAC users, but not by other AAC users.

- Do not differentiate between part-time and full-time AAC use. Describe the person's communication needs and preferences across contexts.

- When an AAC user's ability to speak matters, consider using 'intermittently speaking', 'intermittently non-speaking', or minimally speaking.

- 'Communication disability' is most preferred. Fewer AAC users dislike disability terms (13%) than similar terms such as 'difference' (42%), 'disorder' (46%), 'deficit' (78%) or 'impairment' (48%).

- Disorder terms are more likely to be disliked than disability terms.

- Avoid severity ratings and terms such as 'significant', 'severe' and 'profound'. These are reductionist and dehumanising terms that overshadow the individual's specific needs. They instil fear and pity and may influence supporters to limit access to robust forms of AAC due to assumptions around the person's capabilities.

- Avoid the term 'pedantic' to describe communication and a processing style that favours specificity and accuracy of information. An individual's choice of conversational topic should not be denigrated based on its popularity or other's judgements of 'social acceptability'.

- 'Speech deficit' or 'communication deficit' are widely not preferred. 'Speech disability' is preferred over 'speech impairment'.

- Avoid euphemisms such as 'special needs'.

- Avoid terms such as 'complex' needs. This is an arbitrary term that places blame on the person with a communication disability for communication problems rather than acknowledging the failings of the communication partner, the lack of access to alternative modes of communication and the impact of the environment.

A Brief History of Autistic People and the Neurodiversity Movement

Trigger warning: The content of this section contains information about both historical and ongoing abuse of Autistic children and adults and may be upsetting for some readers.

The following chapter was also included in our book *The Adult Autism Assessment Handbook* (Hartman et al., 2023, Chapter 3, pp. 28–44). We felt it would be valuable to reproduce this information here for readers new to our writing, as understanding the history is vital to supporting Autistic children into the future.

3.1 A Brief History of Autistic People and the Neurodiversity Movement

Since autism was first introduced as a term in 1908 by Swiss psychiatrist Eugene Bleuler, Autistic children, adults and their families have been plagued by flawed and damaging myths, assumptions and untruths about them. These have been perpetrated by a great many professionals who, while possibly well-intentioned, failed to examine their own biases and so subsequently this prejudice had a lasting negative impact that reverberated through the century and continues today. Thankfully, alongside this, there have been many determined advocates and parent advocates who (at great personal emotional cost) have helped bring this once considered rare and judged as shameful 'diagnosis' to both better understanding and an increased recognition of prevalence.

Autistic children were initially, and for a very long time, seen as having a childhood psychiatric disorder, a subset of childhood schizophrenia marked by a detachment from reality. Up until exceptionally recently, any literature (research or otherwise) to do with Autistic neurology was focused solely on children, with Temple Grandin (the first Autistic advocate to speak openly about being Autistic) even in the 2000s needing to remind conference attendees that she had not 'recovered' from autism, but was in fact still, of course, Autistic.

3.1.1 The 1940s, 'Bad Parenting'

In 1943, Leo Kanner, an American child psychiatrist, published a paper describing a group of 11 children who he later said had 'early infantile autism'. These children were described as being intelligent and displaying a desire for aloneness, repetition of actions and vocalisations and an insistence on sameness. He also noted that the children's parents were highly successful and intelligent. In his 1943 paper entitled 'Autistic disturbances of effective contact', Kanner described autism as a rare childhood disorder. He separated autism from Bleuler's childhood schizophrenia as the characteristics of childhood schizophrenia include 'normal' development followed by a state of regression, while Kanner's description of Autistic children is characterised by a state of self-absorption which is present from birth.

In 1944, Hans Asperger, a German scientist, worked in the Heilpädagogik clinic under Erwin Lazar, a physician who had an innovative approach to helping children which (even by today's standards) would still be considered innovative. Lazar did not see the children as sick or damaged but instead believed their 'burden' originated due to neglect from the society that had failed to provide suitable teaching methods for their unique styles of learning (Silberman, 2016). Lazar's clinic utilised an approach developed from the 1800s theory of Heilpädagogik 'therapeutic education' which sought to help each child find their own potential as opposed to treating psychological issues in isolation. The approach was one of compassion to foster environments where children could develop the skills to interact in conditions of mutual respect. During his time at the clinic Asperger examined more than 200 children who displayed the 'Autistic thinking' previously identified by Bleuler. Asperger also identified Autistic thinking in several adolescents, adults and mothers of the children too (Silberman, 2016). Asperger wrote about a small group of boys who were similarly described to Kanner's group of children with the exception of not presenting with echolalia, but instead 'talking like grown-ups', and having additional fine and gross motor difficulties. This group of traits and characteristics was to become known as Asperger's syndrome.

Asperger also recognised the biological aspect to 'Autistic pathology' (as he described it). He acknowledged that it ran in families and was not uncommon and he warned his colleagues that it was very unlikely that one single gene could be responsible for such an elaborate system of traits and that it was more likely that the 'Autistic pathology' was polygenetic. Asperger coined the term Autistic pathology. Autistic characteristics included social awkwardness, precocious abilities and an obsession with routine and rules. He acknowledged that Autistic pathology remained present throughout an individual's life and involved a broad spectrum of people, from the most talented and intelligent individuals to the most disabled. Asperger's work was published in German in 1944 and was not translated into English until 1981 by Lorna Wing (Wing, 1981).

In the late 1940s, psychiatrists argued the cause of autism was 'cold' parents (particularly mothers) who did not love their children enough. This theory became known as the 'refrigerator mother' theory, which was popularised by Austrian psychologist Bruno Bettelheim. Bettelheim was heavily influenced by Sigmund Freud who theorised that emotional or behavioural difficulties in children are all caused by the child's upbringing. He was also heavily influenced by Leo Kanner's observation that Autistic children had professional successful parents who he judged as not being as emotionally present for their children as stay at home parents. Unfortunately, even Leo Kanner, who had initially felt that being Autistic was something a child was born with, adopted this theory and with continued support from both Kanner and Bettleheim, it was for decades the prevalent theory of how people 'became' Autistic, with the recommended course of action being institutionalisation for the child and long-term psychoanalysis for the parents to investigate why they could not correctly nurture and care for their children. Parents, especially mothers, were stigmatised and shamed, and children were ripped from their families to spend the rest of their lives in horrific, dehumanising conditions in institutions, often in adult psychosis wards where they were beaten and given electroshock therapy (EST) in the name of 'treatment' (EST in fact still continues today in some US states and other countries with Autistic and otherwise disabled people).

Much of Bettleheim's work (not just the 'refrigerator mother' theory) has been discredited since his death, but this did not halt decades being lost in relation to a valid and meaningful understanding of Autistic people. Not only did it influence what people thought was the cause of Autistic neurology, but because of the recommendation of institutionalisation for Autistic children, it had an enormous impact on what people thought was the natural lifetime developmental progression for an Autistic child. As most diagnosed Autistic children were sent to institutions, naturally all of the research data and anecdotal practice-based information about Autistic children and how they develop into Autistic adults was based on how Autistic people appeared after a life of trauma, abuse and institutionalisation. Understandably, many of these children (and subsequent adults) presented with trauma responses, such as self-harm, reduced communication and hitting out.

3.1.2 The 1960s and 1970s, Genetics and a Spectrum

The idea that to be Autistic is a fate worse than death can be directly linked to the perception of how Autistic adults in these institutions (i.e., wholly inappropriate and abusive environments) presented. Tragically, many Autistic people continue to live long term in inappropriate 'inpatient' units in hospitals to this day. Thankfully, in the 1960s and 1970s, a body of research which included twin studies disproved the 'refrigerator mother' concept and began to show the genetic and biological underpinnings of being Autistic, and over the next two decades it was increasingly recognised that parenting did not cause Autistic children.

In 1964, Bernard Rimland, an American psychologist with an Autistic child who disagreed with the refrigerator mother concept, published the book *Infantile Autism: The Syndrome and Its Implications for a Neural Theory of Behaviour*. Rimland's work had a large hand to play in the move away from blaming parents and was subsequently highly influential in relation to how Autistic children were understood. However, unfortunately, while positive in relation to moving away from the idea of blaming parents, Rimland believed that autism was caused by environmental pollutants, antibiotics and vaccinations (although he acknowledged there may also be a genetic component predisposing children). He also supported chelation, Applied Behaviour Analysis and the use of aversives.

In the 1970s Lorna Wing (a British psychiatrist whose daughter was Autistic and had learning difficulties) and Judith Gould undertook the first epidemiological study of autism (leading to a significantly higher incidence than previously thought) and established in the 1970s the 'triad of impairments' that subsequently came to define autism. Wing was the first person to introduce the helpful concept of the spectrum and the vast range of presentations shown by Autistic people. She highlighted the great variability between Autistic people, noting that autism should be considered dimensionally, and occurs in all ages and in people of all intellectual abilities. It was the first time it was recognised that Autistic people could be of all ages and abilities, including those with lower support needs. She also advocated for parents and professionals to work closely together and for individual rights for Autistic people. In the 1980s Wing also brought the work of Hans Asperger to the English-speaking world, which had significant influence on subsequent framings of autism.

In 1980, 'infantile autism' (described as a 'pervasive developmental disorder') was listed for the first time in the DSM, and established autism as its own separate diagnosis distinct from schizophrenia.

In 1987, the DSM replaced 'infantile autism' with the broader 'autism disorder' and included a checklist of diagnostic criteria. However, autism was still at this time considered to be very rare, and was largely unknown in the general public.

3.1.3 The 1980s, and Applied Behaviour Analysis

Hugely influential in the history of autism was the development and subsequent proliferation of Applied Behaviour Analysis (ABA) as the 'gold standard treatment' for Autistic children. In 1987, the American psychologist Ivor Lovaas published his first study related to intensive behaviour therapy for Autistic children, which was to become known as ABA. In an interview with *Psychology* in 1974 in which he advocated for physical punishment, Lovaas is quoted to have said 'You start pretty much from scratch when you work with an Autistic child. You have a person in the physical sense – they have hair, a nose and a mouth – but they are not people in the psychological sense. One way to look at the job of helping Autistic kids is to see it as a matter of constructing a person. You have the raw materials, but you have to construct the person' (Chance & Lovaas, 1974, p. 76).

We encourage you not to skim over this Lovaas quote as a historical note but instead truly 'sit' with it for a few minutes, imagining it was you or your child being described in such terms (i.e., essentially not human). Really engaging with what was done and said as a reality is to begin to understand the impact that history has had in perpetuating trauma upon multitudes of Autistic people in the guise of us being less than human. Indeed, Lovaas published a study at the time claiming to have 'cured' autism. However, this study has since been totally discredited due to the fact that his method during research was to use aversive techniques with the children in his care.

ABA is based on influential American psychologist B. F. Skinner's behaviourist framework, in which the only target for 'treatment' can be observable behaviour and the only way to target the behaviour is by a controlled experimental design. 'Treatment' success is defined as the behaviour changing in the way the experiment was designed to do. Feelings, thoughts, distress, environment, sensory discomfort, whether the behaviour should be changed and who is deciding the behaviour should be changed and why are not relevant factors in Lovaas's traditional behaviourist framework. A seductive aspect of behaviourism is that it often 'works' at a superficial or surface level in changing short-term behaviour, but we need to ask ourselves to what end, and with what long-term results? Severely neglected newborn babies, for example, will stop crying out to be held but their need for comfort is not diminished, they have just learned that there is simply no point crying for something that will never come.

Despite limited success, Lovaas further developed his programme to target younger children under 5 years of age and advocated for 40 hours weekly of therapy (this regimen continues to be recommended today despite being at odds with a large body of research in relation to how children this age learn best). It is also an entire working week (for an adult) on top of school and the regular business of being a child. How can any child fulfil the job description of being a child subjected to so many hours of direct intervention? Again, despite limited success, the media quickly began reporting about Autistic children 'transformed' into 'apparently normal children' from their engagement with ABA. In the absence of any other well-publicised programme offering hope, worried parents began flocking to ABA to help 'cure' their child, while being Autistic was described to them as 'a fate worse than death'. ABA has since grown to become a powerful, multi-billion-dollar industry in America and worldwide. It has subsequently been widely denounced and rejected by the Autistic community as harmful and traumatic, denying the validity of Autistic experience and fundamentally seeking to change Autistic people into something they can never be, or want to be. It is wholly counter to developing a positive Autistic identity.

The centring from the early days of autism awareness of a behaviourist framework as the 'go to treatment' for Autistic children had a dehumanising impact which still reverberates today in relation to how professionals even begin to understand and support Autistic children. For example, if a neurotypical child experiences a traumatic event and is, for example, speaking less, hitting themselves or running away, the professionals around that child would hopefully know not to implement a behaviour plan with rewards or aversives to shape the behaviour. They should instead know to try to understand why the child was behaving this way and help provide connection, empathy, consistency, safer environments, appropriate child-centred therapy and education to the people around the child in relation to the trauma. However, the Autistic experience has always been described and framed as observable, undesirable behaviours which need to be ameliorated and it is part of the legacy of ABA that it is typically the behaviour of the Autistic child and how to shape it that is paramount, instead of efforts first being made to empathise and understand why the child may be behaving that way, and changing the environment around them.

3.1.4 The 1980s and 1990s, Self-Advocating and the Internet

Alongside the growth of ABA in the 1980s and 1990s, Autistic adults began attending parent conferences about autism and speaking out about their own experiences, often at great emotional cost to themselves. Temple Grandin also began publishing books and speaking publicly during this time. This meant that for the first time, parents and professionals were hearing information from Autistic people directly (Autistic people who had not spent their lives in institutions), about how they view and experience the world. As well as helping to reduce shame and prejudice, listening to these Autistic adults was revelatory for worried parents and gave them hope that the 'diagnosis' was not as life-limiting as they had been led to believe. It also helped them understand for the first time why their children experienced the world as they did, and thus helped improve the lives of a great many children and their families.

In the late 1980s only a very small group of people knew what autism was, and even then, it was a very limited conceptualisation. Then, in 1989 the movie *Rain Man* was released to popular acclaim and with an enormous impact on public awareness of autism as it included an Autistic savant with a photographic memory (a character who while sympathetic and intelligent, is ultimately there to teach the protagonist life lessons before being dispatched back to an institution). Because of its popularity, bolstered by an Oscar for Dustin Hoffman in the title role, after *Rain Man* was released, a great many people (which of course included parents) knew at least one way that Autistic people can present (although it was such a stereotyped and limited portrayal that it perpetuated myths about what it was to be Autistic).

The growth of the internet in the 1990s allowed new communities across the world to connect, communicate and organise. This included the

Autistic community, for whom the medium of the internet may have been particularly well suited given the reduced need to mask or camouflage when communicating, as well as it being less demanding, with less burden on auditory processing, and allowing thinking time, which led to a significant increase in advocacy and activism.

In 1992, Jim Sinclair (the first Autistic advocate to write publicly from an Autistic rights and anti-cure perspective), Donna Williams and Kathy Grant (influential Autistic activists) co-founded Autism Network International, which among other projects published newsletters 'by and for Autistic people'.

In 1993, Jim Sinclair published his hugely influential essay 'Don't mourn for us'. This is a seminal paper which should be read by anyone working in this field. Included is this powerful new framing of Autistic identity:

> It is not possible to separate the autism from the person. Therefore, when parents say, 'I wish my child did not have autism', what they're really saying is, 'I wish the Autistic child I have did not exist and I had a different (non-autistic) child instead.' Read that again. This is what we hear when you mourn over our existence. This is what we hear when you pray for a cure. This is what we know, when you tell us of your fondest hopes and dreams for us: that your greatest wish is that one day we will cease to be, and strangers you can love will move in behind our faces.

> *(Sinclair, 1993)*

This was the start of the growth of a strong Autistic advocacy and Neurodiversity Movement.

3.1.5 The 1990s and 2000s, and the Neurodiversity Movement

In 1996, Autreat was established, the first retreat and conference specifically for Autistic people, which inspired other similar retreats globally.

Also in 1996, an email list called Independent Living on the Autism Spectrum was established by Martjin Dekker, an Autistic computer programmer from the Netherlands. Of significance to the development of the concept of neurodiversity, the list described autism's 'cousin conditions', for example, dyslexia and ADHD.

Singer (an Australian disability and public housing activist) has been attributed to having first coined the term 'neurodiversity' in her sociology honours thesis, in which she wrote about the liberatory, activist aspects of the concept, and the potential for it doing for the neurodivergent what feminism and LGBTQIA+ rights have done for these groups. Botha et al. (2024) point out, however, that neurodiversity as a concept/term was developed collectively amongst Autistic activist communities.

With increased access to information about disability activism, the young adults who had been diagnosed as Autistic in the 1990s began looking at the disability rights community and recognising themselves. Thus, for the first time a bridge began to grow between the growing Autistic community and the disability rights community.

The 1990s and 2000s continued to see the growth of an increasing number of advocacy groups, including the Autism National Committee, The Autistic Self Advocacy Network, Autistic Women, the Academic Autistic Spectrum Partnership in Research and Education and the Non-Binary Network.

Alongside this growth of activism, in the 1990s came the broadening of the diagnostic criteria for autism, and in 1994, Asperger's syndrome was added to the DSM, expanding autism to include people with less care needs. Also, at this time more statistically reliable tests to assess autism became more widely accessible, with an assessment no longer only accessible to those with a connection to a tiny group of experts (although while statistically reliable these tests did not capture the full breadth of the Autistic experience). These factors, alongside the *Rain Man* effect, meant that diagnostic rates of autism began to soar (and they have continued to soar since then).

Unfortunately, what should have been seen as positive (i.e., that children were being correctly identified and so could finally begin to be understood and supported appropriately) was framed by organisations such as the American charity Autism Speaks as an epidemic to be scourged. Prominent, frightening and damaging media campaigns were released by Autism Speaks in which autism was described as 'taking over your child'. This terrified families and the damage of this framing continues to reverberate today every time the increased rates of autism are published. It also brought in a lot of money for the charities and for research. Unfortunately, much of this money went (and continues to go) towards searching for a cause rather than greater understanding or the provision of better supports.

3.1.6 Controversy

In 1998, the now disgraced Andrew Wakefield, a UK doctor, published a case series suggesting that the measles, mumps and rubella vaccine may cause behaviour regression and pervasive developmental disorder in children. This idea spread rapidly worldwide and immediately MMR vaccinations began to drop. Although there were quickly multiple studies published refuting Wakefield's study, the link between autism and vaccines was set in people's minds. Wakefield's papers have since been retracted, and he has been held guilty of ethical violations, scientific misrepresentation and deliberate fraud which appears to have taken place for financial gain. Over the years, a great amount of wasted resources and funding has gone into refuting Wakefield's tiny paper which could have been put to much better use for the Autistic community.

Worryingly (and worth bearing in mind when analysing research publications in general), it was not academic vigilance which highlighted these issues with Wakefield's study, but journalistic investigation.

Throughout the 2000s, the Autistic community continued to grow in confidence and numbers, speaking out about what they wanted and needed, namely control over their own lives and an end to the focus on cure and pathologisation of their ways of being. What had previously been acceptable began to be unacceptable. An early example of this was when in 2007 the NYU Child Study Centre released advertisements in the form of ransom notes (echoing many previous publicly unchallenged campaigns from Autism Speaks). These ads took the form of ransoms saying 'We have your son. We will make sure he will not be able to care for himself or interact socially as long as he lives. This is only the beginning.' It was signed 'Autism'. The ad campaign was quite rightly accused of using some of the oldest and most offensive stereotypes to frighten parents, and of including untruths and heavily biased ableism.

While during previous Autism Speaks campaigns the Autistic community did not have a voice, now Autistic advocates were mobilised. Spearheaded by Ari Ne'eman (author, PhD candidate in Health Policy in Harvard University and an American disability rights activist who co-founded the Autistic Self Advocacy Network), Autistic advocates sparked a huge protest much to the surprise of the NYU Child Study Centre. Ne'eman (with the support of the majority of American disability rights organisations) undertook a highly successful letter writing campaign which was picked up in many major media outlets in the

USA, including *The New York Times*. This was the first and most public time that a major organisation needed to reckon with a community that was not looking for cure or scaremongering, but societal changes. The ads were pulled within three weeks.

3.1.7 The 2000s to Today, Steps Forward and Back

In 2013, the DSM-5 folded all sub-categories of autism into one umbrella diagnosis of autism spectrum disorder, with Asperger's syndrome no longer seen as a separate diagnosis.

In 2019, Greta Thunberg, Autistic Swedish climate activist, was named *Time* magazine's Person of the Year. Thunberg has from the start spoken openly about being Autistic (Asperger's syndrome specifically), saying that instead of a hindrance, it has helped her see things from outside the box and has therefore been key to her ideas and success as an activist. Thunberg's high profile has had an enormous positive impact on the general public's perceptions of Autistic people and has also helped greatly increase awareness of the presence of Autistic girls and women.

In 2020, the Centers for Disease Control and Prevention reported that the rates of formal identification of their neurology from professionals were at that time 1 in 54 children.

Today, there is a thriving Autistic and neurodivergent culture and community. Alongside an increased openness of Autistic adults to talk about being Autistic, more and more prominent public figures such as Elon Musk, Sir Anthony Hopkins, Wentworth Miller (actor) and Melanie Sykes (presenter) are also openly talking about being Autistic. With reduced societal stigma, more and more parents/caregivers of Autistic children are recognising that they themselves are Autistic and are accessing diagnosis as well as joining their voices with autism activism. Companies are finally beginning to see that this is something they must address in relation to hiring, disability and equality, with training in neurodiversity affirmative practices fast becoming a booming business.

There has also been an overdue explosion of public Autistic activism, openly Autistic professionals and therapists, Autistic-led and co-produced research, and new Autistic-led organisations and charities.

The following are just a few of the great many Autistic activists and scholars, and Autistic-led organisations. This is a small, illustrative and by no means exhaustive list.

- Thriving Autistic – Thriving Autistic is an Autistic-led non-profit, founded in Ireland in 2020 by one of our authors. It is the world's first global team of Autistic and otherwise neurodivergent health and social care professionals working to support the international Autistic adult community: www.thrivingautistic.org.

- Autistic Staff School Project – The Autistic School Staff Project is a multi-phased research endeavour that started in 2019 and focuses on the experiences, needs and strengths of Autistic education staff across a range of roles in schools. Dr Rebecca Wood is the principal investigator of the project. One significant output of the project is the publication of an edited book that gathers the diverse and rich experiences of Autistic Education staff. The project has an informative website that can be found at: www. autisticschoolstaffproject.com.

- Autistic Doctors International – Autistic Doctors International is a peer support, advocacy, research and education group for Autistic doctors. Founded in 2019 by Dr Mary Doherty, Irish Consultant Anaesthesist, it has members in Europe, the UK, the US, Canada, Australia and New Zealand. See www.autisticdoctorsinternational.com.

- Therapist Neurodiversity Collective – Guided by Autistic and otherwise neurodivergent therapists and mentors, Therapist Neurodiversity Collective is an international therapy, education and advocacy collaborative for therapists, therapist assistants and students. One of its mission goals is to provide free public access non-behavioural-based, trauma-informed, Neurodiversity Paradigm aligned therapists. www. therapistndc.org.

- Ausome Training – Ausome Training provide Autistic-led neurodiversity training and mentoring to parents, teachers and professionals.

- AsIAm – AsIAm is an Autistic-led charity based in Ireland. They work to create a society in which every Autistic person is empowered to reach their own personal potential and fully participate in society. They believe that by developing the capacity of the autism community and addressing the societal barriers to inclusion they can make Ireland the world's most autism-friendly country. AsIAm started in 2014 and is today Ireland's most influential autism charity. See www.asiam.ie.

- Damien Milton – Consultant, author and lecturer at the Tizard Centre, University of Kent, project leader of the National Autistic Taskforce, and chair of the Participatory Autism Research Collective. Milton's development and research into the double empathy problem has been hugely influential in relation to a modern understanding of the interactions between neurotypical and Autistic people.

- Dr Wenn Lawson – Influential psychologist, lecturer and one of the earliest authors writing about their own Autistic experience.

- Dinah Murray – Key figure in autism studies, who with Wenn Lawson and Mike Lesser developed the theory of monotropism. She was an early and passionate campaigner and activist.

- Emily Lees – UK-based speech and language therapist championing Autistic children, young people and adults and one of a growing number of openly Autistic therapists. www.autisticslt.com. She advocates and campaigns for autism acceptance in order to transform the way professionals assess and support Autistic children and young people through neurodiversity affirmative understanding and supports.

- Sarah Selvaggi Hernandez – An Autistic occupational therapist, author, public speaker and advocate. She was also the first openly Autistic person elected to serve in a government position in the United States. Sarah is passionate about occupational science, sensory processing and Autistic identity. Her vision remains centred on the creation of identity-affirming Autistic contexts to support neurodivergent development. She runs the popular social media site The Autistic OT.

- Kassiane Asasumasu – Multiply divergent Autistic activist credited with coining the term 'neurodivergent', and passionate advocate for the Neurodiversity Movement being inclusive of all neurodivergencies.

- Dr Nick Walker – American professor of psychology, author and educator, who is best known for her work on Neuroqueer Theory. Walker has written about how the long-term well-being and empowerment of Autistic and otherwise Neurodivergent people hinges on their ability to create a paradigm shift away from the pathology paradigm and towards the Neurodiversity Paradigm, while emphasising the need for change within individual beliefs as well as systemic cultural changes.

- Lydia X. Z. Brown – Prominent American Autistic disability rights activist and public speaker, who has lectured on neurodiversity, disability, racial justice and the connections between the queer, trans and disability experiences.

- Morénike Giwa Onaiw – American author and educator who is the editor of *All the Weight of Our Dreams*, an anthology of art and writing created entirely by Autistic people of colour.

At this point, a phenomenal amount of research funding has been pumped into searching for the genetic and other 'causes' of autism, with the most recent large-scale studies involving millions of children indicating that autism is predominantly inherited, with gene sequencing studies implicating over a hundred different genes. Despite disproportionate attention from the media and a scared general public in relation to environmental causes (e.g., factors such as the mother's weight or nutritional intake) these studies indicate that environment does not have a significant impact. The Autistic community are extremely frustrated with this ongoing focus on cause, with the implication of future wide-scale eugenics should a cause be found. The high rates of Down syndrome pregnancies being terminated means this fear is not unfounded.

In a striking example of the emerging power of the Autistic community to shape their future, Spectrum 10k, a large-scale UK-based research project which claimed to be investigating the genetic and environmental factors that contribute to autism and related physical and mental health conditions (but the methodology suggested a possible sub-division of the Autistic community which is in direct opposition to Autistic-identified research priorities), had been put on hold after outcry from the community. Advocates highlighted a lack of meaningful engagement and co-production with the Autistic community, and that the aims of the study and its research area were at odds with community priorities, and queried whether the ultimate goal of the project was cure, i.e., eugenics. What the community needs and wants now and going forward are high-quality trials of clinical and community supports which aim to minimise barriers, improve quality of life and nurture individual differences.

Given the history of treatment of Autistic people by the neurotypical perceived majority, the Autistic community is justifiably angry about being continually spoken over by neurotypical professionals when it comes to matters pertaining to them. In 2024 electroshock therapy is still being given to Autistic people in the Judge Rottenburg Centre in the USA despite continual outcry from the community and the United Nations calling it torture. ABA continues to be dominant despite being opposed by all Autistic advocacy groups. Many current proponents of ABA claim that 'their ABA' isn't like Lovaas's. But the principals remain the same even if the current delivery may look somewhat different. Fundamentally it is about denying the validity of the Autistic experience. Research on Autistic people continues to be largely ableist and with no real Autistic engagement, and researchers continue to know little about the lives of Autistic adults, women, the intersectionality of minority communities within the Autistic community and the effects of related conditions such as epilepsy.

AUTHOR REFLECTIONS ON COMPLIANCE-BASED BEHAVIOUR THERAPY

The authors of this book have provided training (and have spoken to) for many professionals trained and working within compliance-based behavioural frameworks such as Positive Behaviour Support or ABA. A few themes tend to frequently emerge.

First, it is often our experience in our trainings that those with a background in ABA, who are excited about the concept of the neurodiversity affirmative model, can see the value of a human rights approach. There is a clear struggle to reconcile their training background and the positive impact they believed they were making with the overwhelmingly negative reception of their modality by the Autistic adult community. They often question us as to the legitimacy of Autistic peoples' objections. They often purport that 'new' ABA is different and there is much of value in their training. On each occasion, when we unpack this argument with an open curiosity, it becomes evident that the 'parts' of ABA they assert are helpful and respectful turn out to be simply good practice from a different modality (e.g., breaking a task down into manageable chunks). It would appear that this good practice has been packaged and 'sold' to the practitioner as an ABA strategy exclusively.

Another factor that often raises its head is a misunderstanding of the Autistic developmental trajectory and neuro-normative therapy goals.

Goals must be set by a person themselves. Goals of compliance or 'fitting in', 'masking' or suppressing natural Autistic expression such as stimming are harmful to Autistic people's mental health and a potential risk factor for mental health difficulties throughout life.

In the USA particularly, we often hear from practitioners that undertaking ABA is the only way to get insurance billing and therefore access mental health support because insurance companies won't fund other therapies. So therefore, practitioners tell us that that they are not actually utilising compliance therapy, they simply bill it as such.

There can also be a confirmation bias when considering ABA with children. Therapists believe the child can have only achieved progress with a desired goal because of ABA without considering the fact of the Autistic developmental trajectory and the likelihood of the child achieving the goal naturally, or with the support of another therapeutic method (e.g., occupational therapy).

The main concern we have for the ABA community is twofold.

1. Those trained in ABA and who have invested time working in the field must hold the tension that their work has been harmful, if they are to adapt. This is an incredibly difficult thing to ask most humans to do. It takes a great deal of self-awareness and openness to listen to the community you believed you were serving and to hear the harm caused.

2. There are many wonderful, well-intentioned ABA trained therapists and practitioners who, when introduced to and excited by the human rights-based Neurodiversity Movement, do not know where to go with their training. They are left at a loss as to how to move forward. This is a conversation in our opinion that needs to happen within the behaviourist community. ABA associations and leadership organisations must listen to and engage with the communities they purport to serve and humbly change course. It has up until recently been far too easy to dismiss Autistic adults' grievances as a small group of unhappy people, but the issue is clearly much wider now. Autistic adults have the support of a growing group of professionals

such as the authors of this book, a mix of neurodivergent and neurotypical psychologists, the respected Therapist Neurodiversity Collective, the entire team at Thriving Autistic along with many more organisations now recognising the persistent harm and trauma caused by the ABA community in refusing to engage with Autistic voices.

NOTE ON COMPLIANCE-BASED BEHAVIOUR APPROACHES (E.G., ABA)

These approaches are fully rejected by the Autistic community and those working within the Neurodiversity Paradigm. Despite some recent reported industry changes and a great many kind and well-intentioned practitioners, ultimately the end goal of ABA is an Autistic young person and adult who meets neuro-normative standards such that they are 'indistinguishable' from their neurotypical peers. Compliance-based behavioural methods (including Positive Behaviour Support and ABA) have significant negative long-term effects on people's mental health (Anderson, 2023; Ram, 2020; Wakefield & McCarthy, 2020). As clinicians, we should question the authority of knowledge sources, from whom they were produced and whose epistemic position was privileged. Here, we deliberatively include an Autistic written blog recognising that all sources of knowledge are valid. They are incompatible with a human rights model emphasising the vital importance of self-advocacy and self-determination. If a method is based on compliance through behavioural means, it is not neurodiversity affirmative.

The history of Autistic people is full of trauma and pain. How the Autistic experience has been conceptualised has from the start been problematic, with endorsed 'therapeutic' approaches leading to dehumanising treatment and trauma. These models continue to pervade Autistic experience in the present day despite tireless work and advocacy by the Autistic community and their allies. When undertaking assessments, clinicians need to remember this history and the damage it has inflicted and strive to do more to change their lens so that history does not continue to repeat itself.

3.2 Common Criticisms of the Neurodiversity Movement

Concerns regarding the Neurodiversity Movement come from within as well as outside it. For example, there are valid concerns by Autistic advocates that a growing number of clinicians and companies are aligning themselves with the movement by branding themselves as neurodiversity affirmative, or 'embracing neurodiversity' when they are not. Often in these cases clinicians or companies may use the language and branding of the Neurodiversity Movement and talk about strengths as a sales and marketing pitch, but under the surface their systemic processes and thinking are still very much the same as they were before and rooted within the medical paradigm. This has been termed 'neurodiversity-lite'.

Traditionally, throughout history, when any previously powerless group comes together and starts asserting itself, it is common for the dominant majority group to find it difficult to change their thinking and language about the minority group. The majority group also traditionally resists giving up power and the status quo and equal rights need to be hard fought for. There are parallels and similarities here to other movements such as the LGBTQIA+ and feminist rights movements.

Here are some of the most common criticisms that have been levelled at the Neurodiversity Movement and Paradigm.

Criticism 1: The Neurodiversity Paradigm claims that autism is not a disability, but just a different way of looking at the world.

Critics argue that the Neurodiversity Paradigm sanitises the Autistic experience. Embracing neurodiversity and acknowledging the very real challenges that living with a different neurotype can bring are not mutually exclusive. Autistic advocates and neurodiversity proponents are crying out for support, funding and accommodations, and so this criticism is a profound misunderstanding of the movement.

The Neurodiversity Movement started within, and continues to be part of, the broader disability rights movement. It has from the very start advocated and fought for a broad range of supports and equal opportunities for Autistic people. Most neurodivergent and Autistic advocates identify as disabled and share the ideals and goals of the wider disability movement. Many of the original proponents of the Neurodiversity Movement had a range of other disabilities and high support needs in addition to being Autistic.

The Neurodiversity Movement is fighting for everyone's supports needs to be met, and for funding for this. It is fighting for equal rights and an equal voice and position in society for everyone, including those with high support needs and who are non-speaking.

As an example, there has been a strong focus within the Neurodiversity Movement on the rights of non-speaking Autistics to have equal access to communication, e.g., with the provision and use of augmentative and alternative communication (AAC) devices in the same way that physically disabled people have rights to access wheelchairs.

While within the Neurodiversity Paradigm being Autistic is clearly not looked at as a disease or a disorder and is not something that needs or wants to be cured, it is still understood for the most part that being Autistic is disabling within the context of the social model of disability. Under the social model of disability, it is society that disables individuals by being designed for the perceived majority and not including adequate and appropriate supports for all who need them.

It needs to be remembered that there are a great many people talking about neurodiversity publicly. As with any complex topic that involves a lot of people, there will be diverging opinions and different understandings and interpretations of what the Neurodiversity Movement and Paradigm are all about (both within and outside of the Autistic and neurodivergent community). Before accepting a criticism as true, it is important to do some further research into the topic rather than listening to individual people on social media.

Criticism 2: The Neurodiversity Movement is only relevant for a small sub-section of 'high functioning' people

Note: The use of 'high functioning' here is only for illustrative purposes as the authors of this book do not use this stigmatising terminology. It is used as a common example of a criticism.

A large part of the issue here is the misunderstanding that Autistic and otherwise neurodivergent advocates all have 'low support needs' and are only speaking to and advocating for people like themselves. There is an assumption that if someone has spoken out articulately, or they have a job or a family, that they couldn't possibly have high support needs. But this is not the case. Many Autistic people who are, for example, professionals, parents/caregivers and in happy relationships still identify as being disabled and still struggle greatly in other areas of their lives. This is because their needs fluctuate and change over time depending on context and resources. So, someone could enjoy communicating verbally early in the day, but later in the day rely on AAC to communicate. Many people have high support needs in one area but need less in another.

In fact, within the Autistic community there is a huge resistance to the division of Autistic people based on their support needs, and a strong desire to support and protect all members equally. There continue to be huge efforts made within the community for all members of the community to have their views and opinions documented and counted in relation to their collective future. Another large part of the issue here is the misunderstanding addressed already, that the movement focuses on strengths and sanitises disability. The Neurodiversity Movement aims for equal rights and prominence for all Autistic and otherwise neurodivergent people, and always has.

Neurodiversity is about disability rights and the Neurodiversity Movement is the bridge between the worlds of Autistic and otherwise neurodivergent people and disability activism. Disability activism was never about advocating only for those who are less visibly disabled. Disability activism's remit is to bring everyone along.

It is interesting to note that as a group, people with higher support needs are more generally ignored; their wishes for how their care is managed are discounted as them not knowing what is best for themselves. But when individuals with lower support needs talk about what is needed for their community, they are faced with the criticism that they do not speak for the whole of the Autistic community. This begs the question, what will it take for the neurotypical majority to listen to the Autistic community?

Criticism 3: The Autistic community and the Neurodiversity Movement are against all therapy and research

In relation to research, the Autistic community (including a great many Autistic researchers) very much welcome and value research into many areas related to them. This includes research into Autistic well-being, the Autistic developmental trajectory, aging and areas that can cause distress and which have traditionally been under-researched (for example, sleep, and the provision of appropriate communication supports). The Autistic community also wants research that meaningfully involves Autistic people from the start and supports community priorities in relation to research. This should be a basic standard when it comes to research with any minority group.

In relation to therapy, again, the Autistic community welcomes support that respects Autistic identity and community priority goals (i.e., quality of life). Autistic parents/caregivers recognise that children may need to be supported in learning skills. They don't want compliance training, neurotypical social skills training or ABA, but there are a great many other, respectful supports which they absolutely do need and want. This includes increasing sensory self-awareness, adapted mental health therapies to foster Autistic well-being and individualised personal assistant support, for example with phone calls, consistent meals and managing life admin such as paperwork. A huge part of the Neurodiversity Movement and what Autistic advocates are fighting for is increased supports, for example the provision of speech and language and occupational therapy.

For an in-depth exploration of the history of Autistic people and the Neurodiversity Movement, the book *NeuroTribes* by Steve Silberman (2016) is recommended.

CHAPTER 4

Learning from Lived Experience

4.1 Introduction

In this chapter, in order to support clinicians' shift in thinking in relation to the Autistic experience and the work we undertake with children, we take the time to reflect on the stories we are told about ourselves and how these shape us. We also provide lived experiences from Autistic parents and professionals, about their experiences of their child's assessment process, and also their experience of discovering their own Autistic identity later in life and how that has helped shape their practice.

4.2 Stories and How They Shape Us

We all get told stories – as children, the bedtime story is a precious point of connection for both adult and child, enjoying closeness, sharing of imagination, providing a space for discussing ideas. As we grow older, we learn to read, and access more stories ourselves. We soon learn that stories exist not just in books, but in the narratives that society tells us about ourselves, others, the 'right' way to look, act and behave. These narratives are typically dominated by what is perceived to be 'normal behaviour' at that particular time, and frame how we see ourselves and our position in the world. There has been a much-needed shift in children's fiction written by neurodivergent authors, such as Elle McNicholl, featuring main characters who are Autistic or otherwise neurodivergent. These stories present a re-framing of Autistic experience, providing both an intensely enjoyable reading experience but also a springboard for discussion of how others treat people perceived as 'different' (e.g., Addie in *A Kind of Spark* (McNicholl, 2020) makes it her mission to achieve a memorial to the women killed in the Scottish Witch Trials merely for being different). Wider society and clinicians have much learning to do from thinking about the stories we tell our children, be that in fiction or the dominant narratives that prevail about how to be in the world.

Many young people come to us with a veritable library of negative stories that they have been told (either implicitly or explicitly) about their ways of being ('you're weird', 'you never listen', 'you can't do X', 'you need to be Y'), only to leave the assessment space being given yet another negatively framed story: they are someone who has autism, and the story told about what autism 'is' is often deficit-laden. Put simply, this can feel akin to being told we have something like head lice – the having implies a condition, disorder or something unpleasant that needs removing (head lice need removing, with careful scrutiny, combing, chemical shampoos...). This is the type of narrative that leads to 'intervention' based on neuro-normative goals and neurotypical developmental trajectories. This is the approach we seek to challenge in this book. Unlike head lice, autism does not require treatment or combing out – being Autistic runs through our neurology in the same way that words or streaks of colour run through sticks of sweet seaside rock (long coloured candy sticks typically with the name of the place 'written' inside). Any effort to pull the writing out of the rock is not going to end well for anyone concerned.

> Neuro-normative refers to social, cultural and personal norms which assumed neurotypicality as the 'norm' in how to think, feel, behave and communicate (Herrán Salcedo, 2021).

For many Autistic children, young people and adults, the dominant, deficit-laden rhetoric surrounding 'diagnosis' and deficit means that when they are identified as Autistic, they may be presented with stigmatised and negatively valanced accounts of what being Autistic is. Such damaging frameworks can create false perceptions of that person in both how they see themselves and how others perceive them (Hobson, 2011). The path to formal discovery of identification is typically based on struggling and distress. Our ways of being are seen as problematic and pathological, and we carry the burden of that. Deficit-based identification processes mean these narratives can be internalised and impact well-being (Farahar, 2023).

Assessed within a deficit-based frame, an 'autism diagnosis' can become a negative part of the child's story, both in the story that they create for themselves and how those around them re-story the young person as 'disordered'. As Bernadi (2023) observes, an autism 'diagnosis', and the negative narratives surrounding this, in effect creates a new and 'forged' identity. When it is delivered through a medical-based, deficit-laden approach, autism 'diagnosis' can be situated akin to chronic illness, instigating a drive for 'correctional' therapies (Bernadi, 2023). Parents/caregivers and those around the young person must navigate, and try to reconcile, the different narratives that they see surrounding each young person around Autistic experience; one that is deficit-laden against another that celebrates and welcomes Autistic ways of being and does not see this as problematic. For example, from her study involving teaching assistants, teachers, special educational needs coordinators, deputy head teachers, ten Autistic children, ten parents, and ten Autistic adults, Wood (2019b) reported that there was a disconnect between the deficit-based descriptions of autism that participants felt unable to question and the actual child they knew.

> FFS – No, my son does not 'suffer' from autism. He is Autistic. I am literally seeing red...what a f***ing let down this letter is.

> *(Anonymous, personal communication, 2023)*

Another telling of this story is that we are Autistic, being Autistic is part of our fundamental neurology and is part of the beautiful and vital diversity of life. As we will explore in Chapter 5, this is the story told by the Neurodiversity Paradigm which underpins how we approach collaborative discovery of Autistic identity with the young people with whom we have the privilege of working. Our collective shift to neurodiversity affirmative practice has reflected a move from a pathologising epistemological approach to an empowering one (Jackson-Perry et al., 2020, p. 133). As clinicians working within a neurodiversity affirmative frame in collaborative identification of Autistic identity, we exist as both part of the 'system', and yet push back against it. There are different ways to approach formal identification of Autistic experience that do not mean repeating a rhetoric of deficiency and deficit, whilst still adhering to the diagnostic criteria (see Hartman et al., 2023, for a detailed guide to conducting neuro-affirmative, respectful identification of Autistic identity in adults).

Writing this book has been a process of reflection on our personal and professional experiences, exploring our responses, even our rage (c.f., Bertilsdotter Rosqvist & Nygren, 2023), as we realised how epistemic violence has affected the knowledge base around Autistic experience and how this impacts on how the majority of assessments are conducted currently.

When families come to us for an identification piece, they offer us the most precious gift of sharing their family stories and the opportunity to work with their loved young people. By then many families will most likely have fought to be heard, to secure that appointment with us – and the way to do that typically focuses not on the wonders, the beauty, the sheer magic of this unique young person carving out their own way of being, but on focusing on stories of what they don't, can't, won't do (and this is usually from a neurotypical gaze on development, what is 'expected', what is the 'right way' to play, communicate, engage in relationships). It takes great courage to offer up one's precious young person for the most intense scrutiny. And so, we offer two personal stories: one about the identification process for our own young person, and one about being identified Autistic ourselves. We do so in the spirit of honouring and respecting the gift of trust that families give us. We share our experience as a reflection of the rawness of the process, because this is what we seek to support you to move away from. The discovery of Autistic identity, how it is identified, framed and shared with the young person becomes a fundamental part of their life story. As clinicians, we typically have the power to be the narrator in that chapter of the child's story (in how we conduct the identification piece, frame Autistic experience and collaboratively discuss Autistic identity with the young person and their family). Our narrator role may be brief, but as we know from any book, each chapter leads on to the next, and the next and the next, and the threads we establish in our chapter will echo through all subsequent ones. We encourage you to be co-author with the young people and families – collaboration is vital, discovery should be a co-created positive experience which fosters self-understanding and community.

4.2.1 Story 1: Perspectives of a Parent and Professional: My Personal Experience

DR ANNA DAY

Where do I start? Where? When? How far back do we need to go to make sense? I will circle, and for that I do not apologise. I don't think in a linear process, I bounce, endless tabs open, random pop-up ads seeking my attention. This made the identification process difficult. I think in tangents, I take side streets, I linger with intent, circling round my thoughts because that guides how I get to the end. The clinicians want straight answers, clear ticks to the boxes, but I don't communicate like that. And even though they know I am Autistic, I must mask, mask, mask and create a linear story that I don't even hold in my own mind, let alone have the ability to articulate. I'm filtering, sieving through what I need to tell them, trying to find how to articulate it in the way that they want me to, which doesn't fit with my way of communicating. So, I look anxious, because I know I need to 'perform' the expected way of narrating my child's story and experiences and so I must edit internally as I go. All the time I'm doing this, I can see my child through the one-way mirror sitting with the speech and language therapist. I can see her distress; I can read her through the mirror and yet I can't reach her. Nor can the therapist. Are they trying, I wonder? Are they trying to connect with her in how she relates to people or based on neurotypical conventions? I don't yet know the language of Milton's work on double empathy, but I feel it. I see the mismatch in action, I feel it viscerally. I can see her drawing our cat over and over and over because she, I, we, love cats, love drawing them, reading about them, worshipping them. I can read the therapist's face as she makes notes, frowning slightly. She doesn't join in the drawing. She misses a precious moment of connection – which is later documented as repetitive play and lack of interest in communication.

They said she'd be able to see me, but how can she when she is shutdown and can't raise her head. I want to put my hand against the mirror, or tap, do anything to connect – but that's against the rules. The rules said she had to go alone – and I think this makes no sense because she is surrounded by bright lights, with someone she's only just met, and pleaded desperately with her eyes not to have to go. And I feel I am letting her down because her eyes beg me to stay. But I mask and I play by the rules, and I talk and mask and edit myself to the paediatrician and wait for it to be over.

The usual assessment questions start with pregnancy. But that's not my start. What I don't say – because they didn't ask, and I don't know how to say it – is that these aren't the right questions to understand our story. They ask about any other children. And that's not the right question. Because the right story starts with a very brief chapter that didn't make it past Chapter 1: Pregnancy. And that is a fundamental part of my story, the endless hiding in sunglasses walking the streets in tears before the joy of my second child. I manage to tell them I lost my first child. They jot down 'miscarriage', only child. Our story is already being filtered.

We gloss over how long it took to get this appointment. The endless, relentless game of pass the parcel around all the different local services, bouncing to a soundtrack I have long since tired of. It screeches in my mind because everyone repeats the same: we are not the right service. We finally pass the door into one assessment – but after an observation in school the clinician declares my child can't be Autistic because she picked up a glove and gave it to the teacher therefore demonstrating she had 'Theory of Mind' because she must have been concerned for the child who lost it. In a long walk back from the city centre to home, I have a protracted conversation with the clinician on my mobile explaining my child likes putting things back where they belong, she is a secret worker at our local superstore, re-arranging shelves when items are out of place – she loves sorting and organising and this is nothing to do with being concerned about the glove's rightful owner – and info dump about the problematic nature of that construct anyway. But I am wrong, and she is right. My child is not Autistic, not remotely. Many years later, that therapist becomes involved again briefly, and apologises for letting my child down because of her own lack of knowledge about the diversity of Autistic experience. That lack of knowledge cost us years of missed support and understanding – and yet I embrace her apology because it means that she learnt, and reflected, and changed her practice.

We circle back to The Assessment. Eventually the speech therapist comes back with my child, and we must swap so she feeds back to me whilst my child is again sent with a stranger, the paediatrician, where she remains, untouchable, through that mirror. The therapist tells me my child 'wouldn't' engage and 'wouldn't talk' so she couldn't score the formal measures and so she can't declare if she is Autistic or not because the measure can't give the answer. Despite the paediatrician returning and declaring it is likely she is Autistic based on my reports (and it feels like passing an exam), they declare Someone Else needs to see my child at home where she may be more comfortable, and they need her to talk. And so, we wait a bit more. Finally, another speech therapist visits us at home. This time, she asks just a few questions of my child, ones that she can draw or write or go and get a toy or anything else that she wants to use to answer. And from this she recognises that there is no doubt my child is Autistic. We wait a few weeks for the formal letter. And when it comes, I dance because we share our neurology, I knew we always did but finally the 'system' recognises this.

But when I read the letter, it's about the wrong child.

This letter is about a child who is 'disordered', 'non-communicative', has 'complex speech and language difficulties', 'plays repetitively', 'perseverates just drawing cats', 'doesn't play imaginatively', 'is highly anxious', 'resists change'. She has a 'disorder'. They suggest genetic testing because 'something else may be wrong'. And so, it goes on. And on. Each line becoming more and more wrong.

Who is this child?

This is not my child.

My child is a ray of sunshine that bursts forth from clouds of grey. My child is the most perfect little human there has ever been, full of giggles, love, hugs, humour, who loves to read, to spin, to play together, who cares deeply about animals (particularly cats, of course), who is the best person to hang out with, who creates dark and funny stories.

Their version is not my child. Their 'post-diagnosis' course for parents/caregivers keeps trying to fracture my version of my child. They repeat stories of deficit, disorder and lack of interest in others. I think I annoy them. A lot. I debate their narratives of disorder, indulge my granularity and highlight the issues with the literature they present. It doesn't go down too well. I'm supposed to listen about the 'difficulties' my child has in communication – but they don't listen when I try and explain how Autistic people communicate. They tell a story that many parents/caregivers will have been presented with, about having expected a luxury holiday in one country only to have to settle for a 'meh' holiday elsewhere. They may not mean to, but somehow, I am being told to settle for a two-star holiday somewhere I didn't want to go to. And I want to shout at them that my child is my five-star luxury resort. She is exactly as she should be. She is herself. She is.

Many years later we have a medical appointment. My child is largely non-speaking. She sits beside me, needing medical attention, and yet the doctor speaks about her, not to her as if she were not there. She may not speak back but there are many more ways of communicating than just words. Can the doctor hear her I wonder? I can hear her, and yet she does not speak.

She can hear the doctor; she processes the impact of being spoken about as if she is not in the room. I am asked if an upcoming appointment is 'for the autism'. I want to cry at these words. I wish to launch upon a long monologue. But I restrain myself. At least as much as I can. This is the opposite of how we speak about our shared neurology at home: being Autistic is what we are, not something that needs treating. I tell the doctor this because to stay silent is not in my nature and my child knows this. I speak up, for my child, for all the future Autistic young people this doctor will see in the hope that some words may sink in. She stares at me. Am I being too articulate to be Autistic? Or am I so Autistic I cannot see that I must require treatment 'for the autism' also?

Some people fit in. When you or your child fit *out*, it is both glorious…and entrapping. Because too often services do not listen, and they do not provide the care that Autistic people need. Too many Autistic young people have been let down by services throughout their lives, battered from pillow to post in an endless bureaucratic dystopia because they do not fit the right box. Isn't it time that services start thinking outside the box? Shatter those boxes. Find queer spaces to do things differently. Autistic rights are human rights.

4.2.2 Story 2: Perspectives of an OT: My Personal Experience

KATIE KERLEY

As a child raised in an accepting household of quirky people, I think I was cocooned from the feeling of being different in many ways. The security and surety of home was a haven I could always return to no matter what happened in the world outside. I was blanketed in the rhythms and routines of an environment that catered to me.

I felt it outside my home sure, but I also surrounded myself with like-minded souls who understood and accepted me. Nonetheless, stepping out of my comfort zone and into the wide open world, I often did feel that sense of being 'other' and therefore I performed many roles, and was adept at code switching to fit in with different groups. I played the part of a nerd, a goth, a girly girl etc. I think pretty convincingly but then I don't really know how it was received by people I was not close to.

I have the dual experience of having been both the assessor and the assessed, so I have been on both sides of the assessment table. This has given me a lot of insight and empathy in relation to the thoughts and feelings that someone may be experiencing prior to, during and after assessment.

I vividly remember a psychologist friend saying to me beforehand 'What will you do if they say you are not Autistic?' and feeling a small amount of panic that I could be wrong about who I am or that I might not be seen for who I am. This is a question I often ask people who come to see me. The answers are often so sure and so definite, ranging from 'well that would be wrong' to 'if that's the case then I clearly don't know myself'. I felt this way too, but still a small seed of doubt was sown. I think a lot of us late-identified Autistics have this little shadow of uncertainty and imposter syndrome looming over us. Maybe because we have had years of masking and people believed our performance so wholly that we lost who we were behind the mask. In the end, confirming that you are Autistic, it's kind of like a discovery and a rediscovery all in one.

I think it's important to mention something here. I am not proud of this, but I have been 'trained' in identifying an Autistic person as part of a multi-disciplinary team for quite a long time, and I have worked with Autistic children in some capacity for almost two decades by now, and I still did not see myself as being Autistic for years. I just didn't consider it. Even though I seemed to have a strong affinity and sense of kinship with both Autistic children and adults. I already knew I was dyspraxic and possibly ADHD, so surely this accounted for all my traits and quirks? It was only when I expanded my work to include Autistic adults that I started to very vividly see myself mirrored back. And the amazing thing is that my clients identified this in me too. Many of them said, 'it seems that you are Autistic too…are you really not?' At this point, I wasn't sure…

I also attended almost every webinar put out by Ausome Training (an Autistic-led neurodiversity training organisation, offering education and support for Autistic people, families, healthcare providers and educators) over a certain time span and was deeply passionate about doing so. I felt so many feelings during these webinars! I would be pacing, heart racing, intermittently scurrying over to my laptop to frantically type in the chat. Why did I care so much and why did I feel such intense emotions listening to Actually Autistic people talk about Actually Autistic experiences? Over time, my suspicions about myself solidified into a clearer view and I thought during the COVID-19 lockdowns that it was time I confirmed it officially. I considered this then, and still do to this day, to be one of the best gifts I could give to myself, to invest in absolutely confirming who I am.

This left me with a dilemma, where to go and what to do? I had read so many diagnostic reports from my clients and heard their experience of being confronted with a blunt, medicalised and pathologised document describing them as if they were a lab specimen or a case study. I did not want this for myself, even though I knew I would see through the stark language and maybe see it as a means to an end. A necessary ugliness to endure in order for me to confirm my identity.

Months into this predicament (I can be such a ruminant!), a young woman came to see me for an OT assessment. She had recently been identified as Autistic and kindly shared all her documentation with me. Among the documents was a letter from a psychologist at The Adult Autism Practice addressed to her, informing that she was indeed Autistic and warmly welcoming her to the Autistic community, saying that 'Autism is a different neurotype, and a valid way to be in the world', among other wonderful affirming things. Nothing medical or pathologising. This is exactly what I wanted my experience to be.

I experienced the usual anxiety and jitters prior to the assessment nonetheless (I think most people experience this to a lesser or greater extent) but was excited and eager to get started.

All of my communication preferences were checked beforehand and respected. I was given a variety of ways to express myself, including in writing and in conversations. I found the whole experience overwhelmingly validating, and while this was obviously very positive, I was not prepared for the emotions it unlocked. I had a big cry after my final session. I wasn't sad, I don't think, I can't explain it accurately, but it was a strange concoction of relief, validation and maybe grief at not knowing sooner.

Nor was I prepared for the complete exhaustion! I am not by nature a tired person, in fact quite the opposite, but I found myself needing a nap after one of my sessions. This is something I actually hadn't hugely considered for my own clients and is now something I advise them about – the fact that you may feel very tired and need to rest, so let it happen if it needs to. I recommend that if the assessment is in the morning, that children don't go to school in the afternoon afterwards, and that they do what their mind and body needs them to do, be it rest, game, read, run around and blow off steam, whatever.

It's funny, but I feel like acknowledging and confirming my Autistic identity has made me a better OT. I didn't intend for this, or even expect it, but my own identity has become a tool for me – a therapeutic use of self I didn't foresee. I think it's important that I openly talk about this for many reasons. One being to destigmatise the topic and another being to relate and empathise with the children and adults who come see me, and also to let them know (before they even say a word to me) that I may be a kindred spirit and they are safe with this.

I never realised that so much of my shared joy in the clinic came from shared neurodivergent experiences, that I enjoyed stimming and echolalia and deep dives into niche topics not just because my client's joy is rewarding to me, but also because this is my joy too!

A particularly beautiful experience I had was with a girl who was then 8 years old coming to see me in the clinic. I had been part of this girl's Autistic identification process. I felt a particular kinship with her, and also us Autistics often don't massively care for social hierarchy so I, and many of the children who come see me, consider ourselves to be peers. Anyway, I told her that I thought I was Autistic and that I was going to have my own assessment soon. She responded with 'well I think you are Autistic, and I hope the person doing your assessment is as nice to you as you were to me when I had mine'. I'm not ashamed to say that I was close to tears hearing this.

On that note, isn't it interesting that this child identified me as Autistic too?? This is not as uncommon as you might think. We seem to have a sense for recognising each other. I love the old Irish saying 'Athníonn ciaróg ciaróg eile' – one beetle recognises another beetle. And we do recognise each other! I remember during my initial training to do autism assessments asking if other people 'just knew' when a person is Autistic, and people stared at me blankly. I now know what that was.

This is so strong that many of us are drawn to other neurodivergent folk and develop communities and relationships. I am blessed to have an Autistic life partner who really gets me and eclectic neurodivergent friends. I don't know if I could build and share a life with a neurotypical.

Autistic culture is so rich and varied and yet hardly anyone outside of the community knows it exists! But it does, and it takes many wonderful forms.

I often say that I can 'feel' when I meet another Autistic person, be it socially or in the clinic. But I absolutely cannot write this in a report and it is absolutely not best practice!

Neuro-affirmative identification processes are not only valuable and desirable but protective of a person's sense of self and self-worth. Many assessment processes set up an Autistic person to fail as a neurotypical, rather than to succeed as an Autistic. Often, they are a measure of distress when a person does not live up to neuro-normative standards.

Furthermore, more often than not, Autistic people are identified through their struggles rather than their successes. I had the good fortune to choose my process at a time in my life when I wanted to, not because I had to. Not everyone has that luxury. Only identifying autism when a person is struggling sends a message that being Autistic is a struggle. To be clear, I am not saying I or other Autistic people don't struggle; we do, but we don't only struggle. We also have joy and peace and achievement and rich and diverse lives.

If this is the start of the identification journey, how can we expect Autistic young people to thrive, flourish and bloom as their Autistic selves?

Neurodiversity affirmative identification processes say, 'I see you for you, you are who you are supposed to be, you are not a broken neurotypical but a complete and whole Autistic being.' We owe this to the next generation of Autistics. We already exist in a world where we are an often invisible (sometimes visible) minority, and this world does not always suit us. Positive and affirming identification processes enable young people to navigate this world more comfortably and, dare I say, more boldly.

Doing neuro-affirmative assessment also feels better for us clinicians. I promise this is true! It is so much better to know you are equipping a young person and their family with validating information. Not pushing a box of tissues towards them and saying, 'I am so sorry', and continuing to feed into the tragedy narrative. We can send families out into the world with tools to make their way on their own unique journeys. As the people who help identify and confirm that a child or young person is Autistic, we can stop feeding the notion that autism is something bad and help forge a better path. The whole world will be better for it.

CHAPTER 5

The Neurodiversity Paradigm and Neurodiversity Affirmative Practice

5.1 Introduction

In this chapter, we summarise key principles of working with Autistic children and young people within a neurodiversity affirmative framework. We explain our understanding of the Neurodiversity Paradigm (the underlying philosophy) and Neurodiversity Movement (a human rights, disability and social movement). Our emphasis is on working with Autistic children and young people, but the underlying principles apply equally to working with any neurodivergent person.

5.2 What Is the Neurodiversity Paradigm?

Neurodiversity is a social justice movement which posits that the way neurodivergent individuals (e.g., Autistic, ADHDer, dyslexic) experience and interact with the world is part of natural diversity. This movement moves away from the medical model which pathologises disability as something 'wrong' with the individual and aligns closer with the social model which proposes that it is society and the barriers posed by systems that disable people, not something inherent to the person themselves. Bertilsdotter Rosqvist et al. (2020) explain that the Neurodiversity Paradigm encompasses lived experiences, how knowledge is produced, an ethical stance and countering a neurotypical gaze with a neurodivergent gaze.

The term neurodiversity refers to the vast variety of human brain types, how brains are structured, how they process information and interact with the world. Biodiversity means the biological variety and variability in the world. We can see in nature the rich diversity of every living thing. If ecosystems and species were not diverse, the world simply would not survive. All types of brain are considered to be part of neurodiversity. People whose brains are considered different to the perceived majority are considered neurodivergent. This includes autism, dyspraxia, dyslexia and ADHD. It can also include people with cluster headaches, acquired brain injury, PTSD, depression, Tourette's and OCD. The Neurodiversity Movement is a human rights, disability and social movement started by Autistic advocates. Botha et al. (2024) point out that whilst the term has often been (incorrectly) attributed to the work of Judy Singer, it developed collectively amongst Autistic activist communities. The Neurodiversity Paradigm is the philosophy behind the Neurodiversity Movement. This tells us that:

- All ways of being in the world are as valid as another.

- Being neurodivergent is a naturally occurring brain difference which leads to a different way of experiencing the world. It is not a 'disorder' or 'condition'.

- Being neurodivergent is fundamental to everything about that person, who moves through the world and experiences it as a neurodivergent person.

- No neurodivergent person needs to spend their lives trying to meet neurotypical (non-neurodivergent) standards. There is no one way of being in this world.

- We do not have a 'condition'. For example, being Autistic is part of our identity, a community and a culture.

- Difficulties in life arise because we are living in a world that does not always recognise or meet our needs. The challenge is in our environment, not ourselves.

- Non-neurodivergent people very often have not understood that neurodivergent people have different sensory needs, communication styles and experiences. This is where things can lead to challenges for us.

- The Neurodiversity Paradigm acknowledges that Autistic functioning (or flourishing) is driven by the relationship between the individual and their environment, consistent with Beardon's golden equation (Autism + Environment = Outcome; Beardon, 2017).

Neurodiversity is simply a beautiful part of human experience. It is a valid and important way of being. It can offer great beauty (but also challenges when our needs are not met by our environment and systems surrounding us). Sadly, neurodivergent children and young people are often told that they cannot do things, that their way of doing things is not right, or that they should be doing things differently.

The Neurodiversity Paradigm tells that our story is full of strengths that should be celebrated. That we can be creative thinkers that spot details others simply cannot, that our passions for certain topics and activities can lead to us being incredibly knowledgeable, that our ability to focus on something intently is a skill that can give us great joy. It tells us that our way of being in relationships is beautiful, that neurodivergent people often connect with each other through in-depth information sharing and find great friendship in doing so. It tells us that we do not need to change how we are; our preferred way of communicating is just as it should be for us, and that simply because a neurotypical person cannot see the wonder in how we play, relate to others or experience the world it does not mean it is not there. The Neurodiversity Paradigm holds space for both the strengths and the needs that come with being Autistic. It is not a position of being 'positive' about being Autistic. Such a position denies the challenges that many Autistic people face interacting with a world that is not made for and does not understand our neurology.

We refer you to Wise (2024) for a detailed discussion of how the Neurodiversity Movement emerged to recognise all the work that Autistic activists, advocates, academics and the wider community have done to progress thinking about Autistic experience. We also refer you to Chapman's (2023) *Empire of Normality* which locates the histories of the neurodiversity and disability movements within the wider societal context of capitalism. See the two boxes below for an occupational therapist's and a speech and language therapist's view on neurodiversity affirmative services.

PERSPECTIVES OF AN OT: NEURO-AFFIRMATIVE SERVICES

KATIE KERLEY

I established Horizons Therapy Services along with my business partner Margeurite in 2018. I was not neurodiversity affirmative then, in fact I had never heard of the term. I was practicing in a way that I look back at now and shudder: social skills training, modifying behaviour, altering play, assuming I knew what occupations mattered to my clients without thinking too deeply. Things I would be ashamed to do now. I didn't know better then but I do now.

Some things I have learned on my own journey towards neuro-affirmativity in my own practice:

- We have a responsibility to ensure that we are always evolving and responding to communities we work with.

- We have not only learned but we have to unlearn – which sometimes can be harder. Times change and so will we.

- It is important that we:

    - make sure each person is treated as an individual and supported to be the most satisfied and authentic version of themselves

    - modify the environment to support engagement and comfort, including the physical, social and cultural environment

    - promote a pro-neurodiversity culture

    - provide communication means and opportunities suited to each individual

    - provide access to robust and reliable means of assisted communication (e.g., AAC) when needed

    - stay up to date on current information from research and from the neurodivergent, disabled, mental health and LGBTQIA+ communities, and change with updated information

    - contribute to the education of university students and the future of our professions – this way we can ensure that future generations of clinicians will be neuro-affirmative and continue to evolve therapeutic practices.

Due to current evidence and information and to ensure person-centred best practices we do not:

- teach social skills or run social skills groups

- make assumptions about what occupations are meaningful based on neurotypical expectations

- use or recommend behaviour modification including Applied Behaviour Analysis (ABA), Positive Behaviour Support (PBS) or any external reward-based strategies.

Being neurodiversity affirmative as an occupational therapist really harks back to our theoretical foundations – being person centred, focusing on meaning in everyday life and enabling people to what they want to do.

I think the key word for us, more so than 'occupation', is 'meaning'. Things that are meaningful to neurotypicals may not matter to Autistics and other things might matter so much more than we expect.

PERSPECTIVES OF AN SLT: CONDUCTING NEURODIVERSITY AFFIRMATIVE ASSESSMENTS

ELAINE MCGREEVY

The medical model operates under the pathology paradigm (Walker, 2021), which treats cognitive, learning and neurodevelopmental disabilities as atypical, disordered, impaired or dysfunctional. Professionals using this paradigm look for deviation and prescribe treatment. SLTs recommend 'dosage' (Frizelle et al., 2021) to remediate disorder. By contrast, the emancipatory Neurodiversity Paradigm views cognitive diversity as the norm. Chapman and Botha (2023) say that to achieve an inclusive society where neurological minorities are honoured and included necessitates using a neurodivergence-informed set of principles. SLTs can adopt Chapman and Botha's (2023) recommendations to practice within a neurodivergence-informed paradigm.

First, in reconceptualising dysfunction as relational rather than individual, the SLT can use the double empathy problem (Milton, 2012; see Section 6.10) to re-frame and address communication breakdowns, recognising that these occur within social interactions that are continually negotiated and mutually constructed, especially relevant where unequal power relations are at play. To support the neurodivergent child, the SLT focuses on the environment, relationships and communication partners.

Second, through their practice and interactions with the child and family, SLTs can emphasise neurodivergence acceptance and pride. The SLT will draw on an evidence base informed by those with lived experience and will adopt community-preferred language and terminology. SLTs should critique research that centres neuro-normativity and recognise limitations in the evidence base due to lack of research that does not account for the 'full range of human communication including that of people with communication disabilities' (Jagoe & Wharton, 2021).

Third, SLTs should be diligent about cultivating a relational epistemic humility regarding different experiences of neurodivergence and disablement. Recognising the individual and their family as experts in their own experiences, able to contribute to and have agency in their own assessment, will help address the power imbalance that often exists between professionals and families and children receiving support within medical model systems.

5.3 What Is Neuro-Affirmative Practice: How to Work in This Way

Working within a neurodiversity affirming frame means moving away from deficit-based formulations of Autistic experience, understanding being Autistic as a neurotype, recognising the value of diversity, honouring and respecting Autistic ways of being, advocating for systems and environmental change, and not seeking to change the Autistic person's way of being (e.g., rejecting neurotypical social skills training and compliance-based approaches). It means engaging with and committing deeply to the underlying philosophy of the Neurodiversity Paradigm, not merely adopting the language of the Neurodiversity Movement, making superficial shifts to practice but without challenging the underlying ethos of the pathology paradigm driving practice. Chapman (2023) explains that this 'neurodiversity-lite' approach leaves the dominant paradigm unchallenged despite an apparent shift.

In clinical work and educational spaces, a neurodiversity affirmative approach is one which respects and honours all forms of communication and ways of being, incorporating the young person's experiences and opinions in developing supports and goals that are meaningful to them; values sensory needs and using respectful and neurodiversity affirmative language; supports the Autistic young person to cultivate their Autistic identity; and actively seeks to counteract the deficit-based narratives surrounding Autistic experience to support young people to thrive.

We summarise key principles below:

- Re-frame Autistic experience from a disorder to a neurotype.

  The medical model of disability, and all classification systems arising from this model (e.g., the DSM-5-TR and ICD-11) are inherently based on neuro-normative assumptions. Being Autistic is a valid, different way of experiencing the world, not a disorder, and has a distinct developmental trajectory.

- Stop pathologising Autistic ways of being.

  Current autism identification (assessment) procedures and tests are based on pathologisation of Autistic ways of being. For example, being adept at social chit chat is considered an arbitrary 'gold standard' way to interact, with a dislike of this communication style viewed as a 'deficit'. Within Autistic culture, however, communicating in depth on one topic is a much more valued method of communication. Turn taking still occurs in 'info dumping' but at a slower pace than the perceived neuro-majority consider as the 'right' way to interact.

- Supports should target needs and challenges that Autistic people experience, not Autistic ways of being.

  Post-identification support for Autistic children and teenagers should focus on self-advocacy and self-determination. There is no need to 'treat' their neurology. There is nothing to treat. Instead, focus on priority areas for support such as adapting both the physical and social environment to better fit their needs (e.g., sensory needs, monotropic attention, communication styles). Autistic ways of being should be validated, a positive Autistic self-identity cultivated, mental health needs attended to, alongside supporting an understanding of specific perception and sensory differences, empowering self-advocacy and supporting those close to the child to appreciate Autistic experience through a neuro-affirmative lens.

- Ensure that the Autistic voice is at the centre of everything you do.

   This does not mean a tokenistic 'listening to' – an implied power dynamic of the perceived neuro-majority 'allowing' notional space for the voice of a marginalised group but continuing as before. The Autistic community must have the agency and power to choose for themselves how their experience is explored, understood, identified and supported. As a professional working in this area, this means committing to learning and engaging with the Autistic community's voice, culture, Autistic-led research and publications, and community priorities for language, future research and support.

- Respect Autistic culture and identity.

   We have an Autistic culture, communication and identity. Respect the symbols and concepts that we identify with (e.g., gold infinity symbol, double empathy, monotropism), and those that we firmly reject (e.g., the puzzle piece, compliance-based behavioural approaches, 'Theory of Mind'). We have distinct ways of being in, exploring and learning about the world. Learn by listening to us and seek to explore our culture (respectfully, not from a 'zoo' perspective).

- If you have the power, employ Autistic and otherwise neurodivergent team members. If you don't have the power, advocate others to do so.

   This call to action is for all people regardless of their neurology. Many Autistic and otherwise neurodivergent people are employers and leaders too. Being neurodiversity affirmative does not just mean changing your language to be more respectful of the community, but making systemic changes across workplaces, healthcare systems, communities and society so that Autistic and otherwise neurodivergent people have the equal rights they deserve. This requires community allies as well as advocates. It is a basic human right to have a voice and a 'place at the table' in equal decision-making about community needs, and diversifying teams in this way also leads to better care and support.

- Recognise that there is immense value in diversity.

   There is inherent value in diversity in and of itself. We can see the significant negative impact that a reduction of biodiversity causes to ecosystems. As with biodiversity, all humans are part of a tapestry of neurodiversity, and we are all connected to each other. We need all kinds of people and minds in order to flourish as worldwide societies. Being neurodiversity affirmative is to see and celebrate the value of this diversity.

- Recognise that there is value in living a disabled life.

  To see the value in disability and living a disabled life requires examining how our views on disability are inextricably tied to capitalist ideals of being 'productive' and 'independence' (i.e., needing no outside help or support again so that you don't cost the 'system' money). Both professionals and individuals may need support in examining their relationship with disability and unpacking what external factors impact on this. Seeing the value in disability and a disabled life requires ongoing reflection and unpacking of ableism for us all (whether disabled or not). Totton (2015) highlights that so-called 'normalcy' is temporary – for some people it is a rare experience, whereas it is a central feature of others' lives. In other words, we all need to challenge the many assumptions we have collectively gathered over a lifetime of both implicit and explicit messaging transmitted from the people and societal structures around us. To change these external messages and forces, we need first to reflect and change ourselves, including our definition of what 'being productive' means and broadening this from only producing something of monetary or other value to society, to include production of something of value to that individual person, or the production of calm, joy or connection with life.

- Ensure that all neurodivergent people (including those with significant intellectual disability and high support needs) have power, a place at the table, and are supported and advocated for.

  Being neurodiversity affirmative means that all neurodivergent people, no matter how high their support needs are, or how they communicate, have an equal voice and agency in relation to their own lives and communities. The Neurodiversity Movement was born out of the wider disability movement and has always (and continues to) encompassed, embraced and advocated for the voices of all disabled people.

  Traditionally, little effort has been made by researchers or clinicians within healthcare systems to access the voice of non-speaking or sometimes non-speaking Autistic people, with or without an intellectual disability. But it is possible to capture these voices. There is a large online community of non-speaking or minimally speaking Autistic adults (with and without an intellectual disability) who interact online on X, other social media platforms and safe online spaces. They often speak out there about what is important to them, how they want to be spoken about, their priorities for research and how they want their care managed. These voices need to be listened to and taken seriously in terms of service planning and supports.

• Reject compliance-based behaviour approaches, e.g., ABA.

Behaviour-based compliance approaches are fully rejected by the Autistic community and the Neurodiversity Paradigm. Compliance-based behavioural methods (including PBS and ABA) are incompatible with a human rights model emphasising the vital importance of self-advocacy and self-determination. Besides this, the fact alone that the Autistic community rejects them should be enough. If a method is based on compliance through behavioural means, it is not neurodiversity affirmative.

• Reject neurotypical social skills training.

Neurotypical social skills training is fully rejected by the Autistic community and Neurodiversity Paradigm. Neurotypical social skills training encourages neurodivergent people to hide their true selves (which decades of psychological research has shown us is a core element of positive mental health) and instead promotes masking. It leads to internalised feelings of shame and ableism and the person's core ways of being and interacting are presented as something to hide and change. It ignores Milton's (2012) work on double empathy: any difficulties in cross-neurotype communication are mutual and are not located in the Autistic person alone (see Section 6.10). The emphasis should be on both Autistic and neurotypical people developing understanding of each other's ways of being and working together on best ways to best interact with each other. There needs to be a mutual respect for the diversity of communication between humans.

• Advocate for systems and environmental changes.

Systematic, cultural and environmental factors are major barriers for the Autistic community in relation to achieving good quality of life and mental health resulting in Autistic people being misunderstood, misdiagnosed, mischaracterised, rejected and not listened to as a group.

Professionals seeking to make positive changes for Autistic people need to move beyond just assessment (or identification as we call it) or individual therapy and engage in the more wide-reaching work of combatting systemic injustices by advocating for change within the systems around their clients. This means (if you are not Autistic yourself) learning to be a true ally and using your privileged position to stand with Autistic people in helping to change these systems.

- Support fostering a positive Autistic identity as a priority goal.

  Fostering a positive Autistic identity should be the number one goal for all professionals working in this area. Support the children and young people coming to you to have pride in their culture, value their own personal communication style and recognise and increase their own personal strengths. Help them to promote their own self-autonomy and self-advocacy. Perhaps most important of all, link them in with Autistic peers and community. Help them to understand what it means to be neurodiversity affirmative and the social model of disability, and identifying for themselves what the components of a good and valuable life are, and how they can advocate for these things. Support them in understanding the importance of environmental fit to their overall well-being.

Murphy (2022), an early years educator, has developed The Neurodiversity and Ableism Reflection Tool, aimed at supporting early years educators in their re-learning process towards becoming neurodiversity affirmative practitioners. She breaks down this process into two stages:

1. Becoming neurodiversity informed.

   Spending time becoming informed about the concept, movement and approach; involves new learning and ways of being.

2. Becoming neurodiversity affirmative.

   Murphy (2022) explains that this means affirming, empowering and embracing difference, whilst supporting and adapting to address areas of need in our everyday practices and beliefs.

   Murphy (2022) distinguishes between three learning zones. In the Comfort Zone, practitioners reflect on their neurotypical gaze (McDermott, 2022) and making this visible. Remaining in the Curious Zone means being at risk of perpetuating and failing to acknowledge biases in the creation of knowledge and how these can add to the marginalisation of neurodivergent people. The process of re-learning involves deliberately leaving the Comfort and Curious Zones to enter the Learning and Growth Zones. This is not, and should not be, a linear process but one of continued reflection and moving between zones fluidly as we seek to become neurodiversity affirmative practitioners. We summarise these zones briefly below but refer to Murphy (2022) for a full description.

- Comfort Zone. This includes:

  - prioritising what we know over what we could learn
  - using outdated language (e.g., referring to a child as 'high functioning', using person-first language)
  - following usual practices and systemic norms without question
  - adopting an 'expert' position
  - not questioning oppression and oppressive practices.

- Curious Zone. This includes:

  - feeling defensive when new knowledge contradicts what we thought we knew
  - holding onto outdated language and terminology, relying on a position of 'but this is how we have always done it'
  - being curious yet still uncomfortable with new knowledge
  - experimenting with 'neurodiversity-lite' (e.g., superficially using language of the Neurodiversity Paradigm without a real shift in practice), that is, engaging with the Neurodiversity Paradigm in a tokenistic way.

- Learning Zone. This includes:

  - being able to reflect on our discomfort as we recognise what we have learned about autism may have been inaccurate/biased
  - listening and learning from disabled people, questioning ableist practice
  - spreading the word about neurodiversity affirming practices
  - understanding the intersectional model of disability, including privilege and oppression
  - experimenting with language with more confidence and making room for mistakes and learning

- – seeking out views of Autistic/otherwise neurodivergent people.

- Growth Zone. This includes:

  - – speaking up for Autistic rights. Taking opportunities to challenge oppressive language and practice by colleagues
  - – effectively managing guilt about previous practice choices and using this to drive your practice forward
  - – actively dismantling neurodivergent and disability myths with your colleagues and peers
  - – being aware that any fragility is ours to address. Not attributing it to the Autistic people with whom you are working, but owning it
  - – asking about language preferences. Being flexible
  - – combining lived experience frameworks with inclusive, evidence-based practice
  - – taking steps to change practice that does not affirm identity
  - – engaging, interacting with and centring disabled and neurodivergent voices
  - – being compassionate to others at the different zones of growth
  - – using language and terminology accurately but in flexible ways knowing things can change.

We encourage you to reflect on your own learning process and identify where you might be as a practitioner. How does this compare to your previous practice? Has it changed as you have been reading through this book? What might need to happen in the future to keep developing as a practitioner and keep reflecting on which 'zone' you may be in? As Murphy (2022) points out, neurodiversity affirming practice means we need to keep journeying beyond our comfort zone.

5.4 Conclusion

In this chapter, we summarised key ideas of the Neurodiversity Paradigm in order to support clinicians to understand why it is so important to shift to a neurodiversity affirmative approach to the identification process. We explained the Neurodiversity Movement as a human rights, disability and social movement which is underpinned by the philosophy of the Neurodiversity Paradigm. Understanding the tenets of the Neurodiversity Paradigm as opposed to what Walker (2021) describes as the 'pathology paradigm' is crucial to ensure that professionals truly commit to a paradigm shift in how they approach the identification process in order to avoid a 'neurodiversity-lite' approach in which clinicians adopt neurodiversity affirmative language but without a deep understanding of the reasons why. This too often means that assessments remain underpinned by a deficit-based model. We also summarised what neurodiversity affirmative approaches 'look like' in practice and presented guidance for practitioners to reflect upon their professional development, drawing on Murphy's (2022) framework.

CHAPTER 6

Understanding Autistic Experience

6.1 Introduction

In this chapter, and before we begin with the practical 'how to' undertake an identification with children in later chapters, we aim to support clinicians by providing information and reflections on the Autistic experience, as it is an area that has been extensively written about and yet written with so much inaccuracy. This is because a huge part of the journey to becoming a neuro-affirmative practitioner is not only to change our assessment practices, but also to begin questioning our own assumptions and knowledge about Autistic experience. We encourage clinicians to continually reflect on the knowledge we hold and how we came to hold it, and will discuss the rationale for this. Areas covered in this chapter include looking at the concept of label vs. identity, monotropism, double empathy, examining the information we hold about the Autistic experience and how we came to hold it, the notion of 'normal', a brief overview of sensory needs and a discussion of executive function.

6.2 Label vs. Identity

There are many people within society who hold the view that 'labelling' only leads to negative consequences. Parents and caregivers, and those within a child's wider circle, (e.g., teachers, grandparents etc.), often comment that 'labelling' a child would be detrimental to them as it may attract stigma or stereotypes about a young person. While it is true that much of society has outdated and inaccurate beliefs in relation to what being Autistic means (Underhill et al., 2019) and there still can be stigma attached to being Autistic (Jones et al., 2015), there are also documented benefits to understanding Autistic identity and sharing this with others (Sasson & Morrison, 2019). For neurotypical young people, being aware that their peer is neurodivergent leads to better understanding of the differences between them and greater opportunity for better interaction from a double empathy perspective.

For schools, the LEANS project (Learning About Neurodiversity at School) provides a curriculum for 8–11-year-olds which teaches about neurodiversity (Alcorn et al., 2022). There is evidence that university students demonstrate more positive attitudes towards a person who finds social interaction and neurotypical communication challenging when they are aware that the person is Autistic, than when they are incorrectly labelled as neurotypical (Brosnan & Mills, 2016; Matthews et al., 2015).

A perception about the damaging effects of 'labelling' is often used as a reason not to pursue exploring whether or not a young person is Autistic or otherwise neurodivergent. However, there is clear evidence that children who learn that they are Autistic at a younger age have a heightened quality of life and well-being in adulthood, and they are empowered by having access to support and a foundation for self-understanding that supports them to thrive in adulthood (Oredipe et al., 2023). Providing a framework to interpret experiences through identification as Autistic gives rise to self-understanding, self-compassion and coping strategies (Arnold et al., 2020; Crane et al., 2019, 2021). This research is clearly borne out every day in the work that we do with children and adolescents. Furthermore, Autistic adolescents whose parents were open with them from a young age about their Autistic identity tend to describe themselves more positively than peers who have not been told they are Autistic (Riccio et al., 2021), and those who learn about it earlier tend to view it as a positive or neutral aspect of themselves (Mogensen & Mason, 2015) rather than something shameful.

When working with young people and their families, clinicians will often meet parents, caregivers and occasionally other professionals, teachers etc. who express a reluctance to 'label' a child. When this occurs, it is important to work closely with those expressing such views to further understand their reluctance in order to move forward. It must be considered that a biological parent of an Autistic child is likely to be Autistic themselves and may be unaware of this. They may have grown up within a family and/or a society full of stigma and false negative beliefs about Autistic identity, and they may have endured significant pressure to mask their own experiences. They may subconsciously or consciously fear that if their child is identified as Autistic, they will endure similar stress. Other professionals, teachers etc. may hold outdated views and false beliefs about Autistic identity, or they may view the increase in identification of Autistic children and young people as a negative occurrence. It is important to take time during the process to understand and challenge such views and to support the adults within a young person's life to explore the benefits to having an understanding of identity, whether the young person is Autistic or neurotypical in their neurology.

There is clear evidence in relation to the benefits of learning about Autistic identity at a young age. When the 'Autistic' label is not there, other labels will exist anyway in its place and these inaccurate labels from a child's peers are likely to not be helpful, supportive or kind. Furthermore, being incorrectly labelled by parents/caregivers and wider family as 'neurotypical' when a child is not neurotypical can be extremely damaging and can lead to higher levels of masking and mental health challenges. The experience of growing up labelled as neurotypical and then subsequently being identified as Autistic as an adult is associated with a strong and complex emotional impact (Huang et al., 2020). Wrong 'labels' have the potential to harm, whereas the correct identification reduces harm and provides a pathway to supports.

Understanding or knowing one's neurology is essential in building a positive sense of self and identity. Without this, it is impossible to have a stable sense of self or a framework within which to understand experiences. There can be a false belief amongst parents and caregivers that not undertaking an assessment piece means that their child is not Autistic as they have not been formally identified as such. However not having the correct 'label' does not change the underlying identity, it just makes it more challenging for a young person to understand themselves and their experiences, which they usually know are different to their neurotypical peers. Even though for some it may initially be overwhelming to discover that they are Autistic, with access to the right supports and understanding a young person can develop a positive sense of identity that is based on authenticity and acceptance, and that encompasses their strengths as well as the challenges they experience.

6.3 Examining the Information We Hold

As clinicians and practitioners, we need to examine how we came to have our knowledge base of what we think is the Autistic experience and where we obtained the knowledge we now hold. What biases do we hold? Are we Autistic or not? What lies behind the current dominant deficit-based framing of knowledge about autism? In fact, we should question continuously the authority of knowledge sources, from whom it was produced and whose epistemic position was privileged (epistemic refers to knowledge; what we refer to here is whose knowledge was given prominence in the literature that shaped our views on the Autistic experience, how was it collected, and whose knowledge was ignored?). Can formal measures based on criteria developed from a neuro-normative understanding of Autistic experience ever be a truly valid measure of Autistic identity?

We encourage clinicians to critically examine the current diagnostic criteria for autism in the context of the power and privilege within which they were created (e.g., to what extent were Autistic people involved in the creation of DSM-5-TR criteria; did those involved in writing diagnostic criteria reflect people from multiply marginalised groups?). Whose voices are reflected in those criteria? Whose voices were not heard? Who defines notions of normativity? Who has the systemic and epistemic privilege to contribute to diagnostic criteria (e.g., are Autistic researchers, advocates, clinicians involved, and if not, why not)?

> For information about work being done by Community Against Prejudice Towards Autistic People (CAPTAP) to campaign for change in DSM criteria see www.captapnetwork.wordpress.com/revising-autism-diagnosis.

Examining our positionality (by which we mean our own societal and cultural experiences; educational privilege; reflecting on how our own neurotype may affect how we approach the assessment process and how we have gained our knowledge about Autistic experience; being aware of belonging / not belonging to communities of people with whom we are working etc.) is crucial in becoming aware of how it may bias your knowledge and approaches to your clinical work. To counteract this, we need to constantly examine who has the power in any clinical situation we are in, and also our own biases and possible prejudices, and continually be aware that as professionals our narratives about Autistic experiences are likely to be taken as fact and not challenged by the young people and families with whom we are working. This means there is great responsibility on us as assessing clinicians to get this as right as we possibly can, with the information we have at this time.

6.4 Whose Voices Are Heard, and in Which Circumstances?

There are increasing numbers of Autistic researchers, academics and advocates working to (re)construct knowledge about Autistic experiences. However, the dominant narratives (e.g., in diagnostic criteria) surrounding Autistic experiences continue at this time to reflect the perceived predominant neuro-majority (i.e., neurotypical people).

Research around Autistic experience has often excluded those who are non-speaking or who have a co-occurring learning disability. Whilst a full discussion of the ethics surrounding the construction of knowledge about Autistic experience is beyond the scope of this book, it is crucial that at all times we remember that when considering approaches to identification of Autistic experience, the validity of commonly used measures and the underlying research base, it is essential to be aware that Autistic people who do not use spoken language or those with co-occurring learning disabilities were most likely excluded from the research process (Hens, 2021). If we are to understand the full diversity of Autistic experience, we need to develop both research and identification approaches that incorporate the diversity of these experiences; we need to include those who do not use spoken language and those who either do or do not have a co-occurring learning experience. This includes changes in approaches to research and in the clinical space. For example, many Autistic people do not use spoken language, so research methods need to be developed which incorporate the experiences of those who are non-speaking (Hens, 2021).

As stated above, shifting our approach to identification involves understanding the processes involved in the construction of diagnostic criteria and knowledge production around Autistic experience and considering underlying epistemology (the process of knowledge creation). Fricker (2007) provides a full description of the injustice and violence that occurs in the production of knowledge; for example, Autistic people not being believed simply because they are Autistic. This means that Autistic people may not be fully included in research processes (either as participants, research not meeting accessibility or communication needs, or having their authority as academics doubted because they are Autistic). Someone's knowledge may be dismissed because they belong to a minority group (testimonial injustice; Chapman & Carel, 2022), or a community's vocabulary (e.g., to describe their own experiences) may be distorted because they are a minority group, meaning they do not have language with which to describe their own experience (hermeneutical injustice; Chapman & Carel, 2022).

We encourage you as professionals looking to become fully neurodiversity affirmative in your work to seek out Autistic-led research, work by Autistic scholars, research that is guided by the priorities of the Autistic community, and to read material by Autistic authors, both academic and non-academic (e.g., blogs, social media), being mindful that it is a privilege open to only a few to have a 'formal platform' from which to disseminate ideas.

6.5 The Notion of 'Normal'

Narratives of deficiency surrounding Autistic ways of being necessarily assume that there is a 'normal' child, and for this reason in this section we examine briefly how this notion developed. Of course, when considering any notion of what is 'normal', we need to consider who has the power to define what 'normal' is and to what 'normal' is compared to. It is typically those that claim to be 'normal' that have the power to define what is not normal (Totton, 2023).

What comes to your mind when you reflect on the word 'normal'? Does it bring up an image of a normal distribution curve in a statistical sense, where only those in the middle are 'normal' and either side are 'abnormal', perhaps on one side of the distribution curve seen as different in a negative, deficient way, and on the other side, different in an eccentric, artistic, socially valued way? What other reflections come to mind (e.g., epistemic authority, neuro-normativity, hetero-normativity, power relationships, intersectionality)? Do you conceptualise 'normal' as binary ('normal' vs. 'abnormal'), or as existing on a spectrum ('very abnormal, within a socially devalued frame, through to very normal, within a social valued frame')? Can you hold in mind multiple intersections of identity, multiple marginalisations and how we might be seen as 'normal' in one sphere and 'abnormal' in another? How does this impact on your personal construction of what being Autistic is?

For those interested to read more, see Chapman (2023) who outlines the intellectual and social history of mental health and concepts of normality, and explains that coinciding with the rise of capitalism was the development of new statistical methods (allowing mental and cognitive abilities to be ranked in relation to a statistical norm) and mechanistic understanding of the body which permitted 'normality' to be 'scientifically legitimised' (Chapman, 2023, p. 63).

6.6 Construction of the 'Normal Child'

Waltz (2020) explains that the construct of the 'normal' child has existed for only about 100 years and must be seen as having developed within the particular social and industrial context of those times, whereby a 'normal child' was constructed as an 'aspirational production goal for parents' (Waltz, 2020, p. 18) within the industrial context of that time. This included societal structures such as Child Guidance Movements, a context within which Kanner, Bowlby and other child psychiatrists worked, and it was there that early workers in autism theory, 'diagnosis' and practice worked. Chapman (2023) explains that this expanding interest in childhood development in the early 20th century divided children based on their 'apparent normality' compared to newly created, standardised developmental norms (Nadesan, 2005, p. 58), and developmental 'normality' became more constrained by standards of new norms of 'developmental milestones'.

> Chapman (2023), a neurodivergent philosopher, argues that 'normal' became linked to understanding productivity within the context of capitalism, within which the pathology paradigm thrived.

Hens (2021) points out that it was once institutions such as compulsory education, child psychiatry and psychological research gained an influential role in society ('laying down the contours of normality'; Hens, 2021, p. 57) that the concept of autism could develop and be accepted. Whilst we stress that there are different developmental trajectories for Autistic and non-autistic young people (of no less value because those trajectories are different to what is taken as the gold standard based on neuro-normative assumptions and standards), nonetheless Autistic children are inevitably compared to the dominant understanding of what 'normal' development is (Brownlow et al., 2023, p. 21). Waltz (2020) explains that within that context, parents were faced with demands and challenges to teach their children to regulate emotional expression and behaviour within strict notions of what was 'normal', based also within a context of adulthood itself becoming 'more complex in many ways, which meant that children and young people must adjust accordingly. Emotional health itself was redefined, becoming harder to achieve'; Stearns, 2004, p. 49). Waltz (2020) proceeds to point out that regardless of the actual young person that parents had, they were encouraged to follow prescribed ways to raise their child aligned with this false notion of a 'normal child', with the Child Guidance Movements drawing upon fear of 'abnormalcy' to drive parents to aspire to this artificial ideal. It is within such contexts that compliance-based behavioural-based approaches could thrive because parents were driven to aspire to 'normalcy', which equated to neurotypicality.

The box below summarises the PEOP Model which promotes a person-centred approach within occupational therapy.

PERSPECTIVES OF AN OT: THE PEOP MODEL

KATIE KERLEY

The Person-Environment-Occupation-Performance Model (PEOP) (Baum et al., 2015) is a conceptual framework that was initially developed in 1985 to help move occupational therapists away from a mostly biomedical way of thinking and brought us into a more person-centred approach. These person-centred models that enable us to consider the whole human being in their environmental context, and engaging in an occupation, fit well with neuro-affirmativity. The PEOP has the following categories:

The Person

We acknowledge that people are complex, multi-faceted beings. We also do not seek to change who a person inherently is, or to change their natural way of being. When addressing the person in therapy, our aim should be to support, and to develop skills, comfort, confidence and autonomy, not to alter identity.

Within this category, we consider the following:

- identity
- roles
- neurotype
- gender identity
- sexuality
- motor skills
- emotional regulation
- sensory processing
- habituation and routines
- previous experiences

- trauma
- skills and abilities
- interests and sources of joy
- volition, motivation and desires
- morality, spirituality, religion, ethical beliefs
- and more...

The Environment

We cannot view a person holistically without considering the context they exist in. We know that people are immersed in their worlds and it is important that we explore their world with them.

OTs often talk about how environments can either provide opportunities and affordance or barriers.

An affordance does not cause us to do something, but it makes it possible for us to do something. An example of this a sofa which affords us the chance to sit although we may choose not to.

Opportunities are sets of circumstances that make it possible to do something, and access to occupational opportunities fit in with the concept of occupational justice.

We often seek to adapt the environment to make it more suitable and comfortable. This can be physical adaptations for accessibility or for sensory comfort. We can advocate for these changes to happen in environments besides the ones in which we interact with our clients, i.e., home, school, workplace etc.

The environment is more than just the built environment, it is:

- physical environment – the space, buildings etc.

- cultural environment – not only ethnic culture, but also Autistic culture

- political environment – who are the other people surrounding this person, social relationships etc.

- institutional environment – this ranges from the government and government departments all the way to schools, agencies, societies etc.

The Occupations

Anything that occupies your time is an occupation. Occupational therapists often consider certain categories of occupations such as self-care, productivity and leisure. It important that we see the difference between meaningful occupation and being occupied for the sake of it. I often like to say to children that meaningful occupations are things you do either because you have to do them to have a good life or things you do because you want and like to do them.

- We can explore ways to prioritise or modify occupations to make them more doable, as well as explore potential for future occupations.

6.7 What Is Being Autistic?

Put simply, what being Autistic 'is' largely depends on whether we privilege an Autistic person's description from the inside or a non-autistic storying from the outside (although we acknowledge all the work that non-autistic allies are doing in advocating for Autistic rights and for strengths-based conceptualisations of Autistic identity). Being Autistic is just one of many neurotypes (including neurotypical, Autistic, ADHD or otherwise neurodivergent) which each have their own profile of how individuals with that profile interact, experience, and communicate with the world. Note that being Autistic is genetically based.

Autistic individuals are part of a culture and community, albeit a minority group, and being Autistic is part of their identity. There is no one way to be Autistic. There is a great diversity of Autistic experience; no two Autistic people will be the same. There are commonalities in our experiences, but equally there are many differences, for example in our specific sensory needs and experiences, our cultural background or membership of other minoritised communities. Do not use expectations based off one Autistic young person to guide assumptions about the needs or experiences of another (or indeed, base assumptions about how an Autistic adult may be from your experiences of Autistic young people).

We encourage you to be vigilant about falling back on the trope of the white, heterosexual, male presenting boy as the 'prototypical Autistic person', a stereotype that prevails throughout media representations of being Autistic, and indeed will have featured in many clinicians' initial professional training. It is fundamentally unhelpful to think about 'male' and 'female' presentation – this way of thinking reinforces gender binaries and contributes to those assigned female at birth having their Autistic identity 'missed' or misidentified because their Autistic way of being does not align with the stereotypical 'male' presentation that many clinicians still fall back on when thinking about Autistic people. Equally, it means that those assigned male at birth may also not be identified as Autistic because their way of being Autistic does not fit with the cis white male trope. We suggested previously that (Hartman et al., 2023) rather than gendering Autistic experience, it is more helpful to consider internalised or externalised presentations, drawing on Wassell and Burke (2022) who describe an 'externalised' presentation as one that is most recognisable to the majority of people (e.g., stimming openly, being non-speaking, showing distressed behaviour) that is considered different to non-autistic peers, whereas an internal presentation is one in which Autistic ways of being are masked and less visible.

With the benefit of reflection and distance, we are mindful that this in itself creates categories and therefore suggest resisting labelling types of presentation and thinking instead about diversity of Autistic experience. We are not static beings, how we exist in the world varies day by day, and the risk in labelling someone as having an 'internalised' or 'externalised' presentation confines them to one way of being Autistic. This can have a subsequent impact when systems or educators question Autistic identity because the young person does not always 'present' in an internalised way (and vice versa).

As a thought exercise, in Hartman et al. (2023, pp. 61–64) we provided a reworking of diagnostic criteria, positing how 'neurotypical spectrum disorder' (purely a thought exercise, with language used to reflect current diagnostic criteria, not how Autistic people see or want to see neurotypical people) might look if non-autistic people were the perceived minority, as a practice of decentring neurotypicality, inviting readers to question neuro-normativity as the dominant model developed by the perceived neuro-majority. We have reproduced the criteria for neurotypical spectrum disorder below. If you are a neurotypical reader, we invite you to attend curiously and thoughtfully to the discomfort that may arise as you see yourselves described in terms of deficit. Can you cherish this discomfort with compassion and use it to drive a shift in your clinical practice, to support you in catching those moments when it is so easy to be pulled back into deficit-based practice?

Important note: This is not how Autistic people see or want to see neurotypical people. This is purely a thought exercise, with language use reflecting current diagnostic criteria.

Proposed criteria:

- Criteria A: Persistent deficits in social communication and interaction underpin how an individual navigates the social world and interacts with others. Deficits occur in:

  - Social-emotional reciprocity: Atypical social approach and response, e.g., over-focus on sharing emotions, deficits in understanding emotions/communication styles of other neurotypes; inability to tolerate silences; inability to discuss meaningful topics and over-reliance on 'small talk'.
  - Non-verbal social communication: For example, over-reliance and over-focus on eye contact (including atypical use of level of eye contact to gauge interest in conversation); insistence on use of overly animated facial expressions.
  - Reciprocal relationships: Deficits in developing, maintaining and understanding relationships across neurotypes, over-adjusting behaviour to different contexts, over-focus or reliance on peers; impaired ability to understand Autistic social norms.

- Criteria B: Unpredictable behaviours and diversity of interests:

  - Rigid adherence to avoiding routines or rituals, despite their practical benefit, e.g., insistency on taking a different route home 'just because'; different meals each mealtime; finding lack of change or inconsistency particularly challenging which can disrupt preferred chaotic and unplanned schedule.
  - May have multiple but superficial interests.
  - These behaviours can present in different ways from individual to individual and are overly flexible, unpredictable and inefficient.
  - Marked lack of response to sensory input OR lack of interest in sensory input (e.g., unaware of small changes in environment, unaware of potential for pleasures from engaging with sensory objects).
  - These features may present in varying ways for people with

neurotypical spectrum disorder. All individuals with neurotypicalism have difficulties in social interaction and social communication, e.g., insistence on eye contact, inability to 'read' and respond appropriately to the emotional cues of others from a different neurotype.

What does neurotypical spectrum disorder look like?

Social communication and interaction:

- Over-focus on reciprocity.

- Over-focus on eye contact.

- Deficits in social skills and behaviour include the ability to 'read' others, behaviours and expressions, i.e., those with neurotypical spectrum disorder have pronounced deficits in Autistic Theory of Mind.

- Over-reliance on making inferences when drawing conclusions.

- May have personal space difficulties (being unaware or intolerant of others' need for space).

- May have difficulties understanding others / norms of social interaction (e.g., sitting in silence together joyfully, turn taking in information dumping).

- May have too much variation in tone and pitch when speaking.

- May find friendships or making friends difficult outside of their neurotype.

- May have too much (perhaps superficial) interest in others (e.g., spreading gossip).

- May show a 'sheep mindset'.

- May have an over-reliance on gestures and displaying facial expressions.

Unpredictable patterns of behaviour, interests and activities:

• May prefer little or no routine.

• May have difficulties in thinking/understanding – difficulties communicating without reliance on sarcasm, metaphors or figures of speech.

• May display marked lack of repetitive movements OR insistence on denying repetitive movements such as pencil taps, hair twiddling etc.

• May play in a way that over-relies on others, relies on externalising scenarios rather than using rich inner experience.

• May have multiple but superficial interests, or pursue interests valued only by peers.

• Marked lack of response to sensory input or lack of interest in sensory input (e.g., unaware of small changes in environment, unaware of potential for pleasures from engaging with sensory objects).

Check-in points:

• How does it feel being described in a deficit-focused way? Does this feel comfortable?

• Do you recognise yourself in such limited criteria, or are there aspects of neurotypical experience that they do not capture?

• How can you use your reflections to support your clinical work with Autistic people?

• Are you embracing any discomfort, and cherishing it? This will help guide you forward in shifting your lens. Celebrate it gently.

Whilst the deficit-based framing and language used in the diagnostic manuals about autism is problematic, the broad areas outlined can be used helpfully if done so thoughtfully (and continually reflecting on neuro-dominance and epistemic injustice etc.) to provide a framework for understanding how Autistic experience might differ from non-autistic experience.

Whilst current diagnostic criteria are driven by neuro-normative assumptions, it is imperative however that clinicians do follow best practice guidelines in formal identification of Autistic identity, and this does include evidencing how a child / young person's experiences align with current criteria. Whilst this is a tension which may be hard to hold, we do not suggest clinicians abandon diagnostic criteria, but rather use them respectfully and within a neurodiversity affirmative approach whilst acknowledging the systemic injustice driving those criteria and continually advocating for systemic changes in how those criteria are revised.

Autistic children (and adults) use different communication patterns than neurotypical children. Autistic communication is often detailed and motivated by a strong sense of justice and advocacy for Autistic rights, with many having a strong preference for in-depth discussion of meaningful, content- and interest-based topics, rather than 'social chit chat'. This could include 'info dumping' or 'monologuing' about a particular passion in depth. From a neurotypical perspective, such communication is framed as 'challenges with back and forth conversations', or in responding flexibly to others' conversations. However, from an Autistic gaze, this is a respectful, polite and expected way of communication, one that is still turn taking but just in a different time frame of turn taking. Autistic children and adults may show different intonation and facial expression patterns from neurotypical people, and different use or understanding of non-verbal communication patterns.

See the box below for a speech and language therapist's view on Autistic experiences of speaking.

PERSPECTIVES OF AN SLT: AUTISTIC EXPERIENCES OF SPEAKING

ELAINE MCGREEVY

Zisk and Dalton (2019) describe three types of speech experienced by Autistic people. A person with 'intermittent speech' can speak sometimes, but not always. A person with 'unreliable speech' may say things that do not match their preferences or intended meaning.

'Insufficient speech' describes how a person can speak orally and accurately, but not completely. They cannot always communicate everything they wish to using oral speech alone. They discuss the benefits of communication technologies and communication supports for Autistic adults across contexts. Recommendations on communication supports are relevant to Autistic children and young people, many of whom are unable to rely on speech alone to be heard and understood; Steffenburg et al. (2018), for example, found that 63% of children identified with 'selective mutism' were also Autistic.

Many Autistic children and adults have a strong preference for detail and are skilled at finding out highly detailed information or noticing small details that others may miss.

Many Autistic children and adults stim (this could include making sounds, repeating phrases, rocking, hand movements, finger flicking, using fidgets, leg jiggling, listening to the same piece of music over and over), which can be self-soothing, an expression of joy (e.g., stimming freely to a particular piece of music played over and over can be a source of great joy), and a strategy to support energy recovery and cognitive processing. Stimming may involve any of our senses. The multiple functions of stimming are not captured within the limited notions of diagnostic criteria who merely frame 'repetitive behaviours' as departing from perceived normality (and yet everyone stims even if they are not aware, e.g., twisting hair, tapping pens; however, for Autistic people this becomes pathologised). Autistic children might stim because they are feeling anxious, or equally because they are happy. Holding in a stim is painful, like holding back a tsunami of incipient movement or emotion. As Walker (2019) explains, it means repressing the embodiment of our true selves. Children and young people may have not yet learned to repress their stims, and Walker suggests that for those who still stim freely, it is important they are not pressured to conform to non-autistic norms of embodiment.

Encourage and welcome children to stim in all home, clinical or teaching spaces, #FreeTheStim (whilst also recognising that some stims may be harmful (e.g., head banging) and that children and young people may at times need support with finding a stim that is not harmful to them). This will mean that unlike many adults who discover their Autistic identity later in life, they will not have to re-learn how to feel free to stim or have to hide behind a mask that constrains stims. Walker (2019) describes this as an effortful attempt to recover our ability to stim.

For those interested in reading more in this area we encourage you to read Walker's (2019) chapter on 'Somatics and autistic embodiment'.

See the box below for a discussion of stimming as non-spoken communication.

PERSPECTIVES OF AN SLT: STIMMING AS NON-SPOKEN COMMUNICATION

ELAINE MCGREEVY

Stimming, a community-derived term, is a form of interactive, immersive thinking involving the senses. Kapp et al. (2019) found stimming had a self-regulatory function and could be a way to contain or control intense emotions, either positive (e.g., happy or excited) or negative (e.g., anxious or distressed). Stimming, therefore, can convey different emotional states and provide important information for communication partners that can foster connection and shared experiences, and enable co-regulation.

Stimming can be seen as a form of non-spoken communication. Lebenhagen (2020) discusses the importance of ethical listening, i.e., listening to non-spoken forms of human communication, such as non-speaking patterns of sound, gesture, movement, rhythmical patterns of movement and sounds, including the use of silence. She describes how Autistic self-advocate Amanda (Mel) Baggs (2012) challenged non-autistic assumptions of normative communication. The essay, included in the book *Loud Hands, Autistic People Speaking*, calls the reader to consider the limitations of words alone, and reflect on the expansiveness of the many sensory forms of languaging – the language spoken before the existence of words.

Autistic children may experience and show distress differently to non-autistic children. The double empathy problem (Milton, 2012; see Section 6.10) is a helpful frame to understand this; that is, issues arise when neurotypes do not understand each other, running both ways, as difficulties are not located in any one party involved. For example, when highly focused attention (monotropism; Murray, 2019) is misunderstood as a processing and communication style Autistic children may become described as 'obsessive', when it is a communication style associated with Autistic selfhood.

Autistic children (and adults) may play in what is deemed as a 'different' way, e.g., lining up objects, sorting toys. This is often at risk of being dismissed as 'unimaginative' play – but this perspective is based on external observational and the imposition of neuro-normative play. What a non-autistic person sees as 'regimented lining up' of an item (be it blocks, trains, dolls etc.), might be sorting items into sizes (systemising) or equally might have an entire storyline behind it. Maybe those lined up blocks are people queuing for something, or carefully lined up in order of preference (be that colour, characteristics, texture, hair colour, eye colour etc.). Just because a non-autistic person cannot see the imagination and rich internal processes behind our play does not mean it is not there. Autistic children, young people and adults may prefer parallel activities, for example enjoying each other's company whilst doing different activities, or enjoy hanging out over a shared activity (e.g., jigsaws, colouring, building bricks) whilst having random, free-ranging conversations. See the box below for a deep dive into an OT perspective on Autistic play.

PERSPECTIVES OF AN OT: AUTISTIC PLAY

KATIE KERLEY

We need to move away from pathologising Autistic ways of being and an important example of this is Autistic play.

Play is the primary occupation of children, it's how they learn best and also how they get joy. Play, by its very definition, is intrinsically motivated – meaning that the child gets to choose how they play. There is no wrong way to play.

Autistic play is often pathologised. It shouldn't be. Lining things up or stacking them, peering at objects closely, flapping, running, crashing into things – this is all fun! There's nothing wrong with it. Sometimes we just need to shift our perspective. Sometimes we need to join in!

Learning to be child-led was such a mental shift for me. Something I hadn't anticipated as a side effect was how much joy it would bring me, to be child-led. And children know when we are enjoying our time with them and when our heart is really in it!

I used to think being child-led would be chaotic and unstructured, and sometimes it is, but it's more than that too. There are boundaries (on both sides) but we share joy, play together, allow choice and autonomy and notice what they notice.

Gosh, I remember the urge to interact or intervene at all times to feel like I was being therapeutic. How wrong I was. I remember one of my supervisors telling me years ago to 'sit on your hands and stop talking for a minute'. This was great advice, but initially hard for me to do. I learned to step back and observe, squash the urge to intervene. They say occupational therapy is an art and a science – well this was the art for me! Beautiful things happen in the time we step back and let things unfold and let those fizzing synapses connect to each other, forming neural pathways all on their own! Child-led play does this naturally!

An interesting but very valid insight from an Autistic 8-year-old coming to see me recently was 'I spend all day being told what to do and I am just fed up.' It's important that we don't perpetuate this when these young people come to see us, especially when it comes to play.

Occupational therapists talk about opportunities and affordances of objects or environments, e.g., what does it enable or allow you to do? When we jump in too quickly, we steal the experience from our clients. And that is where the art lies!

Many Autistic children have a strong preference for routine, be that at the macro (e.g., general order of the day) or micro level (e.g., order of clothes to put on first when getting dressed). This can relate to their need for sameness, but also interact with, for example, sensory needs. For example, a child brushing their teeth with a specific brand of unflavoured toothpaste relates both to routine (i.e., 'that's the way I do it, anything else feels wrong') and sensory needs ('I hate mint / flavours, the texture or flavour of another brand is not right or tolerable'). The same may apply to food choices – Autistic children, young people (and indeed adults) may eat a carefully selected range of foods and keep to this every day ('same food'). 'Same' foods may be products that are (within manufacturing limits) guaranteed to have the same taste, texture and mouth feel every single bite and every single day. This might be, for example, a specific brand of cracker, oatcake or anything else that meets the child's sensory preferences. 'Same' foods are safe. They are predictable. They are reliable. (And FYI, supermarket own brands do not taste the same as branded items, trying to pass it off as the same will be noticed.)

Compare this to foods such as fruits which, despite being the same fruit (e.g., blueberry) carry an inherent unpredictability to them (e.g., size, degree of squishiness, level of sweetness, firmness). All blueberries are not equal. When the world is chaotic, 'same food' can provide an anchor (unless of course, the manufacturer decides – why, manufacturer, why must you do this?? – to change the recipe). Changes may appear superficial, minor or inconsequential to a non-autistic person, but catastrophic for an Autistic child or adult. Just because you do not perceive it as a change does not mean it is not one. Changes do not have to be big. Tiny changes, e.g., things being moved out of place by a small degree, can feel overwhelming because that is not the way that things are meant to be. Having a routine or plan can serve as a road map in a very confusing world: losing that can feel terrifying and overwhelming.

DEEP CONNECTION WITH ANIMALS

Many (but of course, not all) Autistic children and young people (and adults) have a deep love for and connection with animals. This can be a deeply felt and profoundly connected experience: children may feel more connected to their animals than humans in their lives, for example, naming their animals as their best friends. Respect the importance of their animals to their everyday lives and the friendship and companionship that they offer. Animals can provide sensory joy (e.g., the softness of cat floof against one's face if lucky enough to have a cat who enjoys headbutting and rubbing their face against their human's) or comfort and soothing (a cat lying on a child can feel akin to a weighted blanket and provide deep pressure). Animals can be an immense source of emotional support to Autistic children and young people. For example, despite their mistaken reputation for independence and aloofness, cats form deep emotional attachments to their humans and recognise when they are distressed.

We are aware from our own experience of 'reading / therapy dogs' in schools that otherwise situationally non-speaking children have found words whilst sitting and stroking the dog. Animals do not require spoken words. Many Autistic children and young people will experience understanding from their animals, and they understand their animals.

When life has too much muchness, animals may comfort their children, e.g., grooming them, snuggling them, headbutting endlessly or holding out their paw because somehow they know that sometimes we all need to hold onto someone. A child may feel too overwhelmed to be touched by their guardian yet benefit from contact with their animal. We use connection to animals also as an example of Autistic experience which is not captured in 'diagnostic criteria', despite being an important part of Autistic experience for many children and young people. This may also extend to passion for animal rights (e.g., becoming vegan in response to treatment of animals in the farming industry).

We have chosen to refer to 'animals' in this section because of our own (and our young people's) commitment to animal rights and because the term 'pets' locates animals in relation to humans. Hyper-empathy (see Section 6.10) which is commonly experienced by Autistic children and young people means that mistreatment of animals can be experienced as deeply painful, and children may be very distressed if their animal is unwell or requiring medical treatment. In school, it is helpful for educators to know if a child's animal is unwell as they may be very distressed and worried. Hyper-empathy for animals is not limited to furry, fluffy and cute animals such as cats, dogs and guinea pigs, but may extend to insects, worms or snails (e.g., a child may be very upset if a snail is accidentally squashed or if an insect's habitat is disturbed when a garden is tidied up).

Many Autistic children and young people have strong passions and interests (often referred to as 'special interests' but unless self-describing and Autistic yourself, refer to passions not special interests as this term carries negative connotations of deficit-based diagnostic criteria). Children and young people may acquire a great deal of knowledge about their passions or find them intensely soothing to engage in or talk about. If a child talks at length about their interests, do not 'check out' of the conversation because it doesn't interest you – welcome it as a point of connection and respect their passion, regardless of what it is. Below, Daisy describes some of her passions:

CHILD'S VOICE

DAISY, AGE 14

I love reading, books are EVERYTHING. I hate it when books get hurt or fall on the ground. I smell every book, I want to touch every book, and read every single book I hold. There's something magical about books, they're amazing. Books are my comfort blanket (a term I got from one of my favourite series, Pages and Co by Anna James). I don't like it when people ask me why I like a particular book or anything really: I just like them but don't know why. Part of what I love about my favourite book series, Keeper of The Lost Cities, by Shannon Messenger, is the amount of detail that is included. They're really long books which means there is so much to feel passionate about. In that series there is even a Book 8.5 which is a guide to the details in the series: I really like that the series has so many details there is enough to make a whole guide about them.

Some books are more special and I feel strongest about them because they have comfort blanket characters in them. I really like them, I look forward to every scene with them and it annoys me when the scene with that character ends. They're usually not a main character – it's usually the relationship that they have with a main character. I feel very excited about books, they make me feel really enthusiastic, and I like communicating about the characters and plot even if the other person hasn't read the book and it's really complicated. I really like quoting stuff or mentioning things from books and television shows, like when different books refer to the same characters. Books are my biggest passion but I have lots of other things I really like. I really enjoy animated shows and movies, particularly shows (*My Little Pony, Frozen, Tangled, Ben and Holly, Trolls*) – they might be made for younger children but who cares? Shows should have an age minimum but there's no such thing as being too old for a show or movie. Most of those shows have comfort characters in them. The feeling of comfort blanket characters in shows and movies is really strong, it's complicated to explain how it feels but I just feel so much better when I'm watching them. I was able to brave going to the cinema loads of times to see *Trolls* because I really like the character Velvet, even though going there is a really big deal for me.

I like having stuff from my favourite shows: I have blankets in my room from shows I really like and they make me feel safe. Plain blankets just wouldn't feel the same. I enjoy activities that involve those characters, for example, I wouldn't want to do any colouring unless it has the characters from shows and then I really enjoy doing it. When I feel stressed it helps repeating scenes in my head from shows involving my comfort blanket characters. When I think about those characters it just feels really nice, I don't know how to describe it. I am very passionate about people being inclusive, I never assume things about people, like I don't assume their pronouns – I feel really uncomfortable when people refer to 'gingerbread men', 'snowmen' or 'mermaids' instead of gingerbread people, snow people or merfolk. When I see a book has inclusive characters like a non-binary person or a gay couple it makes me go 'yes' because I want that inclusivity in books. I like criticising children's shows or magazines when they are not inclusive: in children's magazines I hate it when they write 'parent' because not all children have parents looking after them: it should say 'adult'.

I really don't like it when magazines say 'encourage your child to talk about' instead of 'communicate' because words don't have to be spoken. I hate it that people eat animal products such as meat, fish, eggs and dairy: how would people like it if they were treated like that? Some people have allergies, and they might need stuff like that because they can't eat other foods, but I feel so sad for animals that get killed just so people can eat them when they really don't need to. We're not in the past people! There are lots of other plant-based products now. It's the 21st century! I hate it when people call animals 'it' or think they don't have feelings. How would you feel if you were the animal – people treat animals so badly but don't think how they would feel in that position. I hate farms and zoos, and the idea of animals being taken from their home just to be stared at. If I'm honest, I care way more about animals than I care about most people. I'm vegan and that's really important to me. Animal rights is a big passion of mine and I think a lot of laws about animals need changing. I feel very sorry for toys if I see them lost or outside someone's house. Toys are very important to me, and I like to communicate through them. I have loads, we probably have thousands with all of them in our house.

6.7.1 Meltdowns and Shutdowns

A meltdown is the child's bodily reaction to an overwhelming situation. It could be due to a sensory overload or a sudden change in routine or overwhelming stress. As Autistic children often find it hard to voice their needs it can lead to being misunderstood and can result in having a meltdown. Often a meltdown may manifest as crying, shouting, physically hitting out at themselves, others or inanimate objects. However, we might also experience an internal meltdown – not visible to others, but nonetheless as intense and overwhelming as an external meltdown. It is not the same as a shutdown. Imagine being stuck in a burning building, where there are no windows or doors, no one sees the fire raging and yet it is all encompassing and there is no way out. How would that feel? A meltdown is not a temper tantrum, attention-seeking behaviour, bad behaviour or a bad reaction. It is beyond our control.

Shutdowns are also a response to overwhelming stress. They may be far less visible to others but are equally distressing to the child in shutdown. Shutdowns can also happen after a meltdown as an exhausted and a rebooting period as you try to return to a calmer state. A shutdown can leave children unable to talk or communicate, being very closed down in communication ability or physical state, needing to retreat to either a quiet place physically, or 'hide' in their minds to get away from the overwhelm. The child may have limited movement or none at all. A shutdown is not a choice, it is not ignoring others, seeking attention, being rude or dismissive. It is beyond our control.

Children might experience early signs of an impending shutdown or meltdown (e.g., sweating, racing heart). This might also include being more sensitive to lights and noise and feeling overwhelmed. They might experience increased anxiety and racing thoughts, or be stimming more, moving or fidgeting more and speaking faster (or less / not at all). It is not always possible to head off a meltdown or shutdown (and indeed, they can serve as an unpleasant but necessary 'reset') but being able to remove themselves from a situation (preferably with no need to give an explanation) or have support from others can help, as can retreating to bed or a known quiet place, using a weighted blanket or other sensory item (or animal if they have one), using stim toys / fidget objects, and blocking out sound with noise-cancelling headphones.

Phung et al. (2021) interviewed Autistic children and young people about their experiences of burnout, inertia, meltdown and shutdown. Participants spoke about what they wished others knew, emphasising the importance of adults listening to their narratives to better understand their experiences. Participants identified shutdowns, meltdowns, burnout and inertia as whole-body experiences (with a theme of 'I feel with my whole body'), identifying often feeling out of control, such as being carried along on a destructive path. Participants identified different sensations within their body (e.g., vision getting blurry, increased breathing rate).

Participants also identified feeling 'exhausted and / or frozen' (burnout, inertia and shutdown). They identified sensations with their body (e.g., feeling drained, frozen or stuck) or mind (e.g., mind not working, being unable to talk).

Participants made a variety of suggestions for what helped when they felt 'out of control', including knowing the things that can make them 'feel out of control' (e.g., burnout or stress, change in plans, over-stimulation), learning strategies to help regain 'control' (doing a fun activity, positive and supportive interactions, using a personal strategy they created) and understanding the things that can make them feel worse (e.g., negative language and tone, feeling embarrassed, being isolated).

6.8 Understanding Sensory Needs: A Brief Overview

Autistic children and young people's sensory experiences of the world are more intense, and very different to those of non-autistic people (Walker, 2019). Many Autistic children and adults have sensory differences (e.g., needing more or less sensory input which may vary across different sensory domains). These impact on, for example, a child's ability to focus on learning, engage with others and manage the environment around them (e.g., school bells are loud, classrooms can become very loud and are often visually overloading with bright lights and colourful displays, and the waft of food smells from lunch preparation can all combine to make an intolerable learning environment). Different types of sensory input can calm or energise our nervous system. Autistic children do not 'turn down' sensory input the way neurotypical children do. Having a different filtering process and not 'turning down' sensory input can be overwhelming, tiring, exhausting and distressing when in volatile environments that are inaccessible to Autistic perception. Imagine if you permanently lived on a noisy building site, with drills, banging, saws etc., and could not get away – how would you feel living that day after day? Might it take a toll on your concentration, learning and well-being? Equally, Autistic children's perception and sensory processing can be a source of great joy – do you notice all the shifts in lights across the sky, all the different shapes and colours and shades of every leaf, do you feel music running through your body at an embodied level? Sensory input can be stressful, but it can also be soothing, joyful and exciting (e.g., the feel of a brand-new pair of socks is a genuine, utter joy). It is unique to each individual – what one person finds stressful another may experience as soothing.

There are eight senses, and within each sense we may be hypo- (under) or hyper- (very) sensitive which may also vary depending across time, e.g., depending on energy resources, fatigue, stress etc. Sensory inputs can accumulate and lead to overload (e.g., resulting in either shutdown or meltdown – and note meltdowns may be internal or external and you may not 'see it' unless you are vigilant and attuned carefully to the young person's bodily cues).

Experiencing the environment as overwhelming can lead to anxiety about going into demanding sensory environments (e.g., school). This is because of differences in tolerating sensory inputs, and can itself increase anxiety. Imagine you are afraid of spiders and yet every day are being asked to go into a place where you know you will be surrounded, and crawled over, by hundreds of creepy little spider legs (sorry spiders, no disrespect to your beautiful spiderness). This is what going out in a sensory-overwhelming world can feel like as an Autistic person: it can feel so 'peopley', noisy, smelly, bright, invasive, inescapable. Would you be able to keep going in that spider-filled world, knowing you will be covered in spiders, every single day, relentlessly, without it impacting on your well-being? Or would you need some adjustments made?

We have divided the senses into three areas: our environment; our body in relation to the environment; and our body.

6.8.1 Our Environment

- **Auditory:** Hearing and detecting sounds, loudness, detecting sound and pitch, direction and location, speed and timing, foreground / background, identifying different sounds.

  Autistic children and young people may find loud noises very distressing, or equally be very aware of (and distracted by) 'quiet' sounds such as the ticking of a classroom clock. There are specific difficulties with processing auditory information called misophonia which may be experienced by Autistic people (e.g., the sound of someone eating or slurping can provoke an angry / agitated or anxious feeling) and hyperacusis (e.g., being very sensitive to loud noises, and experiencing sounds as excessively / painfully loud at a volume other people find comfortable). Misophonia can also be experienced by non-autistic children / adults. Sometimes parents / caregivers / professionals do not understand why a young person might like listening to loud music on headphones (and find this regulating), and yet find loud places (e.g., schools, shops, parties) distressing. It is an entirely different sensory experience being able to choose and manage sound levels when listening to music of our choice compared to having loud noise inflicted upon us from which there is no escape.

Unfortunately, some clinicians persist in the mistaken belief that children will 'get used to' or habituate to loud noises if they are exposed to them enough, based on neuro-normative assumptions and research based on non-autistic people. This can lead to suggestions that parents / caregivers should keep 'exposing' the child to loud noises (e.g., stay in a loud coffee shop) because they'll get used to it. They will not. They may learn to mask and hide signs of distress, learning that sitting in a loud coffee shop is what they are meant to do, or end up having a meltdown later in the day because they have been so overwhelmed. Clinicians can (albeit whilst being well-meaning) suggest that parents / caregivers are encouraging avoidance in their child if they respond to the child's distress and leave the coffee shop, rather than thinking through an Autistic lens. In our coffee-shop-based example, this could include acknowledging that the sound of the coffee grinding, people talking and milk steamers is overwhelming, and it is entirely understandable that the child is distressed and needs to leave.

Question for whose benefit is it to stay there? Is anyone going to have an enjoyable coffee in this scenario, or is the child going to learn that others do not respond to their sensory needs and distress, become more fearful of being in such places because they know their parents / caregivers will not respond, or learn to shutdown / mask their distress? If the child does actually enjoy hanging out in a coffee shop, for example, reading a magazine with their guardian over coffee / hot chocolate / drink of choice (or explore options relevant to their preferred activities), alternatives could include: leaving the loud shop (even if that was the planned destination) and moving to a quieter coffee shop (result, the planned coffee time still happened, the guardian and young person enjoyed their planned activity and the young person did not experience distress), choosing a different time of day in the future, taking ear defenders / noise cancelling headphones etc.

What can help: (Noise cancelling) headphones, ear defenders, using white (or pink / brown) noise apps, listening to the same song over and over, removing ticking clocks, decreasing sound as much as possible, thinking carefully where sessions take place (e.g., not in a room right next to reception which will be noisy).

- **Olfactory:** Our sense of smell, detecting a range of scents, contributes to our sense of taste and is closely connected to our emotions.

Autistic children may enjoy specific smells and find them regulating or pleasurable, or deeply aversive. Someone without those specific sensory needs / experiences may not notice a smell, but that does not mean that it is not there. A young person who is hypersensitive to smells may notice smells that others without sensory needs do not, so encourage supporters to validate the young person's experience. If they say something smells, do not doubt this. In clinical and teaching spaces, consider whether it is essential to wear perfume / after-shave or whether this might add to sensory overwhelm (or how to balance your own sensory needs – e.g., needing perfume – with those of others). Olfactory needs can impact on engagement in multiple areas of a child's life, including using public transport (often smelly), being in shopping centres (e.g., if there are multiple food outlets) or in school (cooking smells from the canteen, changing room smells, malodorous toilets etc.).

What can help: Finding scented spray, scented oil, smell spray, incense, food items, bubble bath, shower gel that the child likes. Avoiding using strong perfume / after-shave when working clinically and avoiding strong smells in clinical spaces.

- **Visual:** Seeing and detecting objects, colours, movement, images, daylight, contrast, speed and distance, boundary, direction and location.

Visual information can be very overwhelming, for example in cluttered spaces or when overhead lighting is very bright. This may be a level of lighting that non-autistic people do not find challenging, but for an Autistic young person, the light itself can hurt, make our brains feel they cannot work or cause high anxiety in and of itself (tinted glasses can be very helpful). Classrooms in schools, particularly in primary settings, are often highly decorated and stimulating environments as teachers are keen to make their classrooms engaging places to learn. But for an Autistic student, the visual 'clutter' may be extremely distracting or distressing. Equally, some Autistic young people need high levels of visual input (e.g., bright light).

What can help: Sunglasses, tinted prescription glasses (e.g., green, brown, grey, blue tints), baseball cap, darkness, colourful lights, patterns depending on the child's sensory profile.

6.8.2 Our Body in Relation to the Environment

- **Gustatory:** Sense of taste, detects sweet, bitter and savoury flavours, indicates if something is safe or unsafe to eat.

  As well as involving receptors on the upper tongue, soft palate, cheek and oesophagus, our sense of taste and the sensory experience of eating also relies on other sensory systems (tactile – temperature, texture; proprioception – tongue and jaw movements; olfactory – smell; visual – e.g., colour, presentation; auditory – sound of crunching etc.). Autistic children and young people may have a strong preference for bland (often beige) food if they are sensitive to strong flavours, or equally may need spicy flavoured food if they are hyposensitive in this area. If lunch is provided by school, does it cater for all students' taste preferences? If a young person is clear that a food is aversive, do not invalidate their sensory experiences.

  What can help: Strong / bland flavoured drinks, sweets, food. Respecting the young person's sensory experiences, find foods that are similar to 'same' foods and experiment slowly with different flavours (this might include trying a different brand of the same food, e.g., breadstick).

- **Tactile:** Processing touch sensations from the body, discriminative touch, deep and light pressure, pleasant / unpleasant touch, tickle / itch, vibration, temperature, pain etc.

  This plays a role in our perception of shape and form, exploration of surfaces and fine motor skills. It relates to our awareness of location, change in position, and of external stimulation of the skin. Autistic children may be either very sensitive to touch sensations or need more intense input to notice tactile input. Clothing items such as seamed socks can feel intensely distressing and it might take a long time adjusting socks to get them to feel just 'right' (seamless socks can make a huge difference to getting dressed in the morning; for example, one of us recalls having told an acquaintance about seamless socks because their son had meltdowns every morning before school because of the feel of their school socks, but after learning about a particular brand of seamless socks, they made contact to say their son 'is going to sleep in them because he loves them so much' (Anonymous, personal communication, 2022).

  Do not underestimate the huge changes that can be made by small adjustments to clothing. Autistic children and young people may be very sensitive to the feeling of school uniforms (often made from scratchy fabric), labels, waistbands, clothing seams etc. It is important for schools to make reasonable adjustments to uniform requirements to support their students' sensory needs. There are several brands that make adapted school uniforms (e.g., velcro fastening, having polo shirt buttons covered so they do not feel aggravating on the skin, soft waistbands) and once a young person has found clothing that they find comfortable, it can be helpful to buy in bulk, so they always have comfortable clothing. Do not underestimate the distress, agitation and discomfort that arise from having unpleasant sensations against one's body all day because of clothes that feel highly sensory aversive (e.g., think how you might feel having to wear shoes two sizes too small all day – would you feel comfortable and able to focus if your feet were hurting and deeply uncomfortable?).

Remember also that all tactile sensation is not equal – some Autistic children and young people might like deep hugs or firm touch but find light touch very distressing. The feel of food may also impact on food choices – certain textures may be very challenging, or a young person may have a strong need for a specific food texture (e.g., crunchy food, no unexpected lumps in food).

What can help: Fleecy jackets, textured objects, blue tac, wipes, squidgy cube / ball, soft clothing, textured objects, weighted blanket, hot water bottle, bath water, shower, fluffy toys, buying adapted clothing that caters for sensory sensitivities.

- **Vestibular:** Sense of head movement, balance, posture and movement.

This tells us about the position of our head in relation to gravity and our environment. It allows detection of movement (linear / rotational, speed and direction), coordination of body, eyes and head, balance, postural control (static and dynamic) etc. If an Autistic child or young person is over-stimulated by vestibular inputs, they may hold a specific position for a long period of time (e.g., hanging upside down), or feeling distressed if put into a different position (e.g., upside down or in the air). Being very responsive to vestibular input can mean the young person becomes dizzy easily, appears unbalanced, avoids escalators or elevators, or stays lying still to reduce the amount of vestibular input. In contrast, for an Autistic young person who is seeking more vestibular input, they may swing, jump, twirl, head shake, body rock, or flap, which are also ways that can help Autistic people self-soothe and maintain focus.

What can help: Respecting a child's vestibular needs (e.g., not forcing escalator use, finding quiet spaces for lying still in school), welcoming stims in the classroom or clinical space, making sure there are opportunities for regular movement breaks for spinning or jumping etc. (either in the clinical space or at school).

- **Proprioception:** Sense of body position, grading of movement, amount of force being exerted, rate and time of movement.

Proprioception allows us to sense where our body is in space and in relation to all its parts. It is a movement sensation that arises as a result of the individual's own movement, playing a role in fine motor skills, active manipulation and exploration of objects. Young people who find it hard to judge pressure when writing may press very hard with a pen when writing. Not intuitively knowing where our body is in space can result in challenges navigating spaces (e.g., classrooms, pavements where there are lots of people), bumping into things, falling over and finding it tricky to coordinate movements quickly (e.g., when riding a bicycle). Autistic young people might seek proprioceptive input by tip-toe walking, stomping, running, fidgeting, hand flapping, pacing, hanging off pull-up bars, and find ways of exercising that meet their need for proprioceptive input. Unfortunately, educators and others around the young people do not always understand that they are seeking proprioceptive input, and the child may be told to 'sit still' and 'concentrate properly' when they are doing what their body needs to do to meet their sensory needs. Autistic young people who are hypersensitive may prefer wearing loose clothing, avoid being touched, appear to be tired or stiff and be extra sensitive to pain.

What can help: Making sure the clinical space is uncluttered and spreading things out to reduce the likelihood of bumping into things; providing wiggle cushions to sit on and rubber bands on the legs of a chair to provide proprioceptive input when working seated; encouraging the young person to move as their body needs to; providing fidget objects; welcoming and embracing stims; providing materials to doodle with and chewy objects.

6.8.3 Our Body

- **Interoception:** Provides bodily signals of physical and emotional states.

This gives us feedback on what is happening within our body. It plays a key role in the development of self-awareness, self-care and self-connection. It includes noticing physical sensations such as hunger and fullness, thirst, the need to urinate / defaecate, temperature, pain, sensory overload, illness, changes in breathing patterns or heart rates, as well as emotional states such as anger, fear, stress, sadness, happiness etc. Finding it difficult to notice and understand body signals can make it difficult for a child to work out how they feel both physically and emotionally. Experiencing intense feelings or sensations within their bodies but not understanding what they mean can be frustrating, distressing and overwhelming, making it hard for the child to communicate what's going on for them, and making it very difficult to self-regulate or gain support from others to co-regulate. Many Autistic children and young people have interoceptive differences, for example not intuitively recognising thirst, and may either need prompting to drink or rely on visual cues (such as always having a water bottle present) to remind themselves to drink. Alternatively, a child who is hypersensitive to interoceptive input may find input intensely uncomfortable and will try to regulate to avoid those sensations, e.g., by over-eating to avoid feeling hungry or urinating frequently to avoid the feeling of a full bladder. Mahler (2016) explains that body signals can be unclear in different ways. They can be too small (body signals can go unnoticed), distorted (noticeable but not clear enough to give information about the specific type or location of feelings), or too big (too strong, overpowering, or too much at once to make sense of).

What can help: Do not assume that Autistic young people understand their body signals. Understand that urinary 'accidents' can occur because the child or young person does not recognise bladder sensations or only registers the need to urinate when the need has become acute. Recognise that before asking a young person about their emotional state, it is imperative to establish whether they recognise bodily signals, let alone link these with an emotional state. Too often, educators or clinicians assume that Autistic children and young people do understand body signals and start work at an emotional level (e.g., using programmes such as Zones of Regulation) without doing the underlying interoceptive work first to support the young person in developing interoceptive awareness and understanding their body. Children and young people cannot regulate what they cannot recognise.

ALEXITHYMIA

Alexithymia is characterised by difficulties in recognising emotions from internal bodily sensations and is linked to interoceptive differences. Alexithymia is common for Autistic children although not all Autistic children experience it. Non-autistic people can also experience it. Alexithymia can make it difficult for a person to interpret body changes as emotional responses. For example, they might have trouble linking a racing heart to excitement or fear but are still able to acknowledge that they are experiencing a physiological response in the moment. Feeling a sensation and not knowing why can feel frightening and disorientating. Alexithymia can make it difficult for children and young people to both recognise emotions and to communicate how they are feeling to others. This can lead to misunderstanding and confusion as it is very difficult to share, be understood and receive support if they cannot put words to their feelings.

Note that this is a very brief overview, and we urge you to extend your reading about sensory perception and experience (e.g., see Hartman et al., 2023, Chapter 6, pp. 83–111 for a comprehensive overview of sensory processing perception in Autistic adults). We encourage you to liaise with occupational therapy colleagues to support your learning and understanding of sensory needs. We also urge you to read Autistic accounts of sensory needs and how these impact on everyday life and not privilege only professional accounts as a continued commitment to questioning epistemic imbalance and authority.

An excellent resource including discussing sensory needs, hyperacusis etc., is: https://autisticscienceperson.com/2021/07/29/sensory-sensitivities-are-not-preferences-theyre-needs/

6.9 Executive Functioning

Executive function involves a range of processes and cognitive systems and allows us to plan and carry out complex tasks, engage in novel problem solving and to achieve goals. Executive functions are carried out primarily in the prefrontal region of the frontal lobe, with multiple connections to other cortical, subcortical and brainstem regions. Different parts of the frontal lobe are involved in the different aspects of executive functioning.

Online processing of information (such as integrating different aspects of cognition and behaviour) takes place in the dorsolateral prefrontal cortex. This area is associated with executive functions such as planning, inhibition, organisation and problem solving. Emotional regulation takes place in the anterior cingulate cortex. The orbitofrontal cortex is important in impulse control.

As executive function is so central to how our brain functions, any difficulties with it will impact on other cognitive functions such as memory and attention. Aspects of executive functioning include:

- sequencing and multi-tasking

- initiation (e.g., getting going with a task)

- working memory

- flexibility of cognitive processing

- monitoring and impulse / emotional control

- planning organisation

- inhibition (e.g., stopping a task / response).

Executive functioning differences are associated with being Autistic and also with being an ADHDer. It is not a unitary construct so Autistic young people may have strengths in some aspects of executive functioning whilst needing support with other areas. Many studies about executive functioning of Autistic young people do not control for co-occurring intellectual disability or co-occurring neurodivergencies such as ADHD, or consider the different developmental trajectories of Autistic young people and the possibility of a distinct Autistic executive functioning development trajectory (Chown, 2017).

Executive functioning differences can impact on both school and home life, be it in activities of daily living (e.g., sequencing order of clothes to dress, or cleaning teeth) or being able to engage with the curriculum whilst also having to plan workload and move around school with the right equipment for the relevant class. These demands increase with the transition between primary and secondary school and young people's executive functioning needs may become more apparent when the scaffolded primary school learning environment is no longer present (e.g., having to move around school, become more independent in following a timetable etc.). Whilst many Autistic children and young people have the ability to manage the demands of education and subsequent employment, they often struggle with the executive functioning skills that are necessary. Daily executive functioning has been shown to be a valuable predictor of academic progress within young Autistic adults (Dijkhuis et al., 2020) and it is reduced executive functioning, not cognitive aptitude, that leads to the discontinuation of academic study.

We use these executive functions every day, even in 'simple' activities. For example, getting a drink could involve (in addition to the interoceptive awareness of thirst):

- Motivation: I want a drink; I'm going to get myself one.

- Initiation: Get up from sitting, walk to kitchen.

- Decision-making: Do I want water, or squash (and if so, which flavour)?

- Planning, organising and sequencing: Going to the kitchen, getting out a glass, pouring in squash, filling with water.

- Monitoring performance: Adding the right balance of squash to water, not over-filling the glass.

- Flexible thinking: Wanting orange juice but having to make do with squash if there is none left, and switching to consider squash as an alternative.

- Multi-tasking: Paying attention to a parent / carer's conversation whilst preparing the drink.

Going 'off piste' on any of the separate components will impact whether the task is achieved, and so to identify a young person's support needs it is helpful to assess which aspect of executive functioning they need scaffolding. Executive function can be broadly broken down into three types of brain function, all of which are inter-related and need to operate together for the successful application of executive function skills.

1. Inhibitory control

Inhibition involves being able to control our attention, behaviour, thoughts or emotions, so rather than 'acting on automatic pilot' we do what is needed in a particular situation. There are different components of inhibitory control, all of which work together to keep us 'on track' so we can do whatever we need to.

- Attentional control: This allows us to focus on what is important and filter out other information (e.g., classmates talking, clock ticking in a classroom). Many Autistic young people can find it hard to filter out extraneous sensory information (e.g., a ticking clock might make it impossible to focus on what the teacher is saying).

- Cognitive inhibition: This lets us suppress unwanted thoughts or memories, and stop previously learned information getting in the way of what we need to do (e.g., if young people are used to going to a specific classroom, it might be hard to stop (inhibit) themselves going to the usual room on automatic pilot and go to a new room if it has been switched suddenly).

- Self-control / monitoring: This gives us the ability to stay on task despite distractions (and classrooms are typically very distracting environments), not to jump to conclusions based on little information, or speak / act impulsively. A young person who interrupts other students or the teacher may be showing executive functioning differences and should not be mistakenly attributed to being 'rude' or 'disrespectful' (typically activating a consequence in many school behaviour policies).

- Impulsivity: This relates to acting without thought or pause, e.g., blurting out an answer to a question or answering multiple choice tests rapidly. However, it can also have the benefit of making us decisive and carrying out actions without delay.

When we are in a monotropic state, immersed in passions and activities, we are showing intense attentional control by focusing all of our attention on one thing. Autistic hyperfocus can be a great asset meaning students can work and focus intensely and extremely productively on tasks. It means that attention to things of great interest to the Autistic child can be stronger (compared to topics of no interest), and that interest-based learning is a helpful way to harness passions to support learning. However, be aware that children and young people may also prefer their passions not to be 'spoilt' by exploiting those interests for learning opportunities.

Executive functioning is easily affected when we are stressed, tired or not at our physical best, e.g., when we are tired we have far less 'bandwidth' with a knock-on impact on reasoning ability, working memory, problem solving and ability to inhibit responses. Trying to complete complex tasks that require holding in mind more than one idea at a time can easily become overwhelming and result in meltdown or shutdown.

2. Cognitive flexibility

Cognitive flexibility allows us to view things from a different perspective as well as changing how we approach thinking about something. It allows us to adjust to changed demands or priorities, or take advantage of unexpected opportunities (e.g., an unexpected invitation to meet a friend when you had planned to do homework), or to switch tasks. Differences in cognitive flexibility are why many Autistic young people find transitions or sudden unexpected changes very challenging. The flip side is that we are very good at remaining highly focused on tasks without getting distracted.

The other aspects of executive functioning below are all impacted by cognitive flexibility. For example, we need to be able to be flexible when we are organising a task that might require a different approach than we usually take.

Organising and sequencing: Challenges with these can cause issues with thinking ahead about what steps need to be taken, in what order, and then carrying out the sequence of steps necessary to complete the task.

Initiation and activation: We use our executive functioning to 'get up and go' with a task. Initiating a task not only requires our brain to 'get us going' but also draws on other executive functions such as planning, prioritising, organisation, impulse control, attention and working memory.

Sometimes we can feel that our 'get up and go' has 'got up and gone'. Autistic inertia is a common experience, e.g., we know we need to do something but just cannot get going with it (or sometimes once we have started a task, we cannot stop). Autistic inertia is sometimes misattributed to 'laziness' but actually reflects differences in executive functioning.

Working memory: Working memory lets us hold information in mind and work with it (e.g., listening to a teacher give task instructions, use them to plan what we need to do and then monitor task progress). Working memory involves manipulating information, not just remembering it as with short-term memory. It supports our ability to inhibit or stop doing something. We need to hold our goal in mind (i.e., working memory) so we know what actions to take and which we need to inhibit.

Difficulties with executive function can make everyday life very challenging and can cause a lot of distress particularly if we are 'hard on ourselves' and attribute the challenges to 'laziness' or 'not trying', instead of to having some issues with executive function. It is vital to support parents / caregivers and educators in understanding how executive functioning differences impact on activities of daily living and life at school. Clinicians need to consider how a young person's executive functioning impacts on their engagement in the identification process and provide the appropriate supports for the young person. We also highlight that some aspects of Autistic executive functioning can be sources of strength depending on the context and situation. Many 'difficulties' are heightened by living in a neurotypical world that has particular expectations and norms. For example, we suggest that if how the young person approaches tasks does not cause them distress (e.g., focusing intensely on interests rather than switching task) then there is no need to change their usual approach (even if someone suggests they are being too rigid according to their expectations of flexibility). This is particularly relevant in school settings (and of course, during the identification process). Instead, adjustments should be made that support the young person's way of approaching tasks, be that in the assessment space or educational environment.

▨ PRACTICE POINTS

◇ Move away from making assumptions of what being Autistic is or looks like, based on diagnostic manuals or descriptions of Autistic experience written by non-autistic clinicians or researchers.

◇ Always be mindful of epistemic privilege and authority and how these issues impact on what it is you think you know about being Autistic. Remember that research is not neutral; be aware of epistemic injustice and infection.

◇ Actively seek out material written by Autistic authors, bloggers and researchers, and privilege these sources to expand your knowledge. When suggesting reading material to parents / caregivers or other professionals, suggest material written by Autistic bloggers and (age-appropriate) social media accounts to acknowledge the epistemic imbalances that prevail in what is written about Autistic experience.

◇ Commit to a process of unlearning all that you think you know about what being Autistic is – re-learn from Autistic people.

◇ Seek out a wide variety of sources of material to support your learning, e.g., Autistic clinicians and researchers, blogs, social media accounts (X, Instagram, TikTok, Discord etc.). Use these spaces respectfully.

◇ Read biographies by Autistic writers and fiction written by Autistic / neurodivergent authors for young people.

◇ Recognise that Autistic people have their own culture and community. For example, the symbols that we choose to identify with (e.g., the gold infinity symbol) and the ones we firmly reject (e.g., the puzzle piece and the colour blue, which have been imposed by those outside the community). Autistic people have distinct ways of being in, exploring and learning about the world. The only way to become and stay up to date with any of these is by listening to Autistic people (Hartman et al., 2024).

◇ Recognise that self-identification is valid: it is our human right to self-identify our own neurology. We do not need a professional to formally 'grant us Autistic status'. Our neurology is Autistic.

Reflection Point

Supporting a young person and their family to explore their Autistic identity
is a very important and complex process. Going through the process will
shape a young person's sense of self and their identity for their lifetime,
and their experience of the process and what the outcome is has a very
significant impact. The importance of how this process is carried out cannot
be understated and it should not be undertaken by clinicians without due
consideration of a person's experience of the process and also the contextual
factors involved. There has been a significant rise in demand for public
services which has increased demand within the private sector, and there has
been a significant increase in private clinicians offering 'autism assessments'.
An exploration of Autistic identity should only be undertaken by clinicians who
have experience in understanding Autistic identity and also the co-occurring
conditions that intersect with Autistic identity, or those with access to
appropriate supervision.

6.10 Double Empathy

Autistic people have been described as lacking Theory of Mind (referring to
the ability to understand that what another person thinks, feels etc., may be
different to ourselves). Theory of Mind refers to the ability to recognise that
others have different views, emotions etc. than ourselves. Whilst it has been
widely proposed that Autistic children and adults lack Theory of Mind, research
does not support this robustly, given that many Autistic children and adults
can in fact complete tasks which allegedly demonstrate Theory of Mind. While
non-autistic children and adults do not necessarily succeed in these tasks, it has
been suggested that apparent failure is more about how the task is explained
and set up rather than anything to do with Theory of Mind itself. We choose
intentionally not to focus on discussing Theory of Mind as this concept denies
our autonomy, devalues our self-determination and undermines our credibility
(Yergeau, 2018).

Instead, we focus on Milton's work on double empathy which shows that
neurotypical people have as much difficulty 'reading' Autistic people as we
can have 'reading' neurotypical people (e.g., Chen et al., 2021; Crompton et al.,
2020, 2021; Heasman & Gillespie, 2019; Sasson et al., 2017; Sheppard et al.,
2016). In contrast, Autistic people tend to understand Autistic communication
without so many mismatches occurring.

The double empathy problem (Milton, 2012) is a key approach that all professionals working with Autistic children and young people should embrace and familiarise themselves with. It moves away from the familiar deficit-based approach of locating any communication difficulties within the Autistic young person, instead conceptualising these as a result of a communication 'mismatch' between two different neurotypes. This is a key framework for clinicians to understand; we should embrace a way of thinking that sees interacting with others who do not share our neurotype as a dynamic dance (so if you're a non-autistic clinician there will be more work to do on understanding Autistic ways of being, and for Autistic clinicians, there can be more work on understanding non-autistic ways of being and interacting). This is a very brief overview, but it is of such key importance to informing clinical work and re-framing Autistic experience and pushing back against deficit-based conceptualisations of autism that it is vital that you read in far greater detail the ever-emerging research that demonstrates double empathy empirically.

WHAT IS EMPATHY?

There is no clear definition of empathy and there are probably as many definitions of empathy as people working in the area (de Vignemont & Singer, 2006), although the differences are subtle and hard to disentangle. The most typical definition is that empathy is the active process of experiencing the world as you think another person experiences the world (Bloom, 2017). Empathy can be split into two distinct types:

1. Affective empathy: Feeling what another person feels, a shared or vicarious state of being, e.g., suffering when another person is suffering (Nicolaidis et al., 2019).

2. Cognitive empathy: Comprehending what another person is feeling without actually feeling what they are feeling for yourself. One does need to have concern for the others' feelings to understand them (Bloom, 2017).

These two types of empathy are discrete, and it is possible to have high levels of one and low levels of the other (Nicolaidis et al., 2019).

When empathy is referred to in relation to the Autistic experience, it is often hard to know whether the general term of 'empathy' refers to affective empathy or cognitive empathy, a combination of both, or indeed compassion or a general sense of morality.

Empathy can often be an exhausting and draining experience, and Autistic people often describe an experience of hyper-pronounced empathy, usually termed 'hyper-empathy'. Hyper-empathy is an experience commonly described in the Autistic community. Yenn Purkis describes hyper-empathy as when a person experiences the emotions of others near them almost as if by osmosis (Purkis, 2022). It involves being highly attuned to feeling others' emotions, often processing them as one's own and experiencing them intensely. Autistic people may experience hyper-empathy which is not only more intense but also more all-encompassing than the neurotypical experience (Fletcher-Watson & Bird, 2020). It can be overwhelming, painful and at times paralysing to be so attuned to the emotions of others, particularly when those around Autistic children and young people may not understand their experience. Despite this, research to date has largely ignored the Autistic experience of hyper-empathy. Assessing clinicians need to be aware that this experience of hyper-empathy is common for Autistic people.

WHAT IS COMPASSION?

Compassion is when one shows care and concern for another without matching their feelings to another person's feelings. Compassion can often be confused with affective empathy, but whilst affective empathy is feeling what another feels, compassion is a more distanced state from others' direct feelings, with the focus being on concern for others, and a desire to find a way to support them to thrive (Bloom, 2017).

Compassion also differs from cognitive empathy. Cognitive empathy is when one 'cognitively' or intellectually understands how someone is feeling. It does not involve showing concern or care for another's feelings the way compassion does.

Unlike affective empathy, which is biased towards familiarity and short-sighted motivating actions with instant results in the here and now but with little concern for its future impacts (Bloom, 2017), compassion can be applied to the more general, including non-human experience. We get a powerful sense of Autistic morality driven by compassion for example through the work of Greta Thunberg (climate activist) and Dara McAnulty (author and naturalist) for the natural world and life experiences that are new or unfamiliar to us. Amongst the Autistic community, there is immense morality and acts of compassion and concern, and rational action to create a society where we respect our planet, a place where all life can thrive, where human short-term pleasure is not put above the long-term consequences of man-made destruction.

This is an important aspect for professionals to be aware of when engaging in autism identification, for example when exploring children's histories and re-framing the dynamics of human and non-human relationships, including trauma related to the loss of pets, and differing ways in which Autistic individuals are motivated by rational compassion to show care for others, driven by an intense sense of social justice and equal concern for non-human life as much as for human life.

Key ideas of the double empathy problem are summarised below:

- Think difference, not deficit.

- Notions of 'deficit' are defined by the perceived neuro-majority, who drive diagnostic criteria. These criteria arise within the context of the privilege, attitudes and normative assumptions of those who develop them. Put simply, what is seen as a 'deficit' is not an absolute fact: just because one group does things differently to a majority group does not mean their way of being is deficient.

- All communication is dynamic and interactional: any difficulties in communication between individuals of different neurotypes arise from both parties.

- Autistic children experience the world, express emotions, form relationships and communicate differently from non-autistic people.

- These differences are typically located as 'deficits' within the

Autistic child, although non-autistic children experience the same difficulties understanding Autistic experience as Autistic children may have understanding non-autistic ways of being.

- Non-autistic children are the perceived neuro-majority, meaning that Autistic children are often expected to learn non-autistic communication, but non-autistic children are not faced with the same expectations. We see this in schools when Autistic children are given 'social skills training' which are typically teaching neurotypical social skills, rather than teaching all children to welcome all ways of communication.

- Neither communication style / way of being in the world is better or worse. It is just different.

6.11 Masking

When you mask you are hiding a part of yourself. You are fake. That person doesn't exist. Be the real you. Be yourself. Be Autistic.

(DAISY, 2021, AGE 11)

Masking relates to the conscious or unconscious act of hiding all or certain parts of oneself to present 'neurotypically' (Cage & Troxell-Whitman, 2019). Masking can include suppressing stims or body movements, copying facial gestures or phrases used by peers and scripting responses for conversations. Whilst masking may keep Autistic children 'safer', it can equally unwittingly lead them into unsafe situations (e.g., 'going along' with someone's risky suggestions or those that are not in their best interest because to do otherwise would be to drop the mask). Masking for many can be a survival strategy. Both children and adults can do it to feel safe even if this is not at a conscious level.

Writing through the lens of (Black) Critical Race Theory, Simmonds (2023) talks about the tension of supporting Autistic children to be their authentic selves, whilst also managing the tension that promoting unmasking would expose them to conscious and unconscious biases in white spaces. Simmonds writes powerfully about the need to become 'an oppressor' out of love and necessity in order to protect loved ones from losing their lives or being imprisoned. That is, parents / caregivers of Black Autistic children may want to support their children to be their authentic Autistic selves, but feel compelled to promote masking because that is what will keep them safer on the streets or from being misunderstood by police officers etc. and ending up in the criminal justice system.

Too often we hear stories of young people being described as 'fine' in school because educators are either unaware about masking, cannot see behind the mask or the effort it takes to maintain the mask, and do not heed parents / caregivers when they describe how their young person is at home. Not only is this a significant barrier to referral for formal identification, but also to accessing support needed in schools. For example, teachers may present evidence to the Local Authority regarding an assessment of whether an Education Health and Care Plan is necessary, and because on the surface the child looks 'fine', this is what is reported, rather than a nuanced discussion of the effort the child is putting in to get through the school day to appear 'fine'.

We have sat in meetings where teachers have stated that a student is 'fine' in school and that is what will be presented to the Local Authority, whilst simultaneously stating that they know the child is putting great effort into looking 'fine', but do not convey the nuances of this to the Local Authority (or indeed to other staff in school), meaning that the young person does not receive the provision that they need. Lack of understanding of Autistic masking is a significant barrier to referral; lack of awareness can hinder identification of the Autistic experience (e.g., clinicians assuming that a young person who makes eye contact is comfortable with doing so and therefore cannot possibly be Autistic, rather than considering whether this is part of their mask, or exploring how it feels making eye contact). Educators are often unaware of how the child may explode into meltdown and overwhelm when they get home (the so-called 'coke-bottle' effect) from a build of overwhelm caused by masking all day. Over time, continued masking at school can lead to burnout and, for some children, emotionally based school avoidance.

Rice-Adams (2023) explored adolescents' conceptualisations and presentations of self in different contexts. Young people described changing how they presented themselves in order to 'fit in' at school, compared to other places (e.g., home) where they felt safe and free to be themselves. They described school as a place where masking was required to avoid negative judgements about appearing 'strange'. The young people were acutely aware of the need to change their way of being to avoid the judgement of others. Such pressures can add to the stress of being in school, can contribute to meltdowns when the child feels safe back at home, and add to eventual difficulties in attending school.

> Don't you DARE be what they want.
> Don't you DARE be what they expect.
> Don't you DARE be what they say.
> Don't you DARE be anyone other than YOU!!!

(Daisy, 2024, age 14)

Do not expect a child or young person to be unmasked in a clinical setting – you are an unknown person, are you safe? It can be helpful to draw upon a broad range of communication methods to support the Autistic young person to engage in the process as their authentic self. For example, inviting them to write or share poetry or stories that reflect their experiences, using other creative means of expression, engaging through music, or through sharing GIFs etc. that capture inner experience. Words are not the only means by which to communicate. Our job is to support communication in all its forms. Suggested supports for embedding double empathy into our practice and supporting Autistic young people to feel more able to unmask include:

- Support non-autistic communication partners (e.g., families, peers, educators, professionals) to understand that Autistic and non-autistic people communicate differently, and do not impose neuro-normative assumptions in interpreting Autistic communication (e.g., do not frame intense hyperfocus in conversation as being 'obsessed' with something).

- Adopt a position of welcoming and celebrating different interests and perceptions, and understanding that non-autistic and Autistic humour may differ.

- Provide supportive social environments (e.g., recognising that sensory or social needs of the Autistic young person may require socialising to take place in quiet places, or very small groups, and for clearly defined amounts of time).

- Respect Autistic young people's boundaries: if they express a clear limit of what is manageable, do not push it to meet the non-autistic person's wishes.

- Non-autistic people should expect and welcome Autistic young people asking clarifying questions and not interpreting these negatively. Be explicit about communicating thoughts and plans – do not be vague. If suggesting something will happen, ensure that it does (or let the Autistic young person know in advance it will not, e.g., in school if a young person expects their learning mentor to be meeting with them, make sure this session happens or explain it will not, and give a reason).

- Do not teach neurotypical social skills programmes. These promote masking and deny Autistic young people's right to communicate in line with their own neurology and culture. Any 'intervention' should focus on promoting effective communication across all neurotypes, e.g., targeting non-autistic people's knowledge about and attitudes towards Autistic people, as well as non-autistic people's cross-neurotype communication skills. One such programme in the UK and Ireland is LEANS (Learning About Neurodiversity at School; Alcorn et al., 2022). This is a free, teacher-delivered resource package for 8–11-year-olds in mainstream school and aims to improve factual knowledge of neurodiversity concepts, create more positive attitudes and promote inclusive actions within the school community.

6.12 Monotropism

Monotropism is detailed, focused attention on one issue or activity to the exclusion of others. It provides a way to manage perceptual overload (e.g., intense focus on one activity is an excellent way to focus out chaotic, overwhelming environments or reduce uncertainty), whilst also providing an enriching, joyful, beautiful experience. Monotropism as a theory was developed by Autistic scholars Dinah Murray, Mike Lesser and Wenn Lawson (2005; see also www.monotropism.org). It describes intense focus on one area at a time (e.g., issue, activity, immersion in a topic), viewing this as a strength (whereas within a deficit model, our ability to focus intensely can be dismissed as 'obsessive' and is pathologised). Monotropism suggests that Autistic people tend to focus their attention (and everyone has limited attentional resources) onto a focused interest / topic (Murray et al., 2005), compared to neurotypical people who have a more polytropic processing / attentional style (allocating attention to many different things in the environment as well as the immediate task around oneself). See Section 7.5 on interest-led development and Section 16.3 for a discussion of the importance of knowledge about monotropism for educators.

Monotropic attention results in hyperfocus, which can be joyful and extremely productive, but also painfully difficult to emerge from. This is not the case for someone with a polytrophic focus who can switch tasks with ease. The neurodivergent authors of this book have benefited from the wonders of monotropic focus as we write, making us both productive and gaining great joy from being immersed in a pleasurable activity. Monotropism can be a wonderful thing in doing what we set out to, but it can end up being exhausting if the hyperfocus it results in means we do not attend to our other needs or cannot shift out of the monotropic state. Monotropic processing can result in hyperfocus, allowing Autistic people (and also ADHDers) to experience great joy, produce great work and become fully immersed in an activity, becoming experts and having intense knowledge / pleasure regarding a specific area.

Hyperfocus is a state of heightened, focused attention in which one can feel completely 'in the zone', extremely focused and productive. It is a powerful tool – when we can enter it. Hupfeld et al. (2019) explain that during hyperfocus, someone might ignore their personal needs, be completely enveloped in a task, lose track of time, and not attend to the world. Sometimes parents / caregivers or teachers misunderstand the role of hyperfocus: not all learners can produce work ahead of deadlines; they need hyperfocus to complete the task and hyperfocus is often activated because the deadline is there. Welcome all ways of working. @digitallybaffled on Instagram provides some entertaining (and accurate) animations that depict hyperfocus.

It can be helpful to explain Tendril Theory (https://eisforerin.com/2015/08/10/tendril-theory/) to young people and those surrounding them to help promote understanding of why task switching can be both exhausting and need a long time (i.e., imagining intense focus as being a series of 'tendrils' anchoring us into an activity – to shift attention or activity each individual tendril needs to be disconnected and retracted. Only then is it possible to move from the monotropic state). This is also important for clinicians (and educators) to understand – do not expect young people to suddenly shift activity, give notice and time to prepare, and allow those tendrils to retract in the timescale that they need.

6.13 Conclusion

In many ways, because there is such diversity of Autistic experience it is impossible to provide an 'accurate' description of what being Autistic is. Current diagnostic guidelines (used in respectful neuro-affirmative ways) are what we need to follow in the formal identification of children and young people's Autistic experience because it is important that practitioners follow best practice guidelines. However, they do not fully capture Autistic experience. To begin to understand the Autistic experience means ever questioning our own assumptions and knowledge about Autistic experience, recognising that there is 'more' to being Autistic than 'diagnostic criteria' describe, and seeking sources of information such as those discussed in this chapter that are up to date and from good knowledge sources. In this chapter we also summarised understandings of Autistic experience as explained by key concepts such as monotropism, masking and double empathy. It is also important that clinicians consider how any communication mismatches within sessions between them and the child with whom they are working are a result of the interaction between both parties, and do not lie in the child alone. Similarly, understanding monotropism is important for clinicians in appreciating why children may find it difficult to shift activities they are engrossed in during the identification process, and to understand how they usually process information and attend to tasks.

CHAPTER 7

Autistic Developmental Trajectory

7.1 Introduction

As explained in the previous chapter, a core component of the Neurodiversity Paradigm is that it is both natural and important to have variations in neurological development and functioning with humans (Jaarsma & Welin, 2012; Kapp et al., 2019). Humans are not meant to all be the same and while many humans share characteristics, there is significant variation amongst us. The human race has always benefited from neurological variation – different ways of thinking and having different perspectives are what have led to innovation, invention, creativity, design and advancement. If everybody's brain worked the same way, our societies would be a lot further behind than they are today. Differences in neurology include differing developmental trajectories. Many Autistic children will be compared to neurotypical trajectories, being described as 'delayed' or 'late to develop', whereas they are in fact developing in line with an Autistic trajectory.

In this chapter we will examine the under-researched area of the Autistic developmental trajectory, covering areas including the language we use in relation to childhood development, looking at developmental delay vs. developmental difference, speech and language development, interest-led development and monotropism, and cognitive development and the issues around its assessment.

7.2 Language Used in Developmental Descriptions

To our detriment, society has not and does not always recognise that there are variations in neurological development and function, and that this is natural and necessary to our success as humans. In most cultures, value has been placed on neuro-normativity, and this has infiltrated how we conceptualise and understand Autistic neurology and the experience of other neurotypes. This is evident in the language that is used to describe the early development of Autistic children, and the comparisons that are made to neurotypical development. The developmental milestones of Autistic children are often described as being 'delayed' or that there has been a 'regression' in development, but this comparison implies that all children and all brains will develop in the same way and following the same trajectory. It does not allow for individual differences in development, or that development can happen in a different way that is just as valid as the neurotypical developmental trajectory.

The language used in relation to early development is often judgemental and unhelpful, and it primes young children to be pathologised by others as they grow and develop. Before they are identified as Autistic, often the first indicator that a child may be Autistic is in the trajectory of their development as being different from neurotypical development. It is often described in referrals and in discussions amongst health professionals, with parents / caregivers, and amongst research as there being 'red flags' or 'concerns' in relation to development. This type of language perpetuates the idea that there is something wrong with developing differently, and that this difference in development is going to be detrimental to the child being discussed. Use of this type of language implies that it is bad and unwanted to develop differently, and that others should be alarmed. This position is not only inaccurate in relation to Autistic neurology, but it also is harmful to a child as it influences how others perceive them. For parents / caregivers, this use of pathologising language in relation to development causes a wide range of challenging emotions to arise and implies that something negative or concerning is going to happen to their child.

Reflection Point

It is important for those working with very young children and their families to reflect on their position as often being the first healthcare professionals to meet with children and their parents / caregivers. This may be a GP, a public health nurse, a physiotherapist or a speech and language therapist, or any other healthcare professional who happens to be the first person a family meets with professionally. Those who work in this capacity have a significant responsibility to be well-informed in terms of how they communicate with a family, and how they describe the experiences of the children they meet. This early narrative matters hugely to parents / caregivers in navigating the process of exploring their child's experience of the world.

7.3 Developmental Delay or Developmental Difference

In an effort to use the correct language and terminology to describe early development, it is important to understand the nature of developmental trajectories. When professionals describe development as being 'delayed', they are actually stating that in comparison to expected time frames for neurotypical development, a child is developing differently. However, by saying that it is delayed, they are implying that it is a bad thing to develop differently, rather than it being neutral.

Similarly, when professionals describe there being a 'regression' in development, they imply that a child has lost something or has returned to a worse position. Again, they are making the assumption that a skill or ability that a child had is now lost, when this isn't necessarily known. The skill or ability may still be there, it may be the case that it just isn't being used as a child's interest may be focused elsewhere. It can be extremely distressing for parents and caregivers when a child stops using a skill that they previously used, and it isn't fully clear as to why this happens. It can potentially be explained by a shift in attentional focus, or it could be related to additional co-occurring conditions.

In describing a child's early development, it is more helpful and it is an underpinning of neurodiversity affirmative practice to describe development neutrally. Most often when a child first meets a health professional, it is not yet known or clear if they are Autistic, or if they have a different neurotype, or a medical condition etc. Describing their development in neutral terms and without value judgements is more accurate and helpful in terms of the development of their identity and their value. Referring to 'red flags' or 'concerns' in describing a child's development is laden with pathologising and judgemental language that does not accurately describe the differences a child is experiencing in terms of their early development.

7.4 Autistic Developmental Trajectory

There is a distinct lack of research relating to early developmental trajectories for Autistic children. There has been some research investigating developmental trajectories throughout childhood, and this research indicates that there is significant heterogeneity in the developmental trajectories of Autistic children over time (Fountain et al., 2012). In the collective years of clinical practice of the authors of this book, it is clear that there are many differences in terms of early development for Autistic children in comparison to their neurotypical peers. In a longitudinal study of 17,098 Autistic people, substantial variability in average early developmental milestone attainment was found amongst Autistic people in comparison to their neurotypical peers (Kuo et al., 2022). Kuo et al. (2022) also found that more variation in milestone attainment was found within Autistic children with co-occurring intellectual disabilities and in those who were identified as Autistic before the age of 5 years old. This could be interpreted as implying that for those identified later in life there is possibly less variance amongst their early milestone attainment, which could suggest that for some Autistic people, their early development may appear similar to that of their neurotypical peers (however this needs to be interpreted with caution as this is not what the authors explicitly concluded and further retrospective research is required).

Many Autistic children reach communication milestones at different ages to neurotypical children (Anderson et al., 2007). Some use spoken language much earlier than neurotypical children typically do, some don't use spoken language until much later and some don't use spoken language at all. Many experience differences in their toileting milestones (Wiggins et al., 2022), and there may also be differences in motor skills development (Mohd Nordin et al., 2021). It is clear that neurodivergent children experience differences in their developmental processes in comparison to neurotypical development (Prizant et al., 2006), and a different way to conceptualise Autistic development is needed. Hens and Van Goidsenhoven (2023) describe a framework of developmental diversity and propose that atypical developmental trajectories do not necessarily result in lesser outcomes.

Neurodivergent children need for their development to be nurtured according to their own developmental trajectory, rather than being held to neuro-normative expectations of development, as to force them to engage in developmental activities for which they are not yet ready can have significant negative consequences (Black et al., 2023; Hens & Van Goidsenhoven, 2023). Although there may be common characteristics in terms of early development for many Autistic children, there are also many variances. What is anecdotally clear and evident in our own and others' clinical practice is that Autistic development is often non-linear, and that this is different to neurotypical development. Below for those wanting a deeper insight into this topic area, we have included a deep dive of an SLT perspective on speech, language and communication profiles of Autistic children, as well as a discussion of gestalt language acquisition.

PERSPECTIVES OF AN SLT: SPEECH, LANGUAGE AND COMMUNICATION PROFILES OF AUTISTIC CHILDREN

ELAINE MCGREEVY

There is much heterogeneity in the language and communication profiles of Autistic children. Autistic children experience a variety of strengths and challenges in pragmatics (i.e., the use of language in a social context and the ways in which people produce and derive meaning through language), semantics (i.e., word meanings and relations between words), syntax (i.e., the arrangement of words in a sentence according to grammar rules), morphology (i.e., the internal structure of words and parts of words such as word endings that create plurals and tenses) and phonology (i.e., speech sounds) in both spoken and written language. Some Autistic children acquire speech and language skills with ease. In a large sample of Autistic children who were using a few single words at age 4, Wodka et al. (2013) found that 70% of participants acquired phrase and / or fluent speech by age 8 years, with almost half of the children achieving fluent speech. Findings were consistent with a longitudinal study by Anderson et al. (2007) who found that 30% of Autistic children were using no or few consistent spoken words by age 9.

Childhood apraxia of speech (CAS) is a lifelong neurodevelopmental disorder of speech motor programming and planning which occurs with an increased frequency in children and adults with rare gene conditions, intellectual disability, epilepsy and in some Autistic people who use few spoken words. McCabe et al. (2024), in an evidence summary, found that CAS occurs in speaking Autistic children with a prevalence of approximately 1 in 1,000 children, consistent with the prevalence rate for the general population. Non-speaking Autistic self-advocates (e.g., Kedar, 2012) have described the sensory motor differences that underlie what they often describe as a 'body–mind disconnect' and that can involve experiences such as being unable to inhibit or plan motor movements and getting stuck in motor loops or thought loops (NeuroClastic, 2021).

Vogindroukas et al. (2022) cited Shriberg et al. (2011), who found that speech sound disorders ranged between 15 and 20% in Autistic children and concluded there is limited evidence to establish the existence, degree of difficulty and characteristics of speech sound disorders in

Autistic children. The same study summarised fluency differences in Autistic children, ranging from stuttering, cluttering (i.e., a rapid and / or irregular rate of speech accompanied by longer pauses between words, and / or differences in rhythm of speech and / or where syllables of words might be dropped), revisions (i.e., changing the words in a sentence) and repetitions of utterances, and final word repetitions. Cluttering was usually noted in older Autistic children. Ostrolenk et al. (2017), in a systematic review, found a high incidence (84%) of hyperlexia (when a child can read at levels far beyond those expected for their age but not necessarily understand or comprehend what they are reading) in Autistic children.

PERSPECTIVES OF AN SLT: GESTALT LANGUAGE ACQUISITION

ELAINE MCGREEVY

Blanc et al. (2023) outline how Autistic language development often follows the gestalt style of language acquisition which is a natural style of developing language arising from a gestalt cognitive style. This style of language acquisition is distinct from what has been considered traditional language development where the child progresses from using single words to phrases to sentences. Blanc and colleagues describe the work of Peters (1977, 1983) who noticed some young children perceived units or chunks of language as an unanalysed 'whole' which she termed gestalts. Peters described children using gestalts as 'gestalt language processors' and she described traditional language acquisition as 'analytical language processing'.

Prizant (1983) described the role of episodic memory in creating 'situational gestalts', whereby the individual can recall the whole scene from a past event / moment, including sights, sounds, smells, sensations and feelings, reflecting gestalt and fragmented perception described by Autistic autobiographers such as Donna Williams (1996). The specific elements of the gestalt scene, including the chunks of language processed, form a whole gestalt, and cannot be separated. Prizant (1983) was the first to outline the four stages of gestalt language acquisition. After analysis of 15 years of clinical data, Blanc (2012) described two further stages. Blanc et al. (2023) set out the stages of the Natural Language Acquisition protocol with examples of each of the six stages of gestalt language processing:

- Stage 1: Whole language gestalts or delayed echolalia derived from songs, stories, TV scripts and other's language. Some gestalts may be long, intoned strings of language that are not intelligible but hold meaning for the child, e.g., 'daweeodabuhowouahw ouwouahwouwouahwo uddaweeodabuhowouahwou...'. These gestalts are often emotionally resonant and communication partners are encouraged to look for the meaning beyond literal language.

- Stage 2: Mitigations and mix and match combinations of gestalts / delayed echolalia, e.g., 'daweesondabusgoround andround... allthewayto school'. The child learns about the patterns of their gestalt language by using extensive mitigations where they learn to use combinations of gestalt language to communicate a broad range of communication intentions. Each gestalt processor will progress through this stage in their own time.

- Stage 3: Isolated single words and two-word combinations of referential language. After a period of mitigating echolalia and using different chunks of language with increasing flexibility across contexts, the child is able to isolate single words from the gestalts. Now, in stage 3, single word utterances and noun-noun or noun-adjective utterances are produced, e.g., 'Bus', 'Bus, wheels, round'. The words used are referential, that is, related to the literal context, a person, an object, an entity, a quality or a location.

- Stage 4: Original phrases and beginning sentences. The child begins to construct their own phrases and sentences using grammar rules, e.g., 'The bus coming'.

- Stages 5 and 6 mark the development of complex grammar, for example, joining sentences with conjunctions such as 'because, but, if'.

There are important similarities and differences between gestalt and analytical language acquisition, and it is important that clinicians recognise both styles and provide relevant support. Embracing and honouring an individual's gestalt enables supporters to understand more deeply their language and its connection to the individual's meaningful experiences, emotions and sense-making.

7.5 Interest-Led Development and Monotropism

Early developmental differences experienced by Autistic children may be explained by understanding monotropism (Murray et al., 2005; see Section 6.12 for further detail in relation to monotropism and the development and application of monotropism theory, and Section 16.3 for a discussion of monotropism for educators). Monotropism (Murray et al., 2005) refers to the experience of a person as having their attention pulled to a reduced number of interests, which leaves fewer resources for other processes. Monotropism provides a very helpful and accurate explanation for how their developmental trajectory may be significantly different to that of a neurotypical developmental trajectory. Being interest-led in their attention style means that for Autistic babies and toddlers, when their attention is pulled towards something of interest, it is likely that this interest will develop rapidly, to the exclusion of other pursuits. When something is not of interest or captured by a child's attention style, then it will not develop. Similarly, a skill that had been of interest may no longer be of interest or may have been replaced by something of greater interest, and therefore the initial skill may no longer be demonstrated (commonly referred to as 'regression' in pathologising terms).

Murray et al. (2005) capture perfectly the role monotropism plays in early childhood development. They describe how for some infants, 'regression' in language is reported after they have begun speaking. Murray et al. (2005) described how for these children, they may have started to use speech as a way of expressing their interest, and then the way in which language is used in relating to their interest changes, which reduces their likelihood of continuing to use it. They describe how as a child's vocabulary increases, others use words as way of maintaining their interest. Murray et al. (2005) give an example of a child who may be looking at a ball, but an adult wants them to look at a cat. The adult then points to the cat and uses the word 'cat', which the child then learns, and this gives the adult a tool for manipulating a child's interest system. Murray et al. (2005) propose that the disruption of a child's attention tunnel in this way is a painful experience for the child, and language may suddenly become unattractive for a child who is deeply monotropic.

In our view, and as outlined by Murray et al. (2005), monotropism also explains well how some Autistic children may reach developmental milestones much earlier than their neurotypical peers. For example, some Autistic children develop linguistic skills much earlier than their peers and many are hyperlexic, where their reading skills at a very early age are far more advanced than those of their peers. Some Autistic children may focus on language as a prime area of interest to them and attend to it in a very focused way, at the expense of other areas of interest, e.g., spatial and body awareness (Murray et al., 2005).

7.6 Cognitive Development and How It Is Measured

Monitoring and recording development across early and later childhood is important in understanding a child's strengths and abilities as well as their needs in terms of support. Understanding the differences between Autistic development and neurotypical development is a key component in supporting a child's needs and in cultivating a positive Autistic identity. In measuring childhood development and cognitive abilities, various standardised measures have been issued. These instruments are routinely used in assessing the development and abilities of Autistic children, but they are broadly not fit for purpose and need to be used with extreme caution for the specific purpose of identifying whether a child is Autistic or not. We would advocate that they are not used at all for this specific purpose (although as we will discuss later, they can have broader uses in looking at other areas outside of the Autistic experience).

The main issue in relation to current standardised assessments of development and of cognitive ability is that they have been standardised with apparently neurotypical populations. A measure of development or cognitive ability that has been standardised with an Autistic population does not currently exist. This is problematic in relation to what has already been discussed in terms of Autistic developmental trajectories being different to those of neurotypical trajectories, and as regards the nature of an Autistic interest-led attention and learning style. Current standardised measures of development position Autistic children to be pathologised in terms of their development, often being classified as being 'delayed' in comparison to their neurotypical peers, without taking into account that Autistic development is often not linear. Similarly, current standardised cognitive assessments measure one cognitive and learning style – a polytropic learning style which is more typical of neurotypical people. Current tools are often poor estimates of ability within Autistic young people as they do not account for monotropism and interest-led learning. They assume that interests will be broad and similar across different areas, which is not the case for many Autistic children and young people (Garau, 2023).

Most of the standardised tools that currently exist rely on spoken language being the main form of communication that a child or young person uses. Even so-called 'non-verbal' cognitive measures still have some verbal loading and also assume a polytropic learning style. For non-speaking Autistic children and young people, these measures are inappropriate and yield inaccurate measurements of their abilities. Anecdotally, the authors are aware of many non-speaking Autistic children and young people with exceptional capacity and talents across many areas that have not been captured by current assessment tools. This is not referring to 'savant' abilities, but everyday skills and talents in the areas of creativity, attending to detail, detailed knowledge in specific areas etc. There are many examples of non-speaking Autistic adults who have demonstrated significant capacity in many areas, but whose capacity would not be captured by standardised measures of ability. Some people who may be predominantly speaking in their everyday life may not have capacity to use spoken communication in a testing situation, which would significantly impact the outcome.

Undertaking a standardised measure of development or of cognitive ability is unnecessary in identifying whether or not a child or young person is Autistic. These measures may be helpful in exploring the possibility of alternative explanations, i.e., if it appears as though a child is not Autistic but perhaps has a learning (or intellectual) disability, or they can be helpful in learning about some aspects of a child's learning profile (such as their processing speed or working memory) or whether they are dyslexic, but they do not add any information in terms of specifically determining whether a child or young person is Autistic.

Current best practice guidelines across the world also reflect that a cognitive assessment or a measure of development is not necessary in terms of the process of exploring whether a child or young person is Autistic or not (see Chapter 13 for further exploration of best practice guidelines and how a neuro-affirmative assessment approach fits within them). In terms of understanding and measuring the developmental and cognitive experiences of Autistic children, rather than relying on standardised measures, a better approach is to take a broad overview of their interests, strengths and abilities across different areas. For very young children, information about these areas may be provided by those who know them well, e.g., parents / caregivers, teachers, other professionals; as well as joining them in their interests and learning about their capacity through shared play and activities. This will provide much more reliable and bespoke information about a child's learning and development across a range of areas.

See the box below for a discussion of Autistic occupations across the lifespan.

PERSPECTIVES OF AN OT: AUTISTIC OCCUPATIONS ACROSS THE LIFESPAN

KATIE KERLEY

- We may develop differently – we develop Autistically so neurotypical expectations may set us up to fail. This is important for OTs looking at skill acquisition, emerging independence and the development of play. It is not wrong for this to be different for an Autistic child. We often focus on typical developmental trajectories, but the vast majority of this information is based on neurotypical standards of development.

- We often play differently – there is no wrong way to play, provided no one is being harmed. OTs sometimes talk about 'functional play' or 'appropriate play' but what is this? Yes, play is the main way children learn but it looks different for every child, and this is OK. Play is also sacred just in and of itself – play for play's sake. Children have an intrinsic drive to play (adults do too, we just suppress it more). It is a necessity for physical, cognitive and social development and as a source of joy. Play seems simplistic, likely because it is so innate in us, but it is actually so complex. It involves and integrates pretty much all of a child's abilities, and furthermore develops and enhances these abilities (Stagnitti & Cooper, 2009). Stagnitti and Cooper further elaborate that if play cannot or does not happen for a child, then something has gone drastically wrong. The difficulty we sometimes encounter is that Autistic play is not always seen for what it is, and we forget that some of the main components of play are that it is intrinsically motivated and self-determined. We need to allow Autistic play to unfurl in its own way and not intervene or modify it to make it seem more typical.

- Self-care may be challenging for a variety of reasons. This can be due to differences in sensory processing, perhaps the sensation of certain self-care tasks feel noxious, e.g., sensory sensitivity to the tactile component of brushing teeth or the taste of toothpaste. This can also be due to executive function differences that can make planning, prioritising, sequencing and completing tasks difficult. It can be due to Autistic inertia, where stopping one thing and starting another can be hard. A lot of us experience interoceptive differences. Interoception refers to the brain's perception of the body's internal state, transmitted from receptors in all your internal organs – things such as hunger, thirst, breath rate, heart rate, circadian rhythm etc. This allows us to do self-care because this is how we notice what we need and thus act on that need.

- School experiences can be challenging, often due to being in a system that doesn't recognise or cater to Autistic styles of learning.

- It is often harder for Autistic people to find employment. Often Autistic people who are employed are unpaid or underpaid. Barriers to employment include: the way interviews are carried out, workplace culture, lack of understanding from employers and lack of supports and accommodations.

- Our leisure can be different – niche, intense or deeply passionate.

- We have our own community and culture, and this is not always known to neurotypicals.

- We are prone to burnout. It can be unavoidable at times and if we know this then we can plan for it. OTs can support people to minimise the impact, the frequency and the intensity of burnout.

- Stims absolutely are occupations. They occupy time in our lives and serve many purposes for us.

7.7 Conclusion

In conclusion, working in a neurodiversity affirmative way means understanding that there is a distinct Autistic developmental trajectory, even though there is currently a lack of research in relation to it. It is important not to make comparisons between Autistic and non-autistic children regarding developmental pathways, e.g., skill acquisition. Talking about the developmental differences between children in neutral language avoids unnecessarily pathologising what is just an Autistic developmental trajectory. Clinicians should be wary and critical of standardised assessment tools in this regard, as they are not standardised on an Autistic population. We also need to bear in mind that cognitive assessments, while at times helpful for other reasons, are not necessary to help identify whether a child is Autistic or not. We will next look in detail at other neurodivergencies and how these can overlap with the Autistic experience.

CHAPTER 8

Other Neurodivergencies

8.1 Introduction

This chapter provides an overview of some common other neurodivergencies. Whilst this book focuses on Autistic experience, many children and young people will also be ADHD, dyslexic or dyspraxic and are often a mix of many of these. As such, clinicians should be aware that there may be additional explanations for their experiences and that further assessment may be required to support the child (e.g., identifying dyslexia to support their literacy needs at school). The chapter also discusses intellectual disability, giftedness, including differentiating between giftedness and Autistic experience, and speech, communication and language needs.

8.2 ADHD

In Hartman et al. (2023, Chapter 10, pp. 217–222), we provided a description of ADHD based on diagnostic criteria and prevalence rates. There remains little neurodiversity affirmative work around ADHD, and to some extent, we allowed a more deficit-based narrative to pervade our section on ADHD in the adult assessment book. Reflecting on the narrative around ADHD we presented (and driven also by our own identification as ADHD leading to greater exploration of those narratives), we have chosen in this book to focus primarily on ADHD-storying of ADHD.

There is considerable overlap between Autistic and ADHD experiences, and from an identity perspective, it is extremely important that a person has clarity around their self-understanding. There are also key differences between Autistic and ADHD experiences, and understanding potentially competing inner urges (e.g., hyperfocus on one task or topic for an extended period vs. attention switching rapidly between different ideas or tasks) is not only vital in terms of identity cultivation, but also essential in terms of managing self-regulation and identifying strategies of support (Hartman et al., 2023). We do not focus here on 'management' of ADHD, but instead refer the reader to NICE (2023) guidance around medication and other strategies (see https://cks.nice.org.uk/topics/attention-deficit-hyperactivity-disorder/management/).

As we highlighted in Hartman et al. (2023), there is no clear distinction within the ADHD community about preferred terminology. Does an individual 'have ADHD', or do we say that they 'are ADHD', in the same way we might refer to an individual as 'being Autistic', not 'having autism'. For people who are both Autistic and experience ADHD, this lack of clarity on terminology has implications in terms of identity. Self-describing as ADHDer is not uncommon, and others may self-describe as AuDHD if they are Autistic and ADHD. We have chosen to use ADHDer but acknowledge that there is no clear consensus about language use.

Within the umbrella of neurodivergencies, the ADHD community is one of the largest from a prevalence perspective, with estimates of prevalence varying between 2 and 7% of the child population, with an average of 5% (Sayal et al., 2018). It is likely that this is an underestimation, as work is being undertaken to better understand and identify broader ADHD experiences, e.g., the ADHD experiences of those assigned female at birth. Previous diagnostic criteria in the DSM-IV did not allow for ADHD to be formally identified in Autistic people. There is now a body of research regarding the considerable overlap between ADHD and Autistic children (40–70%).

DSM-5-TR criteria for ADHD include:

- Six or more symptoms of inattention or hyperactivity-impulsivity.

- Several symptoms present by the age of 12 years.

- Several symptoms present in two or more settings.

- Symptoms interfere with or reduce quality of social, educational or occupational functioning.

- Symptoms are not better explained by another condition, such as mood disorder.

These may be experienced as combined type, predominantly inattentive or predominantly hyperactive-impulsive:

- Hyperactivity: e.g., fidgeting, being physically or mentally restless, particularly when waiting, subjectively always needing to be 'on the go', (may be talkative), very active lifestyle, restless sleep.

- Impulsivity: e.g., difficulty in waiting in turn, being very decisive and making rapid decisions, contributing to conversations before others have finished speaking.

- Inattentiveness: e.g., not giving close attention to detail, difficulty remembering where things are or needing to spend a lot of time on details of a task to ensure that they are not forgotten, challenges sustaining attention during tedious tasks, difficulty following task instructions, being distractable, problems organising tasks or activities, procrastination, misjudging how long it takes to complete tasks, ceaseless mental activity, difficulty in filtering and / or selecting information.

The DSM-5-TR criteria align with a cognitive deficit view of ADHD which we summarise briefly before moving onto a cognitive difference understanding (c.f. Bertilsdotter Rosqvist et al., 2023).

1. **Cognitive deficit approach**

Through this lens (e.g., diagnostic criteria as set out in DSM-5-TR; see Posner et al., 2020), ADHD is characterised by hyperactivity, impulsivity and inattention (e.g., NICE, 2023). NICE's (2023) Clinical Knowledge Summary of ADHD describes these as 'age-inappropriate' and as resulting in 'significant psychological, social, and / or educational functional impairment'. Diagnostic criteria specify that 'symptoms' should be present for at least six months, and be pervasive in at least two settings (e.g., home, school, social situations).

There are three sub-types of ADHD, which NICE (2023) describes as inattentive (20–30% of ADHDers), hyperactive-impulsive (15% of ADHDers), and combined (50–70% of ADHDers). NICE cites the global prevalence of ADHD in children as an estimated 5%, with US studies (which they note tend to reflect the highest rates of 'diagnosis' and 'treatment') of between 8 and 10%. They also explain that ADHD is more commonly identified in boys than girls (prevalence rates 2–5:1, with clinic populations having a ratio as a high as 10:1). NICE suggests this difference may be attributed to more disruptive behaviour in boys (more noticeable and hence more likely to prompt referral) and more inattentive ADHD in girls (less noticeable and more likely to 'go under the radar'). NICE (2023) also notes that ADHD is associated with other neurodivergencies (e.g., autism, dyslexia, dyscalculia, dyspraxia) as well as other co-occurring conditions (e.g., oppositional defiant disorder, conduct disorder, substance use disorder and possibly mood disorders, such as depression and mania).

See https://cks.nice.org.uk/topics/attention-deficit-hyperactivity-disorder/ for full discussion of a medical approach to ADHD.

2. Cognitive difference

It is difficult to reconcile the above deficit-based description with the fact that several of the authors of this book identify as ADHDers: Did we somehow 'defy' or 'manage' being ADHDers in our writing, or did being ADHDers facilitate creation and writing through intense focus and hyperfocus. We, of course, have the freedom as adults to set our writing schedule – unlike young people constrained by the demands of the educational system that may conflict with how they need to work, concentrate and produce work.

Bertilsdotter Rosqvist et al. (2023) used collective autoethnographic narratives to explore ADHD from an individual and collective point of view and in relation to research accounts and representations of ADHD. In doing so, they contrast the cognitive deficit model of ADHD with a cognitive difference model explaining that within the Neurodiversity Paradigm, ADHD is conceptualised as 'divergent thinking' (divergent thinking ability, attention divergent) and 'variable attention' (stressing the importance of hyperfocus and interest-based motivation).

Hyperfocus describes a state of intense, highly focused attention often ignoring personal needs, becoming completely immersed in the task at hand, a sense of timelessness, not being able to stop and switch tasks, and is frequently described by ADHDers. This description clearly aligns with a monotropic state. ADHD community theorist Dodson (2022) stresses an association between ADHD and an 'interest-based nervous system', suggesting that ADHD does not reflect attention deficit but rather is a 'nervous system that works well using its own set of rules'. According to Dodson (2022), ADHD does not reflect lack of attention, but 'too much attention to everything' and with 'inconsistent attention'. Once in the 'zone' (i.e., hyperfocus), we experience no 'impairments' but getting in the 'zone' is interest-based (as authors, some of us are aware that large sections of text have been written in hyperfocus mode, particularly those that are areas of great passion to us) and it is hard to find the 'zone' for tasks that do not interest us (again, similar to the idea of monotropic states). Put simply, we might be in hyperfocus / a monotropic state writing about an area of great passion, but find it extremely difficult to get going and focus on a boring task (so a child may find it hard to get focus on a learning or homework task that has no interest to them, and find it 'boring', but delve with passion into a topic that interests them and be unable to 'switch off' from that). As Bertilsdotter Rosqvist et al. (2023) explain, boredom 'does not necessarily mean that one does not care or feel unengaged in the issue. On the contrary, a certain task, such as reading a text, could be considered highly relevant, important and interesting, or at least should feel that way, but the inability to control focus and boredom makes it impossible to understand the text' (p. 6). Bertilsdotter Rosqvist et al. (2023) also highlight the interaction between environment and neurology in creating challenges – it can be difficult to pace tasks (e.g., without being drained after an extended period of hyperfocus) and manage time according to neuro-conventionality (either starting a task, or finishing it), and it is this mismatch that can create challenges in the classroom or everyday life. This is important when making post-identification support recommendations as it is helpful for educators to understand that task focus differences may explain a child's engagement in a topic, rather than framing them as being 'bored' or 'not paying attention'.

Bertilsdotter Rosqvist et al. (2023) re-story ADHD as reflecting intensity and variable attention, allowing space for both positive experiences (e.g., happiness, playfulness, creativity), as well as negative (being exhausted, leading to shame or guilt), as well as hyperfocus / variable attention (rather than hyperactivity / restlessness) offering a means by which to unpick narratives of deficit surrounding ADHD. They also encourage reflection on neuro-normative assumptions about how tasks etc. should be done, questioning what 'productivity' might look like, how a work task is finished, its process, and how different ways of working may yield different results. These are highly salient to all those working with ADHDer children and young people, be it in the identification space or in teaching environments. Bertilsdotter Rosqvist et al. (2023) suggest that supporting ADHDers in self-management means identifying when and under what circumstances intensity happens, given that self-awareness offers a choice, an option to explore individual meanings of intensity, its purposes and consequences.

This should be a dynamic process between the young person and their system in order that neuro-affirmative support can be offered (and that does not mean seeking to change the individual's neurology or approach to tasks to fit neuro-conventional norms).

PRACTICE POINTS

◊ In undertaking an identification piece, ADHD should be considered also as a matter of course and screening should take place routinely.

◊ Be aware of the need to consider different methods of gathering information as part of an identification piece where a child or young person may also experience ADHD (this includes their parents / caregivers).

◊ Being mindful that ADHD may not show itself in a clinical setting due to the novelty of the situation etc.

◊ In terms of cultivating identity from a neurodiversity affirmative framework, it is important to support children and young people to re-frame their experiences to consider the benefits and challenges of ADHD.

◊ Where a child is accessing an ADHD assessment within a different service, support and prepare the young person and their parents / caregivers for the likelihood that their ADHD assessment experience may not be neurodiversity affirmative in its approach.

◊ If an identification piece is going to encompass both autism and ADHD from a neurodiversity affirmative framework, the same principles in re-framing autism to a neurodiversity affirmative framework can be applied to ADHD in terms of classification systems, information gathering, assessment tools and identity cultivation.

◊ Re-framing ADHD within a neurodiversity affirmative framework is not just about viewing traits as strengths. It is about recognising the importance of context and noting that a particular trait can be a strength or a challenge depending on the context. For example, 'impulsivity' can be viewed from the perspective of how it helps a child (e.g., by helping a person to generate lots of ideas and motivating them to try them out), but it can also be viewed as something that might hinder the child (e.g., by making it more difficult to plan the execution of ideas).

8.3 Specific Learning Difficulties

This section outlines a range of specific learning difficulties. All these need consideration during the identification process, both in terms of alternative explanations for a young person's experiences / way of being but also in preparing for and conducting sessions. This relates both to the needs of the young person and their parents / caregivers.

8.3.1 Dyslexia

The British Dyslexia Association (BDA) draws upon the definition of dyslexia as described in the Rose (2009) report on *Identifying and Teaching Children and Young People with Dyslexia and Literacy Difficulties*, which describes dyslexia as a learning difficulty which affects skills involved in accurate and fluent word reading and spelling, phonological awareness, verbal memory and verbal processing speed, occurring across a range of intellectual abilities and a continuum. The BDA note that dyslexia can potentially be accompanied by differences in aspects of language, motor coordination, concentration and organisation, as well as visual and auditory processing difficulties, and strengths in other areas, such as design, problem solving, creative skills, interactive skills and oral skills.

Made by Dyslexia is a dyslexic-led organisation aimed at redefining and promoting understanding and strengths of dyslexia. They describe dyslexia as influencing as many as one in five people, and as a genetic difference in the ability to learn and process information (strengths in communication and creative problem solving, and challenges in spelling, reading, and remembering facts). They conducted a survey across the global dyslexic community, with participants reporting that only one in ten teachers had a good understanding of dyslexic strengths, over half said their school fails to understand dyslexic challenges, with a mere 4% of schools screening ALL learners for dyslexia which the report states results in 80% of dyslexics leaving school unidentified (BDA, 2019).

There is little detailed research exploring the connection between autism and dyslexia, but common overlaps include differences in communication. Most research is mixed regarding rates of Autistic people meeting diagnostic criteria for dyslexia. Intriago et al. (2021) suggest that Autistic children are no more likely to be dyslexic compared to their non-autistic peers but note it may be harder to pick up dyslexia for a variety of reasons. Brimo et al. (2021) summarise research regarding the overlap between dyslexia and other neurodivergencies, citing between 25 and 40% of ADHDers as also being dyslexic, but note that the relationship between being Autistic and dyslexic is more complex. They explain that around 12% of children with dyslexia are also Autistic but note the very wide range of reading skills in Autistic children. Clinicians need to be mindful of any literacy support needs during the identification process, and to consider whether a child's literacy needs require further assessment.

As dyslexia relates to information processing differences and can impact on organisation skills, clinicians should be mindful of how best to support young people who are dyslexic during the identification piece, e.g., ensuring all written material, including formal assessment measures, are accessible to them and that adjustments are made as required to support processing of information. Clearly, all individuals will have a different pattern of strengths and needs related to their dyslexia. It is helpful to support individuals to identify their unique pattern of strengths (e.g., strong visual and creative skills, ability to approach problems from a different perspective). Clinicians also need to consider whether parents / caregivers might also be dyslexic, whether formally identified or not, and how best to support their needs in completing any intake forms or other paperwork.

8.3.2 Dyscalculia

Dyscalculia is classified as a specific learning difficulty in the DSM-5-TR (American Psychiatric Association, 2022) and is described as difficulties in producing or comprehending mathematical concepts (e.g., quantities, numerical symbols, basic arithmetic) that are not consistent with chronological age, education or intellectual ability. The BDA describes dyscalculia as a persistent difficulty in understanding numbers leading to a diverse range of mathematical difficulties which are not expected for age or level of education.

There has been less research and resources focused on dyscalculia compared to dyslexia, but it is estimated that between 3 and 7% of children and adults have dyscalculia (Haberstroh & Shulte-Körne, 2019). The Dyslexia-SPLD Trust point out that many adults and children go undiagnosed due to limited understanding of dyscalculia. Dyscalculia can impact on multiple areas of daily life including managing money, following a diary, and keeping track of time. Unrecognised and unsupported it can result in difficult educational experiences and challenges in daily life.

Dyscalculia often occurs with other forms of neurodivergency. Soares and Patel (2015) explain that between 17 and 70% of children with dyscalculia have dyslexia and that 11% will have ADHD. Haberstroh and Shulte-Körne (2019) also cite the overlap between dyslexia (30–40%) and ADHD (10–20%). From a study of 2,241 primary school children, Morsanyi et al. (2018) identified 5.7% as having a profile of specific learning difficulties related to maths, with about half of these having a language or communication difficulty noting that some of these children were Autistic or had ADHD. Overall, however, whilst the literature makes reference to the overlap between Autistic experience and dyscalculia, it is hard to find any specific figures to illustrate this relationship further. Clinicians should be vigilant to the possibility of co-occurring dyscalculia and not assume that lack of diagnosis means lack of difficulty in this area, particularly given the overall relative lack of recognition and understanding of dyscalculia.

8.3.3 Developmental Coordination Disorder (Dyspraxia)

The DSM-5-TR (American Psychiatric Association, 2022) diagnostic criteria for developmental coordination disorder (DCD) include motor performance that is substantially below the expected level, causing difficulties which, without accommodations, significantly and persistently interfere with activities of daily living or academic achievement. Motor skill differences must start in the early developmental period and not be better explained by intellectual disability, visual impairment or a neurological condition affecting movement.

Movement Matters is a UK group formed in 2011 to represent several organisations (including DCD-UK, the Dyspraxia Foundation and the National Handwriting Association). They produced a consensus statement describing DCD as affecting fine and / or gross motor coordination in children and adults, distinct from other motor disorders such as cerebral palsy, across a range of intellectual ability. Differences associated with dyspraxia may vary and change over time depending on environmental demands and life experiences. Dyspraxia persists into adulthood. Social-emotional differences can be present, as well as support needs with time management, planning and organisation which can impact education and employment. The strengths of dyspraxia include being tenacious, creative, empathetic, kind, sensitive and often good at drama / singing / creative activities.

Lachambre et al. (2021) explain that ADHD frequently co-occurs with DCD (co-occurring in approximately 50% of children), as does autism (30 to 50% concomitance). Over 79% of Autistic children have movement difficulties consistent with DCD (Blank et al., 2019) although many of these children may not have had a full clinical assessment. Bhat (2020) notes the importance of motor screening, assessment and intervention for children following Autistic identification given that 86.9% of children in the SPARK study fell into the 'at risk for motor challenges' category on the screening measure used yet only a third were receiving any physical therapy sessions. This study relied on a parent-completed screening measure rather than clinical assessment but did indicate the large proportion of Autistic children who also have motor challenges. Another report from the SPARK study (Bhat, 2020) states that of 10,234 Autistic children aged between 5 and 15 years, 85% had DCD Questionnaire scores consistent with being 'at risk for DCD' whilst only 14% had formal identification of DCD. High rates are reported by Miller et al. (2021) who retrospectively reviewed standardised assessments and parent reports of 43 Autistic children, finding that over 90% met diagnostic criteria for co-occurring DCD.

Motor challenges are common in Autistic young people, but it is not clear how many would reach 'diagnostic criteria' given that many may not have been given the opportunity for formal assessment. There is the risk of diagnostic overshadowing such that motor challenges are attributed to autism without proper consideration and assessment and therefore the young person may not receive the support that they need. Clinicians need to be mindful not to simply attribute motor challenges to autism in the absence of proper clinical assessment by appropriate professionals.

8.4 Intellectual Disability

There is a genetic overlap between Autistic neurology and intellectual disability, with some of the genes for both being the same (Casanova et al., 2016; Zhu et al., 2014). This is also evident in the high co-occurrence rate of Autistic neurology and intellectual disability, with studies consistently showing estimates of around 25% being both Autistic and intellectually disabled (Arias et al., 2018; Bryson et al., 2008; Maenner et al., 2020). It is therefore important to consider both within the context of exploring Autistic identity, and to understand the complexity of the overlap and the key factors in distinguishing one from the other. In recent years, there has been a significant increase in the identification of Autistic neurology, and a simultaneous decrease in the identification of intellectual disability (King & Bearman, 2009; Polyak et al., 2015), which raises important considerations in relation to the conceptualisation of each.

Identifying Autistic neurology amongst the intellectually disabled community requires an understanding of both Autistic experiences and intellectual disability. A separate set of criteria has been created to provide guidance about modifying DSM-5 criteria for the intellectual disability population (Fletcher et al., 2017), however this does not give any guidance on how or when intellectual disability may or may not better account for Autistic experiences (Thurm et al., 2019) or vice versa. Studies have shown that there is variability in rates of Autistic identification amongst the intellectually disabled population, which may be related to the clinician's degree of reliance on standardised tools as opposed to clinical judgement (Richards et al., 2015). When standardised measures are solely relied on to identify Autistic neurology amongst those with genetic syndromes, the outcome is frequently incorrect (Klusek et al., 2014; Wenger et al., 2016). All of the standardised measures that are currently available to identify Autistic neurology are unreliable amongst the intellectually disabled population (Lord, Rutter et al., 2012; Lord, Luyster et al., 2012; Randall et al., 2018; Risi et al., 2006; Rutter, LeCouteur et al., 2003).

It is best practice to use clinical judgement for the differentiation of Autistic neurology and intellectual disability (Thurm et al., 2019) both in children and in adults. The following is advised when exploring Autistic neurology within the context of intellectual disability:

- Gather information about a child's overall level of cognitive ability. This information may be in the form of a formal cognitive assessment, or it may be information from a young person's parents / caregivers or school in relation to their academic skills and progress.

- Consider the motor skills and hearing / vision capacity of the young person.

- Formal criteria in relation to distinguishing between Autistic neurology and intellectual disability refer to determining whether a person's social communication is aligned with their developmental level or not. While this is important to consider (particularly as a child grows older and whether their social communication has aligned with other areas of their development or not), it is not the only distinguishing factor in establishing whether a person is Autistic or not, and it may even be misleading to rely on this alone both in younger and older children.

- Determining whether a child with an intellectual disability is Autistic or not should be explored collaboratively with a child and their family. It is also better to explore this within the context of a multi-disciplinary team as the complexity of the possibility of other explanations or understandings of a child's experiences is greater than it is for children who are not intellectually disabled.

- Consider whether differences in a child's experiences are evident across all areas of their functioning or whether they are specific to particular areas. Differences across broader areas of development are more typical of intellectual disability than Autistic experiences.

- Consider the young person's experience of hand or body movements or vocalisations used for regulation, as well as their interests and their ability to focus on their interests. These areas can be helpful to focus on in terms of whether a child's experiences in these areas better align with their developmental level or Autistic neurology.

- It must be recognised that intellectual disability is as diverse as Autistic neurology is, and therefore having one approach in distinguishing Autistic neurology from intellectual disability will not be helpful or applicable to all.

- Further research is badly needed in relation to the experience of Autistic people with co-occurring intellectual disability in terms of their strengths, the challenges they experience and their support needs. Intellectually disabled populations have been under-represented across all areas of research in relation to Autistic neurology (Russell et al., 2019), and therefore there is a need for further research in relation to the experiences of this population.

- Conclusions should be subject to change / updating as a person grows and develops.

APRAXIA OF SPEECH AND INTELLECTUAL DISABILITY

As discussed briefly in Chapter 7, childhood apraxia of speech (CAS) is a lifelong neurodevelopmental disorder of speech motor programming and planning which occurs with an increased frequency with Autistic children who use few spoken words. There have been many children assumed to have an intellectual disability where only in adulthood has it been discovered that they have Apraxia and have experienced a lifetime of being misunderstood, stuck in stultifyingly inappropriate education without a method (e.g., AAC) to communicate. Noah Seback, as an example, is one of the growing number of Autistic self-advocates and lived experienced experts who has spoken publicly about this topic. He has spoken out about how he was not able to communicate reliably throughout his childhood until at the age of 16 when he learned to use a letter board to spell out what he wanted to say. He has described it as a silent prison in which he had to hear everyone talking about him but was unable to let them know that he could understand, and has spoken out about the importance of presumed competence in this area.

It is very important for all professionals involved in an autism identification process to take into account the possibility of CAS when working with children who have few to no spoken words, and for there to be speech and language support to investigate the possibility.

8.5 Giftedness

Although the experiences of gifted Autistic people are emerging within the literature as an area of interest, there has been very limited empirical research to date about this population (Uddin, 2022), with much of the research being descriptive (Assouline et al., 2012). Much of the research to date in relation to the Autistic community has focused on 'remediating difficulties' rather than developing strengths (Gelbar et al., 2022), and therefore there has been little research investigating the experience of Autistic people who have exceptional abilities. The prevalence of those with savant skills within the Autistic community has been identified, with estimates of 75% of savants being Autistic (Treffert & Rebedew, 2015). There are many myths in relation to exceptional levels of cognitive ability amongst the Autistic population, with many people now being more aware that not all savants are Autistic and not all Autistic people are savants (Uddin, 2022). There is a misperception that gifted people are less likely to need support or have a co-occurring disability. The term 'twice exceptional (2e)' describes gifted children who show giftedness or talent in one or more areas, while also having difficulties or a disability in one or more other areas (Neihart, 2008), e.g., being Autistic, ADHD or dyslexic, or having speech and language difficulties, emotional / behavioural challenges or physical disabilities (Yilmaz-Yenioglu & Melekoglu, 2021).

Autistic children who are gifted in terms of their cognitive ability level have clear and important support needs. They can often be misunderstood and therefore are less likely to have their social and emotional needs met (Uddin, 2022), and they often need additional support with daily functioning. It can be challenging for many families and educators to understand how to support gifted Autistic children (Reis et al., 2022) with the needs of this group overlapping with yet being distinct from the needs of those who are gifted or Autistic alone. Further research is needed in relation to the supports gifted Autistic people require (Foley Nicpon et al., 2011), particularly in relation to navigating occupational domains, as well as their mental and emotional support needs. Initial research in this area indicates that supportive and safe learning environments, flexibility within the curriculum and a strengths-based approach are beneficial (Wu et al., 2019).

It can be challenging to distinguish Autistic neurology from giftedness as both Autistic people and gifted people are likely to interact and socialise differently to their neurotypical peers. Both Autistic and gifted young people are likely to have deep interests and they both may value rules, structure, and predictability. Both can experience challenges in relation to executive functioning and sensory experiences.

In distinguishing Autistic neurology from the experiences of gifted children and young people, the following should be considered:

- Both Autistic neurology and giftedness are neurodivergent.

- Both Autistic children and gifted children may experience differences in how they interact and engage with their peers.

- Consider the depth and intensity of a child's level of interest in particular topics. Autistic children may demonstrate a deeper level of interest or a more intense depth of knowledge than gifted children who are not Autistic.

- Gifted children who are not Autistic may have more intuition in relation to neurotypical social expectations and may intuitively gravitate more towards neurotypical social behaviours than children who are gifted and Autistic, who may gravitate towards Autistic ways of socialising from the perspective of Autistic culture.

- Consider how a young person uses and understands language. Although both gifted and Autistic children may have advanced vocabularies, gifted children may have a more advanced understanding of the language they are using. Hyperlexia (the ability to read far beyond expected age levels but without necessarily understanding what they are reading) is strongly linked to Autistic neurology with almost 84% of hyperlexic children being Autistic (Ostrolenk et al., 2017).

- Children who are Autistic, gifted, or both require support that reflects their unique thinking styles and their individual differences.

See the box below for a discussion of the role of speech and language therapists in identifying neurodivergent language and communication profiles.

PERSPECTIVES OF AN SLT: THE ROLE OF SPEECH AND LANGUAGE THERAPY IN IDENTIFYING NEURODIVERGENT LANGUAGE AND COMMUNICATION PROFILES

ELAINE MCGREEVY

Speech, language and communication needs (SLCN) is an umbrella term for a range of needs and difficulties an individual may experience across one or multiple areas of communication including speech, expressive and receptive language, and pragmatic language. In a study of 4–5-year-olds, Norbury et al. (2016) estimated a total population prevalence of 9.92% for language disorder, defined in the DSM-5-TR (American Psychiatric Association, 2022), as persistent difficulties in the acquisition and use of language arising from difficulties with comprehension or production of language. The authors suggested these prevalence figures are a minimum estimate of the proportion of children in the UK with language needs given that children in special schools and bilingual children were excluded in this study.

Speech and language therapists (SLTs) contribute to a multi-disciplinary autism identification process (NICE, 2017). The SLT identifies and describes the child's SLCN and considers how their profile of strengths and needs is consistent with an Autistic profile and / or other neurodivergent profile such as ADHD, learning disability / intellectual impairment or developmental language disorder (DLD).

There is substantial overlap between the linguistic profiles of children with ADHD, DLD and other neurodivergences (Parks et al., 2023). Georgiou and Spanoudis (2021) found a common profile of language and pragmatic language differences in Autistic children and children with DLD. They cited studies that found children who were initially identified as having DLD were later identified as Autistic. Parks et al. (2023) cited Reilly et al. (2010) who found that social communication difficulties resolved as children aged. SLTs will often have to consider whether language difficulties and differences are related to DLD, or if they are part of the Autistic child's linguistic profile.

DLD is a highly heterogeneous and common neurodivergence where the individual develops expressive, receptive and / or pragmatic language abilities differently from the neuro-majority of same-aged peers, in the absence of an intellectual disability, known biomedical basis or sensory impairment. Hobson et al. (2024) discuss the application of neurodiversity-affirming perspectives for DLD given that individuals with DLD will require support and adjustments to reduce obstacles to communication in education, healthcare and the workplace. The prevalence of DLD has been estimated in monolingual populations at 7.58% (Norbury et al., 2016), 8.5% (Wu et al., 2023), 6.4% (Calder et al., 2022) and 7.4% (Tomblin et al., 1997).

8.6 Conclusion

In this chapter we aimed to provide professionals with an overview of other common neurodivergencies and how these overlap. It is vital that if you are undertaking autism identification work, these neurodivergencies also be taken into account and at the very least screened for. We will look next at the co-occurring conditions of mental health issues and trauma and how these intersect with Autistic identity.

CHAPTER 9

Mental Health, Trauma and How They Intersect with Autistic Identity

9.1 Introduction

This chapter explores mental health and trauma and how these intersect with Autistic identity as clinicians need to be aware of these issues prior to engaging in an exploration of Autistic identity with a young person and their family. Clinicians need to be able to distinguish between Autistic experience, mental health needs and trauma to ensure that being Autistic is not erroneously 'ruled out' because the child has experienced trauma, or that mental health support needs are not wrongly attributed to Autistic experience. For example, many children and young people have great difficulties accessing support from Children's Mental Health Services who unfortunately often persist in conceptualising debilitating anxiety as an inevitable part of Autistic experience and therefore exclude them from receiving support (see the work of advocate David Gray-Hammond on social media regarding the damaging impact on Autistic children and young people when they cannot access appropriate support for their mental health simply because they are Autistic; e.g., Gray-Hammond & Adkin, 2022).

It is also important that clinicians understand other support needs (separate from their Autistic experience) of Autistic children and young people who are going through the identification process to ensure that these needs are provided for, or relevant referrals are made as part of post-identification support. Children and young people also need to understand their identity fully in order to cultivate a positive sense of self, and this includes an understanding of their life story, experiences of trauma and any mental health support needs.

9.2 Mental Health

The topic of mental health is a high priority for research within the Autistic community (Autistica, 2015; Roche et al., 2020). There is good reason for this as it is frequently the case that Autistic people will also meet criteria for co-occurring mental health challenges (Rosen et al., 2018). However, understanding the overlap between Autistic experiences and mental health experiences can be complex. Common co-occurring mental health challenges amongst Autistic people include anxiety, depression and obsessive-compulsive disorder (OCD) (Buck et al., 2014; Hollocks et al., 2019; Joshi et al., 2013), as well as eating disorders (Huke et al., 2013; Westwood & Tchanturia, 2017) with prevalence rates being significantly higher for Autistic people than within the neurotypical population (Griffiths et al., 2019; Joshi et al., 2013; Lugo-Marín et al., 2019; Roche et al., 2020). There is a growing body of evidence to suggest that the majority of Autistic children and adolescents will meet criteria for at least one co-occurring mental health diagnosis, with studies (e.g., Simonoff et al., 2008; Gjevik et al., 2011; Leyfer et al., 2006) repeatedly showing that around 71–72% and up to as high as 95% of Autistic children and adolescents have a co-occurring mental health diagnosis, or will meet criteria for the same. The mental health of Autistic adolescents is of particular concern, with many studies reporting that anxiety remains or increases, and there is a rise in depression (Gotham et al., 2015; McCauley et al., 2020).

For many unidentified Autistic children and adolescents, the first time they engage with services is often in relation to their mental health. The challenges for Autistic young people in adapting to neurotypical environments can significantly increase the likelihood of them experiencing mental health challenges (Lugo-Marín et al., 2019) and the first time they may seek support in trying to understand their experience of the world is often via mental health services. Unfortunately, for many children and adolescents, the presence of mental health challenges often masks the presence of their Autistic identity (Bargiela et al., 2016; Mazefsky et al., 2012) and the lack of knowledge of the clinicians they meet in relation to mental health and Autistic identity often perpetuates this challenge. When Autistic traits are accounted for within Autistic children and adolescents, almost 60% would not continue to meet criteria for their previous psychiatric diagnosis, particularly bipolar disorder and OCD (Mazefsky et al., 2012). This means that a significant amount of diagnostic overshadowing is occurring and Autistic people from an early age are being misunderstood and misidentified as having significant psychiatric disorders, when this is not the case for many. This can lead to potentially inappropriate pharmacological and therapeutic treatments, as well as the potential trauma and psychological damage caused by not having access to a true and correct sense of identity by not being identified as Autistic. Given the exceptionally high rates of unidentified Autistic children and adolescents with co-occurring mental health conditions, mental health teams and services need to be aware of and consider the possibility that the young person they are working with may actually be Autistic.

Autistic burnout is defined as a highly debilitating experience which is characterised by exhaustion, withdrawal, challenges in relation to executive functioning and reduced functioning in general (Higgins et al., 2021). It is thought to arise from the stress of masking combined with trying to navigate a world that is primarily designed to accommodate the needs of neurotypical people (Higgins et al., 2021). Unfortunately, Autistic burnout is anecdotally reported to be a common experience for many Autistic adults, but there has been little academic research to date in relation to Autistic burnout (Higgins et al., 2021; Raymaker et al., 2020). Indeed, Autistic advocate Kieran Rose comments that Autistic burnout is a core experience in the life of an Autistic person, yet nobody outside of the Autistic community appears to know about it (Rose, 2018).

If Autistic adults experience Autistic burnout, it is highly probable that many children and adolescents do too, and anecdotally this is seen in clinical practice where young people are often struggling to attend school, to leave their home or to engage in their interests. There is evidence emerging that Autistic burnout is frequently misdiagnosed as depression, anxiety, bipolar disorder and borderline personality disorder amongst Autistic people (Higgins et al., 2021), which leads to significant harm in terms of inappropriate pharmacological and therapeutic 'treatments' and also trauma and psychological harm for the person. Having a better understanding of Autistic burnout could lead to better recognition, relief, support and prevention of Autistic burnout (Raymaker et al., 2020), and might avoid the current occurrence of Autistic identity being missed.

Conversely, it is also often unfortunately the case that the mental health experiences of identified Autistic young people are not recognised, validated or supported, and the challenges they experience in terms of their mental health are often deemed as being 'part of being Autistic'. A study by Mukherjee and Beresford (2023) cited a lack of access to statutory mental health services for

Autistic young people as one of the prevailing factors influencing children's poor mental health. Furthermore, those who did have access to mental health support reported mixed experiences, with challenges related to the barriers in attending appointments in the clinic setting being highlighted as a significant factor (Mukherjee & Beresford, 2023). There is a significant need for further research and development in relation to mental health supports and services for Autistic people across the lifespan (Maddox et al., 2021).

For most children and young people, learning that they are Autistic at a young age is a protective factor in terms of their mental health and other behavioural and social outcomes (Mandy et al., 2022; May et al., 2021). For some children and adolescents, however, learning that they are Autistic can challenge their identity development and can bring about a significant sense of overwhelm that can impact their mental health (Mukherjee & Beresford, 2023). In the post-identification phase, there is a need for support for young people and their parents / caregivers in understanding what being Autistic means, managing their Autistic needs in relation to regulation, stress etc., and there is a need for guidance for schools on nurturing positive aspects of neurodiversity (Cresswell & Cage, 2019; Mesa & Hamilton, 2022; Mukherjee & Beresford, 2023), all of which will bring about better outcomes in terms of mental health for Autistic children and adolescents.

> For clinicians undertaking an exploratory piece with a young person and their family in relation to whether they are Autistic or not, it is clearly evident that it is essential to have a detailed understanding of the mental health experiences of Autistic people and the diagnostic overshadowing and barriers to accessing support that frequently occur for Autistic people. Clinicians need to be aware of and skilled at distinguishing between Autistic experiences and mental health experiences, and they need to be able to recognise Autistic burnout.

9.3 Trauma

Although there has been a limited amount of research into Autistic people's experience of trauma, the research that has been carried out clearly demonstrates that Autistic people experience very high levels of trauma. A study of 687 Autistic adults found that 72% reported having experienced interpersonal trauma and 44% met criteria for PTSD (Reuben et al., 2021). This is overwhelmingly higher than rates of PTSD in the general population, which are estimated to be approximately 3.9% in a general sample and 5.6% for those who have been exposed to traumatic events (Koenen et al., 2017). Given such high rates of trauma and PTSD among the Autistic population, further research is needed in order to understand the nature of trauma experiences and the supports required.

For Autistic children and young people, there are two types of potential trauma they may be exposed to. The first relates to the trauma experienced from specific events, such as abuse, assault, illness, parental separation, disasters etc. The second type of trauma is that which results from chronic exposure to being misunderstood, having to adapt to neurotypical environments, being denied access to regulation and stimming etc. For those who engage in high levels of masking, this is likely an indicator of trauma. Autistic people are a minority group in a society dominated by neurotypical people. This leads Autistic people to engage in masking as an attempt to avoid stigma and hardship, which mostly results in increased burnout and mental health challenges. High levels of masking amongst Autistic people are associated with higher levels of interpersonal trauma and mental health challenges (Evans et al., 2023).

Not only is the high level of trauma experienced by the Autistic population and the lack of research in relation to understanding trauma and trauma supports of huge concern, in exploring Autistic neurology with a young person there is also the significant issue of diagnostic overshadowing. This occurs when professionals assume that a young person is not Autistic as they have experienced trauma in their lives and that this must be the explanation for their experience of the world. This often-incorrect assumption has led to the misidentification of many people's experiences, and also has led to further trauma from a system that has failed to understand and support a person's experiences. This may also be the case for a young person's parents / caregivers who may have experienced their own trauma relating to being misunderstood by services themselves. It is essential for any professional who is engaged in work to support young people in understanding their neurology and identity to have a deep understanding of the high likelihood of trauma experiences amongst Autistic young people, and also the differences between trauma experiences and Autistic experiences (see Chapter 15 for further information on how to distinguish between trauma experiences and Autistic experiences). Not being aware of this distinction results in a very high risk of further trauma and harm for many young people.

During an exploratory piece with any child or young person and their family, the process needs to be trauma-informed from the outset. It is safer to assume the presence of trauma and to act accordingly, as the impact of doing this will not be harmful, whereas the impact of not offering a trauma-informed process has the potential to add to a person's trauma experience.

What are the aspects of a trauma-informed process?

1. Routinely enquire about trauma and trauma experiences. Ask about significant events in a person's life and their experience of trauma.

2. Be aware that previous experiences within health services may have been traumatic. For many young people and their families, they may have met with other health professionals who misunderstood them, where their communication was not heard and where there were potentially difficult dynamics between them and the clinicians.

3. Be aware of power dynamics. Even if health professionals do not intend for there to be power dynamics or they do not seek to have power, the power imbalance is present. Being aware of this is essential and taking steps to mitigate it and to empower a young person and their family is vital (see Section 10.2 for further exploration of power dynamics within an exploration process).

4. Communicating about previous trauma can be challenging. Particularly within a relatively short process of exploring Autistic identity, for many young people talking or communicating about previous traumatic events they have experienced may be challenging. This also must be considered in terms of potential re-traumatisation if the clinician is not going to be involved in any post-assessment support piece and there will be no continuity in processes. It can be psychologically unsafe to delve into a trauma piece during a short process if no longer-term support piece is available.

5. Autistic neurology and trauma can and do co-occur. It is essential for clinicians to be aware that trauma and being Autistic are unfortunately not mutually exclusive, and that there is a high likelihood of trauma for most Autistic people.

6. Trauma support following the process. Due to the high likelihood

of trauma for most Autistic people, it is essential that further therapeutic support is available to Autistic young people following the process of identifying their Autistic neurology.

9.4 Conclusion

In this chapter we aimed to provide professionals with an understanding of mental health and trauma and how these intersect with Autistic identity. We remind readers that trauma is commonly experienced with the Autistic population: this includes both adverse childhood experiences and other life events as well as other sources of trauma that clinicians may not consider, for example sensory trauma and the trauma of chronic invalidation or being socially excluded or misunderstood. Too often, clinicians conceptualise trauma and Autistic neurology as mutually exclusive; for example, if a child has experienced domestic abuse some clinicians may identify developmental trauma and attribute the child's differences to this only, seemingly unable to hold in mind that trauma experience and Autistic neurology can and do exist. In the next chapter we will look at other important considerations (e.g., power and process, intersectionality etc.) that need to be held in mind whilst working with Autistic children and their parents / caregivers.

CHAPTER 10

Important Considerations

10.1 Introduction

This chapter summarises further considerations not addressed elsewhere in the book that must be held in mind whilst working with Autistic children and their parents / caregivers. These include power and process issues within a formal autism identification process, working with families who have had difficult service experiences, gender variance and GSRD (gender, sexuality and relationship diversity), working with ethnic minorities, children in care and intersectionality and self-identification, and the so called 'widening' of the diagnostic criteria.

All of these areas are central to the identification process, both when thinking about the child and their parents / caregivers, remembering that it is likely at least one parent is neurodivergent themselves, whether formally identified or if they have chosen to share their neurology with the clinician. We encourage you to read Hartman et al. (2023) for a detailed discussion of considerations when working with Autistic adults to understand fully the interweaving threads that should be thought about since working with children clearly involves working closely with those within their system (including understanding and accommodating their own experiences and needs within their young person's identification process).

10.2 Power and Process Issues within a Formal Autism Identification Process

One aspect seen in many medical model assessments is the unhelpful power dynamics that are often present, in which families meet with a (usually non-autistic) 'specialist' and their young person is subjected to a process of being observed, rated, coded and then declared as meeting 'threshold' or not. Social media forums of families going through this gruelling process frequently reflect narratives of their young person not being 'quite' Autistic enough because they scored a point below cut-off on a test instrument, or because they 'made eye contact' and the family expertise in their young person is somehow less important than a clinician who is drawing upon a perhaps outdated understanding of Autistic experience and slavishly adhering to 'diagnostic measures' without critically evaluating the validity of those instruments, or the epistemic environment in which they were created. There is often little sense of collaboration, with the young person, guardian and the professional coming to a mutual, shared understanding of what might be going on for them. Many parents / caregivers have felt a sense of the professional trying to 'disprove' their belief that their child or young person is Autistic rather than showing a warm curiosity for where they are coming from, and working towards a mutual understanding.

Throughout the identification process, we need to attend intentionally to power dynamics with the room when working with both young people and their parents / caregivers. Identification should be a collaborative process with all concerned, but also because families may come to us having experienced a long history of difficult interactions with services where their voices have not been heard, or subject to child protection investigations (and we do not dispute the need for safeguarding concerns to be investigated thoroughly) which were not optional, understood or felt otherwise disempowering.

Differences in power influence families' access to resources, be that knowledge about Autistic experience in general terms, or that there are alternatives to the deficit-laden medical narrative and method of assessment in which the young person and family are passive participants. To ignore power differences is missing half the story. What happens in sessions is as much a product of the clinician as the young person and their guardian. This may be an uncomfortable truth, but it is nonetheless central to our understanding of process. We cannot consider whether someone is Autistic or not simply based on detached reliance on clinical measures, without reflection about our own contribution to that process and how we interacted and facilitated (or not) the overall process. Self-reflection on process and seeking supervision are key. We recommend:

- Focusing on developing self-awareness through personal therapy and clinical supervision to avoid falling into the 'expert' position.

- Acknowledging the 'inescapable presence of expert power' (see Harrison, 2013).

- Recognising that the client is always the foremost authority on themselves, their lives and needs. Do not assume that a non-autistic clinician is more knowledgeable about Autistic experience (no matter how well-read and informed) than an Autistic person.

- Practice humility as you reflect on power and process.

- Be aware that the structure of many assessments privilege neuro-normative communication and needs, with clinicians using tests without critically examining whether they are a valid way of identifying Autistic neurology. If these measures are presented to parents/caregivers as a way of providing a 'definitive' and scientific way of identifying if their child or young person is Autistic, this might look like an open and collaborative sharing of power and structure (in that the parents consent to the process), but it is not if the clinician is not transparent about the limitations of relying on questionnaire and observational measures.

- Consider power to be intrinsic in every interaction, and reflect on how clinical choices impact power dynamics with your client / families and on your power to make changes (e.g., towards working neuro-affirmatively) within your own systems.

- Always be aware that whether we seek to use it or not, we do hold more power and need to be aware of this ('the distance of rank itself translates into the...power to define the situation – to say whose perception is accurate and whose is distorted' (Totton, 2023, p. 77), and consciously attend to how differences (be it neurology, social status, being a member of a minority group etc.) impact on dynamics within the clinical space.

- Make no assumptions about parents / caregivers' communication or information processing style, but rather find points of contact with their way of being.

10.3 Working with Families with Previous Difficult Service Experiences

Families may come to the identification process having had a long history of difficult experiences with services, for example with social care services, education or health services. This may particularly be the case for Autistic parents / caregivers whose communication style is misunderstood by services. For example, we have heard stories of Autistic parents / caregivers who repeatedly raise valid concerns about service delivery in order to advocate for their child or young person and their community, only to have this interpreted as being indicative of mental health needs, or an 'obsession' with some aspect of service. Benson (2023) discusses how neuro-normative assumptions have troublesome implications for social work practice given the 'knowledge' that is created in records and reports which carry the power to significantly harm Autistic parents / caregivers. The imposition of 'compulsory neuro-normativity' can contribute to the identification of 'perplexing presentations' by social workers based on neuro-normative knowledge and standards and the creation of damaging narratives about lives, experiences and identities which parents / caregivers may feel powerless to challenge (Benson, 2023). Parents / caregivers may only find out about the narratives that surround them if they are brave enough to do a Subject Access Request to obtain all records regarding them and their young person (which must be legally provided but are often painful and traumatic to receive). If parents / caregivers have had this experience, they may understand that the narrative presented in official records may not align with their own experience of a meeting, particularly if professionals misunderstand Autistic communication and processing styles. This is understandably likely to result in hesitation to trust or feel safe with the clinician working with their young person during the identification process. No matter how neurodiversity affirmative we are, we cannot eradicate the legacy of difficult interactions with services and the impact that this has on parents / caregivers, and we need to work with this gently and compassionately.

PARENT / CARER BLAME

Being 'too informed' about Autistic experience may become pathologised, with well-researched parents / caregivers being questioned as to why they are 'label seeking', or else professionals may suggest they are trying to 'pass off' poor parenting as autism. Clements and Aiello (2021) described the problem of 'institutional parent carer blame' in their report, highlighting that national and local social care policies in England adopt a default position of attributing a disabled young person's difficulties to parental failings. Their report highlights that many parents experienced social care assessments as focusing on safeguarding / child protection matters and parental 'fitness' rather than addressing the additional support needs that resulted from their child's needs, even when the assessment was around the child's needs and not initiated by safeguarding concerns.

Pohl et al. (2016) reported that one in five mothers of an Autistic child had been investigated by social services. Benson (2023) explored experiences of involuntary social work interventions by Autistic mothers through the lens of neuro-normative scrutiny, finding that neurodivergency in mothers and children were considered 'perplexing', particularly when the children had difficulties attending school. She suggests that relying on neuro-normative scripts and standards means that social workers may fill gaps in knowledge with mistaken and malign interpretations of Autistic presentations and behaviours that perplex them.

10.4 Gender Variance and GSRD

Gender-affirming language is an essential component of any identification process and should be a core component in the operation of any service. Clinicians also need an understanding of divergence of gender identity and sexuality when working with Autistic children and young people. Toft (2023) points out that most research exploring sexuality and / or gender identity in Autistic people focuses on demonstrating that experience and expression of sexuality and gender may differ in Autistic people compared to non-autistic people. This includes more sexual minority orientations or gender non-conforming feelings, particularly amongst Autistic people assigned female at birth (e.g., Hillier et al., 2020; Warrier et al., 2020; Weir et al., 2021). Overall, research suggests that a higher percentage of Autistic people identify as LGBTQIA+ compared to non-autistic people (e.g., George & Stokes, 2018; Pecora et al., 2019). There is also evidence suggesting increased levels of gender variance (e.g., trans, non-binary, genderqueer, gender fluid etc.), for example see Cooper et al. (2018) and Dewinter et al. (2017).

Hartman et al. (2023) highlighted that Autistic people (and this will include Autistic children and teenagers) may have their sexuality and / or gender identity doubted by others because of being Autistic, compounding and replicating other experiences of invalidation throughout their lives; they stress that supporting Autistic gender variant young people with exploring their identities is a key area of progression and continuous concern with the community, particularly given the pathologising of Autistic identity and the impact of ableism in creating barriers to supporting young people with gender identity exploration. Within the identification process, it is important that clinicians are gender-affirming as well as neuro-affirming so that invalidation does not play out also in the identification space.

Toft et al.'s (2020) study of young people (Autistic, with intellectual disabilities or mental health needs) describes the narratives around sexuality and gender in young disabled people which typically involve disabled young people being 'too immature' to be LGBTQIA+ (locating being queer as more complex than being heterosexual), 'incapable' of being LGBTQIA+ because they did not have access to knowledge or understanding to enable them to be so, or having their sexual and gender identity delegitimised due to the projection that their disability informed their sexuality. Toft et al. (2020) highlight that these damaging narratives not only offer no affirmation of the young people's LGBTQIA+ identities, but also lead to a lack of appropriate information being shared with the young people as they negotiate their emerging sexual lives. Such perspectives deny access to sexual health information, support in navigating relationships and consent, as well as being invalidating.

Research (and clinicians) too often takes a position that Autistic LGBTQIA+ people are not capable of recognising their sexuality or gender identity (see Santinele Martino, 2017; Toft et al., 2020). Toft (2023) highlights that most research comes from a position of deficit, examining what it is about being Autistic that leads to a higher prevalence of GSRD in Autistic people, pointing out that this position suggests that LGBTQIA+ identities are also seen as 'deficient' and something to be protected from. Instead, drawing upon Jackson-Perry et al. (2020), Toft argues that research should focus on how sexuality and gender identity are experienced by Autistic (young) people, rather than prevalence rates. Autistic ways of being are inherently entwined with gender and sexuality and, simultaneously, may queer rigid identity categories of sexualities. Young people may be familiar with other terms from social media: for example, autigender, gendervague, neurogender or autisexual have emerged to demonstrate the unique ways in which neurodivergent people may experience gender or sexuality given that all experiences, including sexuality / gender identity, are filtered through the lens of being Autistic (see Valvano & Shelton, 2021). Toft (2023) also highlights Jack's (2012) suggestion that Autistic sexuality / gender should be considered distinctly given that constructions of sexuality / gender are ableist and Autistic people do not and should not fit with these existing definitions.

Toft's (2023) study of 16–25- year-old Autistic young people suggested that sexuality was a social norm they did not either see or feel they need to adhere with, which he suggests aligns with other research suggesting that Autistic people 'do' gender based on what feels normal to them, with a concomitantly more fluid gender identity (Kourti & MacLeod, 2019).

Narratives surrounding Autistic young people's sexuality and gender identity tend not only to be deeply invalidating, but also deny access to information and services surrounding sexual health information and exploration of gender identity. Along with being asked about how they experience their gender, all young people attending for assessment should be routinely asked for their preferred pronouns, and these should be used throughout the process and in written documentation. There will, of course, be situations in which the young person is not 'out' to their parents / caregivers and this needs to be negotiated carefully with the young person, e.g., would they like support in discussing sexuality / gender identity with their parents / caregivers, and how do they wish to be referred to during sessions (e.g., preferred names, pronouns) and in supporting documentation (this might include issuing separate reports in the young person's legal name and in their preferred name)?

10.5 Intersectionality / Ethnic Minorities

Research and clinical literature too often ignores intersectionality, approaching Autistic experience as if all Autistic young people and adults are from similar social groups, cultures, ethnicities, gender orientations and sexual orientations, with standard assessment approaches and measures typically ignoring the multiple identities and experiences that someone brings with them (Hartman et al., 2023). Intersectionality takes into account the complex and multiple identities that a person may have, the combination of which will shape their individual experiences. Race consciousness is central to intersectionality – to apply this concept to intersecting identity markers without race can be potentially harmful and inadvertently centre whiteness. Clinicians need to centre intersectionality in their work. Taking an intersectional approach means recognising that we do not have a single identity or community; we, and the children and the families with whom we work, may have multiple, perhaps simultaneously. Clinicians need to acknowledge, sit with and actively confront our previous practice where we have not actively attended to intersectionality. This also includes being culturally competent (a person's cultural sensitivity and attitudes, cultural awareness and cultural knowledge; Kaihlanen et al., 2019) and attending to how our cultural beliefs and awareness shape our clinical assessments and decisions. Being culturally competent goes beyond simply respecting the different cultures of the children and families with whom we work: it is also about having an understanding of how we work, and responding to the needs of our diverse clients.

Being a white, straight, Autistic cis teen boy will be a different experience to that of a Black, gender divergent, Autistic teen girl. Standardised assessment protocols and diagnostic criteria do not take account of all these factors that impact on both the individual's lived experience, route to assessment, and understanding of the individual's autism in the context of their intersectionality.

> Whilst there is the need for a systemic shift in ensuring that standard assessment measures adequately address cultural diversity, individual clinicians must ensure that they utilise existing measures through a critical cultural lens, unpacking their own cultural assumptions and experiences and how these impact on how they both approach assessments and understand an individual's needs in view of their cultural background and experiences.

There is little information available around approaching identification (including measures) from a culturally sensitive perspective, with research tending to focus on the discrepancies and disparities in 'diagnosis' rather than exploring the causes and maintenance of these (Stoll et al., 2021). Previous research has suggested that the identification of autism in certain ethnic groups can be missed or delayed (Tromans et al., 2021). This means that already marginalised individuals are further marginalised through lack of access to appropriate sources of support (e.g., Straiton & Sridhar, 2022, suggested that Black families encounter a racist system that perpetuates disparities and offers a poor quality of care to families), with longer wait times and a later age for formal identification. Black Autistic children are 2.6 times more likely to be misidentified than white Autistic children and are more likely to be diagnosed with an adjustment or conduct disorder instead of being correctly identified as Autistic (e.g., Straiton & Sridhar, 2022).

Pham et al. (2022) stressed the importance of developing culturally responsive approaches to support racially, ethnically and linguistically diverse families of Autistic young people, pointing out that language or communication barriers, systemic issues and limited training in cultural responsiveness are a significant barrier to service access (and hence formal identification). There is some evidence that (in the USA at least) this gap is reducing. In 2023, the

Centers for Disease Control and Prevention reported that for the first time, the Autism and Developmental Disabilities Monitoring Network found the percentage of 8-year-old children identified with ASD was higher among Black, Hispanic and Asian or Pacific Islander children compared with white children (Centers for Disease Control and Prevention, 2023). Prior to 2016, the percentage of children identified as Autistic was higher among white children than among Black or Hispanic children although by 2018 there was no overall difference in identification rates by age 8 years (in 2018, the percentage of Black and Hispanic children identified as Autistic aged 4 years was higher compared to white children, continuing in 2020 and then being reflected also in the 8-year-old data). The CDC report suggested that this may indicate increased awareness and identification of autism, and great access to services in communities serving Black, Hispanic and Asian or Pacific Islander children. Clinicians need to attend to how these issues may play out in the identification space, for example being vigilant to the misidentification of Autistic Black children and challenging other professionals who are seemingly less aware of these issues or less culturally competent than they should be.

PRACTICE POINTS

◊   Clinicians need to actively acknowledge, and seek to challenge, how their profession perpetuates racism or cultural insensitivity, and embrace a position of cultural humility.

◊   Cultural humility is a process of self-reflection including examination of one's own beliefs and cultural identities, and having genuine regard and curiosity for other cultures, in addition to paying attention to intersectionality. Straiton and Sridhar (2022) provide a wealth of suggested resources to support clinicians to develop cultural humility.

◊   We need to actively reflect on intersectionality and be mindful that includes a broad range of marginalisation.

◊   Clinicians must be mindful of all the complex pathways that individuals and families navigate when accessing services, explicitly naming and holding a space for these to be heard.

10.6 Autistic Neurology – Age for Identification

If a young person is Autistic, it is important that this is identified as early as possible in their life, to ensure that they can access the right supports and understanding in the environments they live, play and learn in. The importance of early identification and implementation of early supports is well-documented (Elder et al., 2017; Hyman et al., 2020). For many Autistic people, indicators of their Autistic neurology can emerge as early as 12 to 18 months of age (Landa et al., 2013; Pierce et al., 2019) and identifications made at 18 months have been shown to be reliable and stable (Ozonoff et al., 2015). Indeed, there have been many studies that have demonstrated that identification of Autistic neurology prior to the age of 3 years old is stable and reliable (Chawarska et al., 2009; Guthrie et al., 2013). However, while the false-positive rate of identification prior to the age of 3 is low, the false-negative identification is higher (Ozonoff et al., 2015) with many Autistic children being missed in very early childhood. For many young people, their Autistic neurology does not emerge until later in their childhood (Davidovitch et al., 2015; Ozonoff et al., 2018). Many children who are identified later in childhood have typical early developmental trajectories (Ozonoff et al., 2018), and 'diagnostic overshadowing' in early life can also play a role (Davidovitch et al., 2015).

10.7 Children in Care

The process of exploring Autistic identity with young people who are in state care needs careful consideration. The vast majority of young people who are in state care have been exposed to traumatic experiences, and given the overlap between Autistic experiences and trauma experiences (see Chapter 9 and Section 15.4.3.3 for further discussion on trauma experiences and how they overlap with Autistic experiences), identifying Autistic neurology within this group requires a careful approach. However, due to the likely presence of trauma, it is vital that this group not be overlooked in terms of exploring their possible Autistic neurology, and identifying whether they are Autistic or not is essential in terms of supporting them through their experience of state care and beyond.

There is a higher likelihood of Autistic young people (and those with other disabilities) being brought into state care than neurotypical young people (Cidav et al., 2018; Hall-Lande et al., 2015). Furthermore, young people who have experienced several adverse childhood experiences (ACEs) are significantly more likely to have to wait much longer than children who have not experienced several ACEs to be identified as Autistic (Berg et al., 2018). As a result of these stark statistics, it is imperative that a robust process is in place of exploring Autistic neurology with children in care where this is indicated.

It can be challenging for young people in care to access a process to explore possible Autistic neurology due to multiple factors, including (but not limited to):

- Geographical reasons: Young people are often placed in care in geographical locations away from their original hometown, which can complicate and sometimes delay access to therapeutic supports.

- Lack of continuity: Often it is parents or caregivers and sometimes teachers at school who may initially notice differences in their child's experience of the world. However if a young person's caregiver and / or teacher changes frequently (as can often be the case for children in care), then there may not be enough time for others to get to know a young person in order to support them with exploring their neurology and to access services that can support them in exploring this further.

- Trauma experiences: As highlighted above, many children in care have experienced higher levels of trauma than their peers who are not in care. Not only does this delay them accessing identification processes (Berg et al., 2018), it can also cause 'diagnostic overshadowing', where a child's experiences are incorrectly explained by their trauma experiences without due consideration being given to the possibility of co-occurring Autistic neurology.

When working with children in state care, the following is advised:

- Clinicians need to adopt a trauma-informed approach to the exploration piece with a young person and their caregivers.

- Clinicians and caregivers need to collaborate with a young person to establish the correct time within which to undertake a process exploring Autistic neurology. For some young people, being unaware that they are Autistic will further add to their distress, while for others their current distress from trauma experiences may be active which may make it challenging for them to engage in an exploration process.

- Consideration needs to be given to differentiating Autistic experiences from trauma experiences (see Chapter 15 for further discussion on the process of differentiating both).

- Young people in care will need support and resources to develop their Autistic identity following the process if they are identified as Autistic. If they are not identified as Autistic, then they will still need support with their sense of self and identity.

- Clinicians need to be aware that when a young person is in care, it may be more helpful to explore their sense of self over time rather than within a short process.

- Support and welfare services need to be aware that if a young person is identified as Autistic, then there is a high likelihood that their biological parent(s) are also Autistic. This has implications in terms of the supports that biological family members may need.

10.8 Self-Identification and the So-Called 'Widening' of Diagnostic Criteria

The Neurodiversity Paradigm welcomes self-identification and the greater understanding of the diversity of Autistic experience that can support Autistic young people in recognising and understanding their neurology. This does not come without tensions, however, as researchers, journalists and clinicians continue to question the so-called 'widening' of diagnostic criteria, pointing out the disparity in 'diagnosis rates' across different region (e.g., Hill, 2024). Such research may be disseminated before it has even been peer reviewed. Whilst any identification piece clearly needs to follow best practice and be robust and reliable, these reports erode the underpinnings of neuro-affirmative ways of working by questioning the widening knowledge base of Autistic experience which has fostered greater understanding of neurology by Autistic people and by clinicians working with them to explore their identity – rather than exploring why some clinicians continue to miss Autistic identity (e.g., due to lack of contemporary knowledge), the position taken is to question why there is 'too much' recognition.

Those wedded to the medical model are perhaps reluctant to cede their power to 'diagnose', rather than embracing that Autistic children and adults are exploring their identity and reaching self-understanding outside of the clinical space (e.g., by watching TikTok). Narratives about the 'dangers of self-diagnosis' abound (e.g., David & Heeley, 2024), rather than celebrating that greater accessibility of information around Autistic experience is enabling young people to take steps to understand their way of being. At the same time, we invite curiosity as to why identification rates appear to vary across services, how practitioners are working across those different settings and what identification protocols they are following.

10.9 Conclusion

In this chapter we aimed to outline areas central to a neurodiversity affirmative identification process, including examining power and process issues within a formal autism identification process, working with families who have had difficult service experiences, gender variance and GSRD, working with ethnic minorities and children in care, intersectionality and self-identification, and the so called 'widening' of the diagnostic criteria. The next chapter proceeds to examine and provide practical advice around conducting a sensory audit of the space in which you see children and families.

CHAPTER 11

Conducting a Sensory Audit

11.1 Introduction

When performing a sensory audit, it is crucial to consider the entire process rather than just the primary space in which the child's or young person's identification process occurs. This means that we must also consider all the other spaces involved in the identification process, such as the materials distributed beforehand, the modes of communication available to access information, arrange appointments and communicate, any online spaces, waiting areas and any other transitional spaces, such as hallways or entrances.

In this section, we will refer to all these different considerations, such as physical environments, online environments, resources, communication and transitions, as spaces, as they are all different spaces in their own right and need to be considered when conducting a sensory audit.

Sensory auditing must be conducted as a continuous process, requiring regular re-evaluation and updates to keep up with the ever-changing spaces. Accessibility cannot be achieved through a one-time checkbox exercise; it demands a continuous effort to be successful.

It is important that all people conducting sensory audits, designing spaces, or working in spaces that children, young people and their families / parents / caregivers come into contact with have an awareness and understanding of the distinct perceptual mechanism of Autistic people, as well as otherwise neurodivergent and neurotypical people when auditing all such spaces. A sensory audit ensures that all of these spaces, resources and communications are accessible to all those who use them.

It is crucial to recognise that one way in which perception can differ across neurotypes is that people have different ways of perceiving uncertainty and different levels of sensory habituation. Therefore, spaces and materials should be adapted / designed thoughtfully with these differences in mind, considering the eight sensory domains: auditory, taste, visual, smell, touch, proprioception, interoception and vestibular. The goal is to create adaptable spaces that are responsive to the experiences of families, parents / caregivers, young people and children. This will ensure that adaptations can be made to meet the diversity of individual needs.

11.2 Sensory Audit Preparation and Key People

As you prepare for an audit, it's important to recognise the effect that space design can have on different perceptions. What may be harmless or unnoticeable sensory stimuli for neurotypical people can profoundly affect accessibility, inclusion, interaction and well-being for Autistic people.

Autistic children and young people often do not habituate to sensory stimuli in the same way as neurotypical people. While neurotypical children and young people may become accustomed to recurrent sensory inputs over time, reducing their intensity with each exposure, Autistic people will often continue to perceive repeated sensory information at the same level of intensity each time. This can be a source of joy and flow, but it can be intrusive or distressing at other times.

To ensure that an audit considers Autistic perceptions of spaces, it is necessary to consult with Autistic individuals and Autistic specialists who can offer insight into their unique mechanisms of perception. Since neurotypical individuals cannot perceive spaces in the same way as Autistic individuals, engaging the services of an Autistic consultant who has an understanding of the diversity of Autistic perception is crucial when conducting audits. By working together and valuing Autistic experience and Autistic perception as different and warranting consideration to the same extent as neurotypical perception, we can create more inclusive and accessible spaces for everyone.

To support accessibility for all people, including Autistic people, we need to take a comprehensive approach that balances reducing sensory overload with providing enriching sensory inputs that are adaptable to the diversity of optimum sensory balance the people using these spaces have. This requires a tailored, adaptable design and an audit checklist that covers all eight sensory domains. Involving Autistic professionals with skills in auditing is critical due to our ability to perceive nuances that may be missed by neurotypical people. Our insights ensure that spaces are accessible and affirming of Autistic neurology.

Given the difference in perception between Autistic people and neurotypical people, it is crucial that you engage the support of an Autistic consultant when conducting a sensory audit.

The term 'sensory' is often associated with occupational therapy, but it actually has a much broader scope. Sensory experiences are a fundamental part of our daily lives, and they are closely linked with our cognition. We rely on a combination of our senses and cognition to perceive and interact with the world around us.

Our sensory systems play a crucial role in shaping our perceptions, and they are closely intertwined with our brain structure and function. This complex relationship has a lot to do with the fields of psychology, neurology and neuroscience. Every aspect of interior design and architecture is meant to engage our senses. If we consider an Autistic consultant, their expertise could span across a wide range of specialities, including neuroscience, psychology, occupational therapy, architecture and interior design.

Given that variety, it is important to find a consultant who meets the following four criteria:

1. A consultant must be Autistic to perceive the level of uncertainty that is unique to Autistic neurology, and which is often overlooked.

2. A consultant should have a demonstrable neurodiversity affirmative understanding of the mechanisms of Autistic perception and how Autistic people perceive uncertainty differently to neurotypical people.

3. A consultant should be aware of the variety and nuances of sensory balances that Autistic people can have and how important stimming is to self-regulation and well-being.

4. A consultant should have experience in conducting sensory audits with a range of Autistic people across various spaces.

Remember, what is often necessary for Autistic people to have accessibility in spaces is often also beneficial to everyone else.

By making Autistic-informed changes to physical and virtual spaces, information spaces and communication spaces, we can make significant strides in fostering inclusive and neuro-affirmative practices.

The following section provides examples and strategies for auditing across different sensory domains. While this is not an exhaustive list, it should help identify other considerations that may be unique to your space.

11.3 Conducting Your Audit

11.3.1 Auditory Assessment

When it comes to evaluating auditory input in a given space, it's crucial to consider two key sources of input that can affect users. First, there are potential risks of excessive noise or specific sounds that can be an unnecessary source of uncertainty, take up energy and increase the likelihood of overload. These noises can create barriers within the space and lead to discomfort, distraction or even harm to individual users. Other sources of auditory input that can cause issues include a radio or TV playing in the waiting area and changes in the noise level when moving through different transitional spaces. Second, there are opportunities to enhance the accessibility of spaces by allowing users to control ambient noises. See Appendix 2 for examples of auditory inputs to consider when auditing spaces.

Provide information beforehand about the auditory environment, how users can adapt the environment to their needs and what to expect, for example if noise levels change on different days or at different times. Empower families, parents / caregivers, young people and children to use spaces in a way that works best for them.

11.3.2 Visual Assessment

When assessing a space's visual aspect, several important factors must be considered. One such factor is the balance of lighting, which must be scrutinised carefully to ensure that it is neither too dim nor too bright. It should create no visual flicker or make no humming sound; again, this will often not be perceived by neurotypical people but can be highly problematic or distressing for Autistic people.

Lighting adjustments are important to help individuals control their sensory environment according to their needs. To achieve this, you can utilise dimmer switches or lamps that allow for the adjustment of both direction and intensity of light.

Another important consideration is visual clutter – too many visuals, whether in information spaces or in physical spaces, can be overwhelming, distracting and exhausting. However, too little visual input can also be problematic. See Appendix 2 for more on getting this balance right. It is important to incorporate different adaptable stimuli, for example using lamps with controllable levels, intensity and colour of light, moveable biophilic design elements, and pops of texture and colour to create a visually pleasing environment that can be adapted for each user's optimum sensory balance.

When auditing a physical space, it is important to consider visual input coming not just from the space in use but also the spaces that are used to get to that space, such as corridors and waiting areas. It's important to assess such visual inputs on the way to the main space, such as the pattern on the floor, reflections as people move through spaces, and the presence of multiple signs, digital screens or cluttered notice boards.

Art on walls can really help lift a space and, when done correctly, provide a good source of input, but beware that too much or too many different types of art can lead to exhaustion and overload. Abstract art or adding children's or young people's art to the walls can sometimes be nice, but it can also become too much, confusing and overloading. Avoid bright primary colours; instead stick to soft pastel colours and soft warm lights. If you have clients who need high visual sensory input for spaces to be accessible for them, consider how you could add objects or art that can easily be put away for others who find such material overwhelming.

Doors can be another source of uncertainty and can lead to / increase anxiety or avoidance. Not knowing what is behind the door, what will happen when you go through it, or not knowing if you will be required to go through it can cause issues with accessibility. Preparation material with maps and wayfinding can provide predictability for young people, children and their families and parents / caregivers before arriving at spaces. See Appendix 2 for more examples of ways to prepare.

Other spaces to consider when auditing are those places which can be seen from the main space, such as the visual input from a window in an assessment room. Are there people who walk by the window, or cars or animals? Is there any surprise stimulus that could be seen from the window and that users need to be aware of? Are there certain times when there is more going on outside windows? Is there a lot of movement? See Appendix 2 for more examples of questions to consider when conducting a visual audit.

It's best to avoid using fluorescent lights whenever possible. These lights can cause significant fatigue, visual strain and even migraines. For neurodivergent individuals, they can be especially painful and have a lasting impact even after leaving the space. In buildings that use harsh, strong fluorescent lighting, it is crucial to change bulbs regularly. As bulbs reach the end of their life, they can start flickering and buzzing, which can intensify issues even more, while neurotypical people might not even notice these issues or are more likely to get used to such input with repeated exposure. Remember, repeated exposure does not reduce the intensity of perception for Autistic individuals and otherwise neurodivergent people as it does for neurotypical people. These lights are a major barrier for an Autistic person entering and using spaces.

Fluorescent light management can be challenging, especially when replacing the lights is not an option. In such cases, you can minimise the issues by using fluorescent light sleeves, filters and covers. These tools can help diffuse harshness and create softer rays, making it more comfortable and less intense for people. Many sleeves available feature imagery of nature, which can create an interesting pop of colour. Avoid any sleeves with stripes, patterns or multiple colours, as this could also be problematic and be a further source of uncertainty.

Another way to improve the lighting conditions is to provide the option of turning off overhead lights and using natural light or softer lighting solutions, such as uplighting and adjustable light direction and intensity lamps. This way, individuals can choose their preferred lighting conditions and use these spaces more comfortably. See Appendix 2 for alternatives to fluorescent lighting.

Another important aspect to consider when conducting an audit is how different areas of the space integrate with one another. This includes assessing how transition spaces and main areas flow together and how colours and lighting can be used to create a smooth transition between different spaces and changing levels of sensory input. For example, painting walls with different tones of the same colour or analogous colours can signal changes in sensory stimulus levels. Use different colours in one area to separate the area into types of activities. Remember to avoid primary colours or plain white or grey walls; instead, use soft colours and stick to gentle pastel tones which move gently through differing tones and shades for permanent elements. Designing areas which help the user prepare for entering new areas can also enhance accessibility, for example designing a seating cubby or a bench / booth on a corridor with a view to a new area, such as an outside space or busier area, where users can sit and observe the new area before going into it. This can help provide time to self-regulate and create predictability and time to adjust when moving between different spaces. In an online environment, a small period in a waiting area can also work; this allows the user to get used to the interface, check their camera and microphone levels and understand how to use text before the call begins.

FROM ONE LIGHTING HELL TO ANOTHER: THE IMPACT OF SUPER BRIGHT LED LIGHTS

In recent years, there has been a shift from fluorescent lighting to super bright LED lights. These LEDs are often touted as being more beneficial for human health, environmentally friendly and cost-effective. However, the way these lights are being implemented raises significant concerns.

While some LED lights come with adaptability features such as masking daylight, colour change adjustability and intensity level control, these features are frequently inaccessible to users and even staff. Consequently, the lights are often set at maximum brightness and left unchanged, failing to mimic the natural variation in daylight intensity. This constant high-level brightness, with no shaded areas or dimming, can lead to several issues.

It is important to note that while fluorescent lights have their own drawbacks, and we are certainly not recommending them, the current use of super bright LED / daylight lights presents new, significant challenges. Unlike fluorescent lights, which allow for darker corners, these super bright LEDs maintain their intense brightness throughout the day and are often installed in multiples lighting up every corner of a space. Prolonged exposure to such high light levels can cause stress, agitation, discomfort, fatigue and even pain. Often, these lights are set up as several squares that fit into the ceiling or baton-style lighting. This intense downlighting can create a feeling of being pushed down, contributing to a sense of unease.

Furthermore, the fixed intensity levels do not accommodate the differing needs of neurodivergent individuals, whose perceptual systems may be more sensitive to such lighting. This is particularly concerning in settings where children and young people spend considerable time, such as schools, libraries, GP practices, hospitals and indoor public spaces. Even residential settings, health services and sports halls are affected.

Addressing the Issues with Super Bright LED Lights

To address the problems associated with super bright LED lights, several measures can be taken:

1. Accessible controls: Install lights with controls that are easily accessible to users. At a minimum, all users should have clear guidance on how to request staff to change the lighting. This allows for adjustments in colour and intensity, creating a more comfortable environment.

2. Dynamic intensity: Ensure that the intensity of the lights mimics natural daylight throughout the day, reducing the strain of constant brightness.

3. Use of diffusers: In spaces where lighting is needed all the time, such as hospitals, install diffusers to soften the light and reduce glare.

4. Selective installation: Avoid using super bright LED lights everywhere. Create a variety of areas within every space with varied lighting, including areas with softer, less intense light, incorporating actual daylight where possible or installing lights with changing directions.

5. Retreat spaces: Provide places where individuals can escape the bright light, such as quiet corners, less intense lighting walkways, and dimmed waiting areas.

6. Avoid cluttered lighting: Avoid cluttering a space with too many sources of light. This can create visual chaos and decrease accessibility.

7. Strategic placement: Avoid installing lights directly above seats or beds. Instead, use furniture and placement to conceal direct sources of light. Concealing the light source can often improve its effectiveness. A light can still do its job, and will often do it better if the light source itself cannot actually be seen.

8. Concealed light sources: Ensure that the light source itself is not directly visible, as indirect lighting can often be more beneficial for those with heightened sensory sensitivities.

Implementing these strategies can create more comfortable and accessible spaces that accommodate the diverse needs of all individuals. Lighting can make or break a space, and adaptability features are great if they work, but without access, they are redundant and useless and continue to add barriers for young people and children.

11.3.3 Olfactory Assessment

Assessment of smells or odours is essential to minimise unpleasant or strong scents. It's also necessary to consider the impact of the lack of smell in remote settings on people's engagement levels. Plants in such environments can enhance sensory experiences by providing fresh, natural scents while also absorbing unpleasant or strong odours. Additionally, they contribute to a biophilic design that promotes well-being.

When conducting an audit for olfactory input, it is necessary to consider the ventilation of spaces and the ability to air them out. This is important because even if a space is under strict control or is only used by a single organisation, human error can occur. For instance, if someone brings in a lunch with a strong spicy aroma, it's essential that ventilation can be activated, windows can be opened and the odour doesn't persist in the space.

In large physical spaces, it is recommended that a well-ventilated area be designed specifically for food consumption. This space should be a separate space with preventative measures to ensure that it is set up to stop smells from travelling to other spaces. It is also advisable to reduce chewing gum or eating during meetings for professionals as this can also linger or be unpleasant in smell and noise. Try to design coffee areas in designated spaces, also. See Appendix 2 for considerations around scented product usage.

11.3.4 Gustatory Assessment

It is important to note that taste assessments may not always be relevant when conducting audits in certain spaces. To determine the relevance of taste assessments, consider factors such as whether the area being audited involves eating or drinking, if there are plain and separate food options available, if plain water is available and if people are allowed to bring their own food and refreshments. These factors will help determine the relevance of taste assessments in the audit process.

11.3.5 Proprioceptive and Tactile Assessment

When assessing proprioceptive and tactile input, it's crucial to consider how spaces are designed to impact the user's sense of body position, movement and effort.

When choosing seating and furniture options, it is crucial to consider stability, height and tactile feedback. Stability is important because it ensures that the furniture will not tip over or collapse under the weight of different users. It is recommended to have a range of different seating options available, such as adjustable seating, to allow the user to reach the ground and maintain good posture comfortably. Provide options that enable them to put their feet up, cross their legs or sit on the floor.

Tactile feedback is the sensation the user receives through physical contact. One way to enhance this feedback is to choose furniture that offers adjustable seating. This allows users to shift their weight and experience different levels of support, which can increase proprioceptive feedback.

While soft and deep chairs might be comfortable for some individuals, they may not be suitable for those who require more proprioceptive input to feel secure. Deep chairs can be challenging for users who need more proprioceptive input and have an uncomfortable feeling like they are sinking and not provided with enough support. This type of soft furniture can pose difficulties for individuals with co-occurring conditions such as dyspraxia or

Ehlers-Danlos syndrome. On the other hand, chairs that are too firm or rigid can be uncomfortable, restrict movement and not provide enough tactile input. Therefore, it's crucial to choose a range of furniture that strikes the right balance between comfort and support.

When conducting audits and designing spaces, it's important to consider the materials used on floors and surfaces. Different textures and materials can provide varying levels of feedback to the user's body. For example, thick carpets may reduce the intensity of movements, whereas hard floors can offer more direct feedback. Uneven surfaces, such as textured floors with raised bumps, can be used to signal transitions, but they can also be a barrier to navigate and should be used in moderation with clear information given about them in advance. It's important for users to understand the purpose of such tools before entering a space.

The arrangement of a space affects how accessible it is for users to navigate it, influencing their proprioceptive sense. Open areas allowing movement, including stimming, stretching, walking or bouncing, can help. Consider whether the environment is free of unnecessary obstructions. Have users been provided with information before attending physical spaces to help with navigation? Have you considered differing heights that individuals may need to navigate, such as steps, stairs and curbs? Have you considered adjustments for those people who have fine motor difficulties or hypermobility, such as easy-to-use door handles and seating options, which provide sufficient adaptable support and reduce fatigue?

Incorporate tools or equipment that can be used to apply pressure or resistance. Items like weighted blankets, weight pads or wrist weights can offer proprioceptive input, which can be calming and grounding for some individuals.

Since proprioceptive needs vary widely, it is important to offer options to adapt the assessment space. Allowing users to choose from a range of seating options or control the layout of their immediate environment can significantly improve their comfort and engagement level.

When dealing with the sense of touch, it's important to choose the right space and therapy tools. This means finding materials that are either soothing or stimulating based on personal preferences.

One way to balance the need for stimulation is by introducing plants and textures that are not overly busy. For example, ferns or lamb ears can provide comforting tactile input. It's important to remember that too little stimulation can be just as challenging as too much. Therefore, the goal is to create a healthy balance that can be adapted for different users.

11.3.6 Vestibular Assessment

Conducting a vestibular audit requires an understanding of the variety of ways movement and balance can impact an individual's experience of spaces. This encompasses evaluating both physical and online environments to ensure they support vestibular needs.

In physical spaces, offering dynamic seating options that allow for movement, such as swivel chairs, balance balls or rocking chairs, can help individuals regulate their vestibular input. This is similar to ensuring that furniture provides adequate proprioceptive feedback but focuses on the need for movement to increase accessibility.

The design of spaces, including corridors and waiting areas, should facilitate safe, easy navigation with opportunities for varied movement. Wide, obstacle-free pathways allow for walking, pacing or stimming that can help individuals seeking vestibular stimulation.

Providing material beforehand that explains what to expect during the visit can help prepare individuals for the sensory environment. This includes details on the physical layout, types of seating available and any vestibular-friendly resources they can access during their meeting.

It's important to include scheduled movement breaks in both physical and online sessions. This applies to families, parents / caregivers, young people and children. They should be made aware that they can take movement breaks whenever they need to. It's not necessary to always sit down in an office for assessments. Other physical spaces like a car, where the vibrational vestibular input of a moving vehicle can help, or going for a walk or a swim in a pool could also be explored. In online spaces, incorporating interactive elements that require physical response, such as virtual reality experiences or movement-based activities, can simulate vestibular engagement. While these suggestions may seem unconventional, we need to think outside the box to ensure accessibility and system change.

Designated movement areas or sensory pathways can be created within physical spaces to encourage vestibular stimulation for those who require it. These pathways may consist of different textures or elements that provide gentle vestibular challenges, such as soft inclines or balance beams and moving seating. These areas can be integrated subtly into corridors or waiting areas, but it is important that they can also be avoided for those who are hypersensitive to vestibular input. Adaptability is key. See Appendix 2 for ways in which visual signs can be used to help navigate spaces.

11.3.7 Interoceptive Assessment

Interoceptive assessments are important to ensure that spaces are designed to support the awareness of and response to internal cues, such as the need for temperature control or hydration. By adapting spaces to meet these internal sensory requirements, we can improve the overall comfort and well-being of individuals.

There are several ways to increase interoceptive accessibility. For instance, clear signage and navigation can be included to direct individuals to the bathroom. A sign that asks, 'Do you need the bathroom? It's this way' or 'Is it too hot or cold for you? You can open or close the window here' could help prompt those who have difficulty sensing internal cues. Similarly, before starting an online or in-person meeting, it is helpful to let participants know where the bathroom is located and that they can take a break and use it anytime they wish.

Providing easily accessible and visual drinking water is also important. This can be done by providing a water cooler in waiting areas or asking individuals if they want something to drink during meetings. Additionally, sending regular reminders available in a variety of communication methods about appointment times can be helpful.

11.4 Assessment of Flexibility in Appointments and Space Settings

Acknowledging and planning for the possibility of changes is crucial in creating a supportive and understanding environment for all users, especially for Autistic individuals who perceive more of the uncertainty that exists in the world and can find unpredictability more challenging. It's important to communicate clearly about potential changes and the measures in place to manage these changes smoothly. This section outlines the importance of maintaining flexibility in appointments and space settings, along with strategies to mitigate the impact of these changes on users.

When conducting an audit on communication space, it is important to assess how you inform users about changes. This is an important consideration as change is inevitable. While every effort might be made to adhere to schedules and keep spaces the same, given that we are humans and not robots, there will always be some level of change that occurs. This might include variations in appointment times, room assignments, or online platform updates or changes.

- Giving advance notice when possible is important, as surprises can be a considerable source of uncertainty and distress.

- Establish clear policies regarding appointment delays. For example, communicate that there may sometimes be a delay of 5 to 10 minutes, but users will never be left waiting longer than 15 minutes without further communication from the service provider. This sets clear expectations and reduces anxiety around uncertainty.

- Provide detailed information or video tours of all therapy rooms or spaces users may encounter. Highlighting if a specific room cannot always be predetermined but ensuring that all spaces adhere to the same accessibility standards helps in preparing users for potential changes.

- Users should be offered flexible rescheduling options in case the changes in appointment times or settings are not suitable for them. This gives families, parents / caregivers, young people and children control over their appointment details and empowers them to make decisions that best suit their needs.

- When changes are necessary, providing materials that help users prepare for the new space or time is crucial. This could include updated maps of spaces, visuals or information about different online platforms.

- Implement mechanisms that allow users to provide feedback on how changes are communicated and handled. Make sure to provide a variety of ways for this feedback. The feedback can be invaluable in refining processes and making future transitions smoother.

- Continuity should be maintained wherever possible, such as trying to keep the same practitioner, even if the space changes. Familiarity with the person can help mitigate the impact of changes in the physical spaces or schedule.

- Communicate changes in a supportive and understanding way. Make sure you provide information on changes in a format which is accessible to the user, acknowledging the potential stress and offering reassurance. Ensuring that the users' needs are a priority will help make the transition smoother for them.

When conducting a sensory audit, it is crucial to observe and ask for feedback from individuals using the space. Optimum sensory balance varies for each person, and adaptability in spaces with multiple users is necessary for accessibility.

11.5 Conclusion

In conclusion, conducting a sensory audit with a neurodiversity affirmative approach is vital for creating genuinely supportive and inclusive environments for all individuals. This approach values Autistic perception and involves Autistic professionals, ensuring that therapy rooms, waiting areas and remote settings affirm Autistic neurology. Such spaces not only avoid sensory and accessibility pitfalls but also enrich the diversity of perceptual mechanisms and experiences of users while fostering a positive atmosphere for exploring Autistic identity.

CHAPTER 12

Making the Identification Process Accessible

12.1 Introduction

The prospect of attending a session for an exploration of Autistic identity can often be overwhelming for many families, children and young people. It is possible that they have been waiting for a long time for this process, and that a child or young person is struggling without access to the supports they need. They may have had challenging experiences in other healthcare settings or have found it difficult to access healthcare environments due to adjustments not having been made for differences in communication or sensory experiences. A young person and their family may be feeling overwhelmed by the uncertainty of what to expect during a process, or the possibility of power imbalances that may be present. Parents and caregivers may feel concerned about how their young person will be 'evaluated' during the process, and whether their needs and experiences will be accurately identified. They may also be overwhelmed by a collection of emotions, from excitement to anxious anticipation of what will happen and what will be the outcome. Although several factors may contribute to the initial overwhelming feeling experienced by most families at the prospect of this process, accessibility within the process and adjustments made to the process can significantly alleviate the level of overwhelm experienced. In this chapter, we outline ways that professionals can do this, for example with discussions about barriers in healthcare settings, communication adjustments, providing information in advance and gathering information appropriately.

> Before undertaking to offer an identification process to any young person and their family, it is crucial that all clinicians listen to the documented accounts from Autistic people about their experiences

of 'assessment'. Unless a clinician has undergone such a process, they cannot fully grasp the experience and the power imbalance that usually exists. They cannot understand the feeling of uncertainty regarding what will happen during the process or in relation to the outcome, and they don't have a sense of what it feels like to be administered certain 'tests'. First-hand accounts of these experiences are extremely important and will help to guide clinicians in identifying the best approach for a young person and their family. Please refer back to Chapter 4 in this book for further discussion of first-hand experiences. Samples from a child's perspective are also included throughout this book, and see also examples such as Emma (2020), Du and McDaniel (2016) and Lockwood (2023).

12.2 Barriers to Accessing Healthcare Settings

Healthcare access refers to the ability to seek services, identify healthcare needs, and use or be offered services appropriate to identified needs (Levesque et al., 2013). Being unable to access healthcare, i.e., due to particular barriers being in place, is likely to lead to healthcare inequalities (Hill et al., 2015). Autistic young people experience higher rates than their peers across a range of different medical conditions (Lai, Kassee et al., 2019), including epilepsy (Spence & Schneider, 2009), allergies (Lyall et al., 2015) and gastrointestinal issues (Isaksson et al., 2017), to name but a few. They are also more likely than their neurotypical peers to experience mental health challenges (Gobrial, 2019; Simonoff et al., 2008). The barriers to accessing healthcare for Autistic people are well-documented (e.g., Doherty et al., 2022; Malik-Soni et al., 2022). Within childhood, some of the most significant barriers to accessing healthcare for Autistic children include the limited availability of services (those to identify Autistic neurology and those providing supports) and a lack of clear referral pathways for supports (Malik-Soni et al., 2022). Babalola et al. (2024) found that sensory perceptual differences, system-level barriers, communication differences, lack of person-centred care, stigma, culture, and professional and parental knowledge about Autistic neurology were the most significant barriers for Autistic children in accessing healthcare.

As has been evidenced above, there are significant barriers for Autistic children in accessing healthcare. Although one of the barriers to accessing healthcare is the limited availability of healthcare services for Autistic children (Malik-Soni et al., 2022), even when a service is available, there can still be significant barriers to a young person in accessing that service. Some of the most significant barriers are:

- Limitations on the services available. In most countries, there are long waiting times to access public system services. Even within the private sector, there can be significant waiting times, and the cost makes private services inaccessible to many.

- Lack of universal design. Universal design is the process of designing and composing an environment so that it can be accessed, understood and used to the greatest extent possible by all people, regardless of their age, size, ability or disability (NSAI, 2024). In most settings, both public and private, universal design adjustments are not in place. This means that environments are not being designed to suit all and are inaccessible to many.

- Unclear or prohibitive referral pathways. It is often the case that referral pathways for Autistic young people are unclear (Malik-Soni et al., 2022) and many services often exclude Autistic people from accessing their service (Gray-Hammond, 2024). Furthermore, most services do not have a self-referral option, which is restrictive given that many parents / caregivers report the need to research pathways to services themselves before informing professionals about their child's needs (Slade, 2014; Thomas et al., 2018) in the hope of a referral being made.

- Lack of neurodivergent professionals. There is a significant lack of openly neurodivergent professionals working within clinical services with several factors at play in relation to the cause of this. First, there are significant barriers and a lack of support for Autistic people in pursuing professional training (across all disciplines). Many attempting it experience inaccessible environments and systems, stigma and exclusion, often leading to burnout, and they are more likely to drop out than their neurotypical peers (Cage et al., 2020). Second, there is a significant lack of neuro-affirmative understanding and acceptance of the diversity of Autistic neurology and support for Autistic people within the workplace (López & Keenan, 2014) which makes it very challenging for Autistic employees to maintain their position in the workforce. Clinical services need to do more to both attract and support neurodivergent clinicians to their teams.

- Clinical spaces not designed for Autistic people. Most clinical spaces have not been designed to suit the needs of Autistic people, particularly within public system services. The location of public services is often in spaces where there is little scope to change or adapt the space, or few resources to do so due to the constraints of public systems. Private clinical spaces often have more scope to be designed for Autistic neurology, but many still are not. A lack of understanding about Autistic neurology, in particular different mechanisms of Autistic perception, means that the needs of Autistic people are often not recognised or understood. Neurotypical people often incorrectly assume that Autistic people perceive the same reality as they do, when often Autistic people are perceiving a lot more of the details that neurotypical people do not perceive.

A detailed summary of Autistic perception is provided in Hartman et al. (2023, Chapter 6, pp. 83–111). Whether the space is a public service space or a private service space, every space can be adapted to be made accessible and it is advised to seek information and / or input from Autistic professionals or a sensory audit from an Autistic professional which can highlight the areas that can be adapted. One aspect of adaptation may be to provide information and support to those coming into the space in terms of what to expect when in the environment and also what steps can be taken to ensure their access to and comfort within the space. For example, if there is a bright light in the room a person is going to come into that cannot be switched off, then a person can be given information in advance to expect this and the option to bring a hat or sunglasses to block the light.

See the box below for a summary of the Autistic SPACE framework (Doherty et al, 2023).

PERSPECTIVES OF AN OT: AUTISTIC SPACE:
A FRAMEWORK FOR MEETING THE NEEDS OF
AUTISTIC PEOPLE IN HEALTHCARE SETTINGS

KATIE KERLEY

Autistic people are more likely to experience long-term mental and physical health challenges (Weir et al., 2020) and more likely to experience barriers in accessing healthcare.

Dr Mary Doherty (founder of Autistic Doctors International and Actually Autistic researcher) has been researching barriers to healthcare for Autistics and challenging the tragedy narrative. Mary has also been doing really important and valuable work in supporting Autistic healthcare professionals in their practice as well as ensuring that Autistic patients and service users are able to access healthcare in a way that is comfortable for them.

Many people of all neurotypes find it daunting or challenging to navigate healthcare and appointments and it can be nerve-wracking to attend a clinic or a service.

She and her colleagues published 'Autistic space: A novel framework for meeting the needs of Autistic people in healthcare settings' in January 2023 (Doherty et al, 2023). They use the acronym 'SPACE' to guide healthcare providers in adapting their services to support Autistic people.

S – Sensory needs

It is well-documented and reported that Autistic people experience sensory processing differences in comparison to our neurotypical counterparts. We can be sensitive in different ways and our experiences tend to be very individualised. Many health settings are environments that are jam-packed with challenging sensory information that makes attending a service more demanding than it would otherwise be, sometimes to the extent that a person may avoid going altogether... think, for example, of very bright white lights in a stark white room, or recurrent beeping noises, unpleasant smells, being touched by a stranger in a possibly noxious way...

This may, in fact, cause distress, which may even result in a communication breakdown. We know that sensory stress builds over time and accumulates, causing us to experience lingering negative effects. An additional factor is that sensory sensitivities are heightened when we are stressed or unwell.

Taking this into consideration, it is important for healthcare providers to have an understanding of what sensory processing means and how sensory stress may impact on a person's experience (see Section 6.8 for an overview of sensory needs). Having our sensory needs acknowledged and considered would go a long way towards helping us feel comfortable and more able to attend these settings.

P – Predictability

A lot of Autistic people thrive with structure and predictability, and unexpected change or venturing into the unknown can be incredibly challenging (see Section 6.9 for an overview of executive function and cognitive flexibility). Attending a healthcare appointment is inherently unpredictable, not least because we often don't know what the outcome of said appointment will be, and often we are interacting with a person we are not familiar with.

Waiting can be difficult, especially if you are there for a specific time and then have to wait for an unspecified amount of time. We benefit from knowing in advance how long things may take, when we will be seen, when we will have results or information etc.

Accessing healthcare is easier when predictability is maximised. Healthcare is often by nature chaotic and unpredictable and we can manage this better when things are explained clearly to us and we understand why. Also, this will likely make us feel more included and more like an active participant in our experience as opposed to a passive recipient of a service we have no agency over.

A – Acceptance

'Autism awareness' has been a hot topic for years but this isn't enough and it never was. We need to be accepted for who we are – not deficient neurotypicals but complete and whole Autistic people. It would be so wonderful to see an increase in knowledge of neurodiversity and acceptance of difference across the board in healthcare settings. Autistic people exist in all aspects of society therefore every medical professional in every field will work with and take care of an Autistic person.

Within the identity of being Autistic, we are a heterogeneous group. We are not all the same. It is so valuable to treat everyone as an individual, Autistic people included.

A personal example is my dentist. I hate 'the dentist' with a deep passion, but I like 'my dentist' because he knows I am Autistic, has talked to me about my preferences and has adapted how my appointments go as a result.

C – Communication

We communicate differently as Autistics, whether those of us who speak, those of us who use AAC or those of us who use a blend. Even those of us with fluent and articulate speech may still find communication difficult.

A lot of us benefit from clear and explicit communication. A phrase I like to say in my own practice is 'clarity is kindness' – the clearer you are the less possibility of misinterpretation and the easier the information is to process.

Expectations for us when it comes to communication are also important – we may find it hard to make eye contact, our posture and gestures may look different, and sometimes this can lead to us and our intentions being misunderstood.

The quality of our healthcare will be significantly better when our communication differences are respected and taken into account, and when communication styles are adapted to suit us. And this will have positive implications for our overall health and well-being.

E – Empathy

There is a nasty and pernicious myth that Autistic people lack empathy. This has been a notion in circulation for decades and it has done us so much harm. We may express empathy differently or we may experience it in different intensities to neurotypicals – some of us experiencing hyper-empathy.

As discussed in Section 6.10, Milton's (2012) work on double empathy describes a bidirectional contribution of any communication mismatches between neurotypes. Not having assumptions made about our empathy is important, but so is treating us empathetically and compassionately.

All of these components in the SPACE framework can come to together to make health and social care more accessible and comfortable for Autistic people.

Alongside this is the overarching concept of 'space' – the physical space (i.e., the built environment and the people in it), processing space (i.e., time to digest information or changes) and emotional space (which may actually be time and space to recover from sensory or emotional overload).

Keeping all of this in mind can enable us to adapt our methods of service provision to make it easier for Autistic people to access our service and ensure that we are being person-centred. Ultimately this will have positive effects on the quality and accessibility of health and social care for Autistic people, which will improve outcomes when it comes to physical health, mental health and general well-being.

12.3 Accessibility Considerations for Young People and Caregivers

The process of undertaking an exploration of Autistic identity with a young person and their family essentially involves gathering detailed information about the young person's experiences. This information is gathered from caregivers, school staff, other professionals, and – most importantly – from the young person themselves. When embarking on an identification piece, consideration needs to be given to all aspects of how this information is gathered and what the potential barriers are to it being gathered. Adjustments and adaptations to how information is gathered need to made, depending on the specific needs of the young person and their family, and choices in relation to how this is done should be offered where possible. A safe assumption to make when considering whether any young person may be Autistic is to assume that if a young person is Autistic then at least one of their biological parents (if not both) are Autistic themselves. Their parent may or may not be aware of their own neurodivergence (and it may or may not come up within the process for their young person). Remaining cognisant that there is a strong possibility a parent could be neurodivergent will lead to adjustments, which will be of benefit to all involved.

In approaching the accessibility of the piece, consideration needs to be given to how much stress a young person may experience in engaging with the process. Regardless of their neurotype, it can be highly stressful meeting with a new person in a new place, with there being uncertainty about what will happen while there and what the outcome will be. Having an understanding of the experience for a young person and implementing adjustments and adaptations to reduce any stress for them will not only lead to a richer piece for the young person, it also gives them a positive experience of the process of discovering their neurology. Consideration also needs to be given to the environment that the process will take place in – whether this is carried out using online platforms, in-person or a combination of both. Environments that are accessible to neurotypical people from a sensory perspective can often be inaccessible to Autistic people, e.g., because of certain smells, noises etc. (see Chapter 11 on conducting a sensory audit).

12.3.1 Communication Adjustments

Accessible communication is one of the most important factors in undertaking a neurodiversity affirmative process with a young person and their family. When communication is not accessible, there is a much higher possibility of the information gathered being incorrect or incomplete. Poor communication is also more likely to lead to disengagement and the increased likelihood of an incorrect outcome. It is important for clinicians to keep in mind that when exploring the possibility of a young person having an Autistic identity, the whole piece is a process of information gathering. The quality of the information gathered will depend on how comfortable and accessible it is for those who are providing the information.

In making communication accessible to all, the following are advised:

1. Spend time learning about different communication styles and different methods of communication.

2. Communication methods that meet the principle of universal design are crucial. A choice of different communication options (e.g., written, spoken, AAC, synchronous, asynchronous etc.) should automatically be made available to all who are accessing the service. It should not be dependent on the person asking for a different method and communication methods should not be restricted to just one type for the entirety of the identification process. Depending on the day, energy levels, or topic of discussion, the young person or family may need to be able to access different communication methods to explore various areas of their experience.

3. Clinicians need to be open to the possibility of needing to learn and adapt communication to a style that may not have been offered before.

4. For all sessions, anyone attending the session who is going to be asked to provide information needs to be offered the option of knowing in advance what information they will be asked to provide. If they wish to know in advance, this can be communicated to them via a communication method of their choice.

5. Throughout the process, a collaborative approach to communication needs to be maintained. A young person and their family need to have control and choice in relation to the communication methods used, and clinicians need to ensure that there is predictability and clarity for both caregivers and young people throughout the process. This means welcoming all styles of communication, for example seemingly 'tangential' or non-linear ways of presenting information (see Chapter 4 and the account of how assuming parents / caregivers can communicate in a linear fashion adds to parental stress in the process). Practical examples of offering this control and choice in communication include asking parents / caregivers and children how they would like to be communicated with, whether they prefer email, phone or voice messages, whether they prefer to meet in person or remotely, if they like aural information to be backed up with a written summary afterwards, if they would like to give information written or orally, and if they are ok with multiple emails or possibly would prefer one email a week from one clinician.

The richness and quality of information gathered during an identification process varies based on the communication method used and whether it aligns with the person's needs. Information is likely to be more detailed, accurate and valid if the communication method aligns with that of the person's style, and this will lead to a more accurate outcome of the piece. See the box below for an in-depth SLT perspective on AAC.

PERSPECTIVES OF AN SLT: AUGMENTATIVE AND ALTERNATIVE COMMUNICATION

ELAINE MCGREEVY

Most people use some form of AAC every day. The American Speech-Language-Hearing Association states that 'AAC means all of the ways that someone communicates besides talking' (American

Speech-Language-Hearing Association, n.d.). Unaided AAC refers to modes of communication that do not require additional equipment such as gestures, facial expressions and Makaton / key word signs. Aided AAC includes the use of a tool or device that is external to the individual such as high-tech communication devices and AAC apps, or light tech supports such as pen and paper, a communication book, photos, a core vocabulary board, or a letter board. Donaldson et al. (2023) report that Autistic people preferred to use high-tech AAC tools such as an iPad with an AAC app and light tech communication supports such as picture-based communication over unaided communication supports (e.g., manual sign systems).

There is a paucity of research regarding the experiences of speaking Autistic children who use AAC. Research to date has examined the effectiveness of using AAC with non-speaking and minimally speaking Autistic children's communication. Ganz et al. (2012), Logan et al. (2017) and Holyfield et al. (2017) conclude that using AAC appears to be effective, however most of the studies targeted limited communication functions such as requesting wants and needs within individual therapy settings. It is therefore important that professionals and parents / carers listen to and learn from AAC users to understand more about the experience of being an AAC user, and sources of community support and resources.

Barriers to AAC

Society privileges spoken communication over other forms of communication. SLT practices have often focused on achieving spoken communication as the end goal with speech positioned at the top of the communication pyramid (Morgan & Dipper, 2018). AAC has often been regarded as a last resort when speech does not develop. Donaldson et al. (2023) cite the work of Binger et al. (2021) who found that only 22% of K–12 public school students with no or highly unintelligible speech had been seen by an AAC specialist. Pressure from families and professionals (e.g., SLTs) for the individual to use speech can result in AAC never being considered. Stigma, lack of social acceptability of AAC, ableism and internalised ableism can lead to the individual feeling unsafe or too uncomfortable to use AAC (Donaldson et al., 2023). Other barriers to AAC are a lack of awareness of communication options, and the cost of dedicated AAC devices. Health service provision may limit the offer of AAC options to an individual, e.g., care pathways dictate that light tech options must be used successfully before consideration of a referral for assessment for a high-tech AAC device. Experiences of working with families seeking high-tech AAC for their child indicate that high-tech AAC is not readily accessible. Parents meet barriers when trying to access referrals to specialist services. If the child or young person is provided with an AAC device, there can be lack of ongoing professional support which can lead to abandonment of the device.

12.3.2 Introducing Clinicians and the Process

As outlined above, for various reasons the prospect of undertaking an exploration of Autistic identity with a young person and their family is usually overwhelming for those involved. Even if it is not, it is safest to assume that it is and to universally offer adjustments to the process that benefit everyone. What is essential for some to participate is often beneficial for those who don't need it. One of the most important considerations within the entire process is how to introduce the process to a family. This sets the tone for the entire piece and is the beginning of a collaborative process. It is an opportunity to establish a neuro-affirming foundation for proceeding – one that is respectful, collaborative and affirming to all.

The first step to beginning a process with a young person and their family is to introduce the clinicians they will meet as part of the process. This helps to reduce uncertainty and provides information about what to expect of those who will be involved. The following pieces are helpful to include as part of an introduction to clinicians process:

- Give the names and professions of the clinicians that a young person and their family will meet. Explain what each profession is.

- Provide a photograph of each person, so that a young person and their family can process in advance what each person will look like.

- A short video of each person can be extremely helpful so that a young person and their family can see how clinicians move and sound when they are interacting. Again, this offers an opportunity to process this information in advance and it reduces uncertainty within the process.

- With introductions to clinicians, be mindful about the balance between 'credentials' and being personable. It is important that young people and families have some information about a person's qualifications, however this can also be experienced as intimidating, and it can promote a power imbalance.

- In teams where there is a high turnover of staff, and it is unclear which professionals will be working with each young person, provide a list of possible professionals that the person might meet and make sure there is one key person on the team that will not change for the duration of their piece.

It is important to offer the option of information in advance of a process beginning, should a young person and their family need to know what to expect. This should be offered as an option, as while many will need this information in advance, some may experience this as overwhelming, and therefore having the option to decline the information is also important. When introducing the process, the following are important:

- Information needs to be offered in a range of different communication methods, i.e., written information, voice-recorded information, picture communication etc., with a young person and their family having the option to choose what method works best for them.

- Information needs to be clear and structured. There needs to be clear information about each part of the process – what will happen, who will be involved, where it will take place, what order appointments will be in etc., as well as notes on possible changes that may be encountered.

- Provide photographs or videos of any clinic spaces appointments will take place in, including corridors, waiting areas and the outside of a building. This provides an opportunity for a young person and their family to process the space in advance and it helps to reduce uncertainty.

- Be specific about times of appointments and how long each appointment will last for. If an appointment sometimes runs late, make sure to mention this as a possibility, e.g., 'It is possible that the appointment before yours will run 5–10 minutes late, but you will never be left waiting for longer than 15 minutes without further communication from us.'

While it is helpful to reduce as much uncertainty as possible, it is also important to build in the possibility of uncertainty within the process. Not everything can be controlled, and if a person has not been prepared for the possibility of something not happening according to plan, then this will be much more challenging for them than if they had been prepared for the possibility.

12.3.3 Information in Advance of Each Session

In advance of each session, the option to receive information about what to expect needs to be made available to a young person and their family. It is important that there is an acknowledgement that this information and these adjustments are available to all – including young people and their parents / caregivers also. Advance information should include the following:

- Who will be at the appointment? Photographs and / or videos of clinicians who will be present should be made available, if they have not already been shared.

- What is going to happen at the appointment? Precise information about what will happen at each session needs to be provided. This should include questions that will be asked or areas that will be discussed.

- How long will the session last for? Give specific information about how long the appointment is expected to last for.

It is helpful to also provide information about environmental expectations and adjustments in advance. This should include:

- An acknowledgement that it can be challenging for a young person and / or their caregivers to be in new or unfamiliar environments.

- Information about any sensory aspects of the space that cannot be adjusted, e.g., a bright light that is on a sensor, internal or external noise that cannot be modified etc. This allows a young person and their family the option to bring their own modifications, e.g., sunglasses, ear plugs etc., and they need to be aware that they are welcome to do so. These could also be provided by the service where possible.

- Information on how a young person and their caregivers can use the room and be in the room. This should include:

  - Eye contact is not expected.
  - Everyone is free to move about the room as needed. There is no expectation for anyone to remain seated. Sitting on the floor, on a table etc. is welcome.
  - The room can be explored.
  - There are no expectations around clothing – comfortable clothing (as determined by the individual) is welcome.
  - Preferred items or comfort items can be brought from home.
  - There is no expectation for spoken communication to be the only communication method used. Written communication is welcome, as are other methods of a person's choice. Silence is ok too.
  - Breaks are available as needed.

12.3.4 Remote Sessions

Many aspects of an exploration of Autistic identity with a young person and their family can be carried out remotely, and offering this option where possible alongside the option of in-person appointments increases accessibility for many (Ali et al., 2023). This is particularly the case for those who find environments outside of their own home challenging to access. There can be many reasons as to why accessing environments outside of home may be challenging. It can often be due to the unfamiliarity and unpredictability of outside environments, but it can also be related to long distances between home and clinic spaces (Burke et al., 2015), or it may be related to parent / caregiver work schedules or childcare needs.

Offering the option of remote or in-person sessions where possible can increase the likelihood of engagement with healthcare appointments (Chen et al., 2023). The occurrence of the COVID-19 pandemic brought about an expedited implementation of a secure online infrastructure that is now accessible to services and to most families, and research is showing that this is a helpful option for Autistic people (Dahiya et al., 2020; Sutherland et al., 2018). The technical literacy of both clients and clinicians plays a role in terms of the use of remote options (Triana et al., 2020), and flexibility on the part of the clinician in terms of using different options and platforms can help to address this (Ali et al., 2023).

For many neurodivergent people, the option of a remote appointment may be more comfortable for them as they are in their own familiar space where they can control the sensory aspects of the environment. Remote sessions also reduce travel time and costs. The focus of an exploration of Autistic identity lies in the richness of the information gathered as part of the process, and the richness of the information will depend on how comfortable and accessible a setting or process is for a person. Offering the option of remote sessions and in-person sessions (where possible during a process), with the choice being left to the person and not being determined by the clinician, can yield much richer information which is exponentially more helpful to the overall process.

At the time of writing, current best practice guidelines state that when exploring Autistic identity with a child or young person, it must be the case that clinicians meet in-person with a young person. While most young people can tolerate an in-person meeting with adjustments and adaptations in place and with the option to acquire information in advance about what to expect, there are many young people who even with adjustments in place cannot tolerate such a meeting. The process of an in-person meeting, particularly in a clinic setting, may just be too overwhelming for them and may be traumatic. A neuro-affirmative approach holds that the option of either an in-person session or a remote session should be offered to a young person, but this is against current best practice guidelines. In situations where an in-person meeting (with adjustments and supports in place) has been attempted but is intolerable to a young person, then a best practice process is not possible. The next best option is to carry out a remote process while acknowledging that a best practice process was attempted and not possible. Although this is not a 'best practice' process, taking this approach reduces the likelihood of a potentially traumatic experience for this group of young people and their families, and yields richer information than meeting a very distressed young person in a clinical setting would give.

12.3.5 Gathering Information

As stated throughout this book, a central component to exploring the possibility of Autistic neurology with a young person and their family is the gathering of detailed information about a young person's experiences of the world. In order to ensure that the exploration piece is accessible to young people and their families, there needs to be various different methods and options for gathering information. Giving consideration to different options for communication and information sharing will yield much richer information, which in turn will ensure that the correct outcome is arrived at and the experience of getting there is a positive one.

Information gathered during an exploration process can either be gathered via spoken or non-spoken methods. Spoken methods include face-to-face spoken communication, voice recordings etc., while non-spoken methods include written information, emails, artwork etc. Information can also be provided in a synchronous manner (i.e., with no delay between it being sought and it being provided – such as face-to-face spoken communication) or in an asynchronous manner (i.e., with a delay between it being sought and it being provided – such as questions being emailed in advance and written or spoken answers provided at a later stage). To obtain the most reliable and rich information, it is advised to collaborate with young people and their families as to which methods would work best for them and which would allow them the necessary time to process what is being required of them.

12.3.6 State Your Position

Prior to undertaking an exploratory piece with a young person and their family, whether clinicians are working in the public system or in private practice it is important for them to state their approach in terms of whether they are neurodiversity affirmative or if they follow a medical model approach. This is highly important so that those attending a service can consider whether the approach taken by the service and the values of the service align with theirs. It is also important to be open and upfront in terms of whether a service is gender affirming or not, for similar reasons in terms of whether clinician's values align with those attending the service and whether identities are validated and respected.

Communicating that a service is gender-affirming can happen in various ways. Having non-spoken symbols of gender affirmation, e.g., pride flags on display, posters in clinic spaces, LGBTQIA+ pins on uniforms and symbols within the environment etc., communicates that a space is safe for the LGBTQIA+ community without the need to speak about it. It is also essential to routinely ask young people about their gender identity and their pronouns, and to use these throughout the process in accordance with their wishes.

12.4 Conclusion

In this chapter, we explained the many ways in which you can make the identification process accessible to the children and families you are working with. The barriers to accessing healthcare settings were examined, as were accessibility considerations, communication adjustments, the use of AAC during the identification process, providing information in advance of sessions, undertaking remote sessions and methods of gathering information. We will next look in detail at best practice guidelines, discussing their use and utility in general and then looking specifically at guidelines regarding Autistic identification.

CHAPTER 13

Best Practice Guidelines

13.1 Introduction

In this chapter, we will discuss the benefits and limitations of best practice guidelines, looking then specifically at a selection of guidelines in relation to Autistic identification.

13.2 Best Practice Guidelines

According to Guerra-Farfan et al. (2022), the main benefit of clinical practice guidelines is to ensure that people receive healthcare that is of proven benefit and to discourage interventions and processes that are ineffective or potentially harmful. Guidelines exist in order to ensure that a standard in healthcare is maintained and delivered. They offer consistency and better outcomes for all, they empower the public and they can be helpful in influencing public policy (Woolf et al., 1999). However, it is also widely acknowledged that guidelines have limitations and that up to 50% of guidelines can be considered untrustworthy (Iannone et al., 2017). One of the most significant limitations of guidelines is that they can be wrong for several reasons (Woolf et al., 1999). First, the evidence may be lacking or misleading and those developing the guidelines may not have been able to scrutinise every piece of evidence to ensure its validity. Second, there are value judgements about what to include in guidelines, and these judgements may be wrong and / or influenced by the opinions and clinical experience of the development group. Third, the development group may have competing priorities in developing guidelines, and the needs of the public / person may not be the only priority. Guidelines that are flawed or that are conflicting can encourage ineffective and / or harmful methods, and they can confuse and cause frustration for practitioners. Outdated guidelines can, and do, maintain outdated practices (Woolf et al., 1999).

Although it is important to have best practice guidelines for processes within healthcare, given the limitations and the issues with guidelines, it is critical to consider guidelines as 'guidelines'. Guidelines are not rules, and their purpose is to offer the best advice. They should be reviewed, understood and followed as advice. It is essential that practitioners are aware of the best practice guidelines in terms of 'autism assessments', but it is equally essential that clinicians are aware of the limitations of current guidelines. Guidelines are only reviewed periodically and often do not align with the most up-to-date research or understanding in a given area. They reflect a fixed moment in time, whereas clinical practice should be dynamic and responsive to emerging knowledge and current understanding. Guidelines may offer a standard framework, but clinical reasoning must be invoked to ensure that a 'best practice' process is delivered to each person and family on an individual basis.

13.2.1 Best Practice Guidelines for the Identification of Autistic Neurology

Across the world currently, a number of different 'best practice guidelines' have been issued by various countries and professional bodies in relation to autism assessment with children and adolescents. These include (but are not limited to):

- 'Autism spectrum disorder in under 19's: Recognition, referral and diagnosis', National Institute for Health and Care Excellence (NICE, 2017) (UK).

- 'Autism spectrum disorder in under 19's: Support and management', NICE, (2021) (UK).

- *Professional Practice Guidelines for the Assessment, Formulation, and Diagnosis of Autism in Children and Adolescents* (2nd edition), Psychological Society of Ireland (PSI, 2022) (Ireland).

- *Working with Autism: Best Practice for Psychologists*, British Psychological Society (2021) (UK).

- *Assessment, Diagnosis and Interventions for Autism Spectrum Disorders: A*

National Clinical Guideline, Scottish Intercollegiate Guidelines Network (SIGN, 2016) (Scotland).

- *A National Guideline for the Assessment and Diagnosis of Autism in Australia: Draft Updated Guideline for Public Consultation*, Goodall et al. (2023) (Australia).

- 'Standards of diagnostic assessment for autism spectrum disorder', Canadian Paediatric Society (2019) (Canada).

Best practice guidelines in the USA are issued independently by each state and therefore a full list of the guidelines issued by each state is not listed here for brevity. Those working in the USA should look for the individual guidelines produced for their specific state.

It is sometimes suggested by some opposers of practice underpinned by the Neurodiversity Paradigm that neurodiversity affirmative practice does not align with best practice guidelines. It is also often the case that those who want to adopt a neurodiversity affirmative approach in their work feel that they cannot do so as they believe that it does not align with best practice. Neither of these positions is true, and it is absolutely the case that neurodiversity affirmative practice aligns with current best practice guidelines across the board.

All of the guidelines listed above emphasise the following, all of which are aligned with neurodiversity affirmative practice:

- The central core component of an autism assessment process is a process of gathering information.

- A process needs to focus on a person's strengths as well as what their needs are in terms of support.

- A process involving a young person needs to be child and / or family centred.

- It is crucial to emphasise that currently none of the guidelines listed above specify that standardised assessment tools must be used. They all state that tools may be considered as aids in gathering information, but they do not state that they must be used.

- Most of the guidelines also emphasise that when tools are used, they should not be used solely, and that clinical reasoning is the most important tool that a clinician has at their disposal when undertaking assessments.

These key aspects of gathering information, focusing on strengths as well as needs and being child- and family-centred are core principles of a neurodiversity affirmative approach, and a neurodiversity affirmative approach is therefore very much aligned with best practice guidelines across the world. Crucially, there is scope within all of the best practice guidelines to gather information without the use of standardised assessment tools. This is a key component of a neurodiversity affirmative approach as there currently are no standardised assessment tools that are entirely aligned with neurodiversity affirmative practice, and learning about a person's inner experiences is best done without 'assessment tools'. Again, this very much aligns with best practice guidelines.

Best practice guidelines for autism assessments across different countries and organisations have been reviewed and updated over time. With each revision, there is further advancement towards a more neurodiversity affirmative approach within guidelines, which is welcome but more is needed. The most recent guidelines of those listed above – the Australian draft guidelines that are currently proposed and are undergoing a review process (at the time of publication), are the first to explicitly state that the assessment process should be 'neurodiversity affirming'. This is a very much-needed direction for guidelines to move towards and reflects the shift in current knowledge and the evidence base in relation to understanding Autistic neurology.

13.3 Evaluation of Current 'Diagnostic' Criteria – What Is Helpful and What Is Not

Prior to beginning any exploration of Autistic identity with a young person and their family, it is important to consider the framework within which their experiences are being considered. Particularly with young people, it is too often the case that clinicians rely on 'scores' or outcomes of individual assessment tools to determine whether a young person is Autistic or not, without giving due consideration to authentic Autistic experiences and to classification systems or current criteria. This can particularly be the case for early career clinicians, or those without access to adequate supervision. Currently, there are two internationally recognised classification systems for Autistic identity – the DSM-5-TR and ICD-11. Each of these systems outlines Autistic experiences within the areas of communication, interaction, connections / relationships with others, body movements, sensory experiences, interests / passions, routines etc.

13.3.1 History of Development of Criteria

The identification of Autistic experiences has evolved significantly within society and within formal classification systems (see Section 6.5 and 6.6 for further discussion on 'The notion of "normal"'). Within the development of the DSM classification, 'autism' began to appear within early editions of the DSM in the 1950s and 1960s when it was mentioned within schizophrenia frameworks. It wasn't until 1980 when the DSM-III was published that autism emerged as a separate experience from schizophrenia, and was termed 'infantile autism'. This was later changed in 1987 to 'Autistic disorder' in the DSM-III-TR, and Autistic experiences were described in much more detail than previous editions, and in particularly pathologising ways. In the DSM-IV which was published in 1994, the criteria were broadened, and four sub-categories of Autistic identity were outlined, including Asperger's disorder, pervasive developmental disorder (not otherwise specified), Rett's disorder and childhood disintegrative disorder. In 2013, the DSM-5 was published which removed 'sub-categories' of Autistic identity and outlined one new category titled 'autism spectrum disorder'.

Within the ICD classification system, the process of classifying 'autism' follows a similar trajectory and time frame to that of the DSM. 'Infantile autism' was first mentioned in the ICD-8 in 1967, around the same time as the DSM-II. Again, it was mentioned within the framework of schizophrenia. The ICD-9 which was published in 1977 framed 'infantile autism' within a grouping called 'psychoses with origin specific to childhood' and, similar to the DSM, it was separated into its own category in the ICD-10 in 1993 titled 'pervasive developmental disorders', with 'childhood autism', 'Asperger's syndrome', 'atypical autism', 'Rett's syndrome' and 'pervasive developmental disorder – unspecified' listed. Alongside the DSM, the ICD in 2013 changed their classification of Autistic identity to 'Autistic disorder', and the latest edition of the ICD-11, published in 2019, changed this to 'Autistic spectrum disorder'.

The changing landscape within classification systems has raised significant challenge, debate, uncertainty and confusion within the Autistic community and amongst professionals. Capturing the nuance of Autistic experiences has proved difficult, and for Autistic people it causes instability in their sense of identity if a group of professionals can decide to change the parameters of their identity (see Section 6.3 and 6.4 for further discussion about who contributes to the professional narrative about what being Autistic is). For professionals, it can be challenging to understand the experiences of a person through such lenses, which can simultaneously be both too broad and too narrow in terms of how Autistic experiences are described within classification systems.

There is a dissonance between formal classification systems and the real-world experiences of Autistic people, and many Autistic people and professionals feel that the current classification systems are quite outdated in terms of current understanding of Autistic experiences. Current conversations and debates in relation to classification systems are focused on whether Autistic identity even belongs within a classification system for 'mental disorders' or 'diseases'.

13.3.2 Issues with Current Criteria

Although there has been much work put into devising classification systems that are up to date, the current classification systems relating to Autistic identity are problematic in a number of ways:

- The landscape of understanding Autistic identity is rapidly changing and evolving as more and more is learned about Autistic experiences from the Autistic community. However, with more than a decade passing between each revision of criteria, classification systems are poor at keeping up with current understanding and there isn't capacity within them to reflect the most up-to-date understanding.

- Of significant challenge is the pathologising, medicalised view of Autistic experiences the classification systems adopt. Autistic experiences are framed as deficits, impairments, deficiencies, deviations etc. as opposed to differences and natural variations within experiences. This is hugely problematic as it frames neurotypical experiences as the better way to be, rather than acknowledging that all experiences are valid and that there are natural variations and differences within experiences that are normal, necessary and helpful to the human race.

- Framing Autistic identity as a 'deficiency' or 'disorder' misrepresents to others what being Autistic actually is. It can also be the reason why many Autistic people find it challenging to understand and relate to their Autistic identity, as the description of Autistic experiences provided within the classification systems may not resonate with them.

- Current criteria do not account for the full range of Autistic experiences, and it isn't clear that the experiences outlined within criteria reflect those of various genders and racial identities. There are many Autistic strengths and abilities, as well as aspects of Autistic cultural experiences that are not within current criteria, or that are framed as 'deficits' within the criteria. Autistic communication, connections and experiences related to creativity, empathy, hyperfocus and a strong sense of justice / fairness etc. are not captured in the criteria, or are framed negatively.

- Although they have followed a very similar trajectory and time frame in terms of their classification of Autistic identity, there are some key differences within each of the current versions of the DSM-5-TR and the ICD-11. One of the most significant differences is that the ICD-11 does not specify the amount or combination of characteristics a person must have in order to meet criteria. It is left completely open for it to be decided whether or not a person's experiences fit or not. This is simultaneously helpful and unhelpful. It is helpful in that there is scope to understand a person's experiences individually and to allow for the nuance within their experience. However, it raises many questions and debates as technically a person may meet criteria on the ICD-11, but not the DSM-5-TR, which has significant implications for their sense of identity. The lack of consistency between classification systems is hugely problematic given the Autistic need for certainty, as the very systems that are supposed to define Autistic neurology are unclear about what the definition is which creates uncertainty for many people in terms of their sense of self.

- The existence of classification systems creates a power imbalance between clinicians and the person attending, as the clinician holds the power to 'decide' another person's neurology. This decision may vary depending on the clinician and their perspective (see Section 10.2 for further discussion of the role of power within the process of Autistic identification).

Although it is clear that there are significant challenges and problems with current classification systems, there does need to be some agreed upon definition in order for Autistic identity to be meaningful. This definition needs to reflect current understanding of the broad range of Autistic experiences, it needs to encompass Autistic strengths, abilities and Autistic culture, and bias towards neurotypical experiences needs to be removed.

13.3.3 Using Existing Criteria as Part of a Neuro-Affirmative Process

Although it is clear that there are challenges in relation to current classification systems which outline criteria for the identification of Autistic identity, the current existing criteria need to be used as part of a best practice framework. While the criteria in their current state do not reflect a neurodiversity affirmative perspective on Autistic experiences, when the deficit-focused and pathologising language is removed from the criteria, the areas themselves are helpful in terms of exploring a young person's experiences.

> ## Reflection Point
>
> Re-framing criteria from a pathologising perspective to a neurodiversity affirmative perspective is essential to a neurodiversity affirmative process. Within this process of re-framing, the exact areas of the criteria are kept, but how they are presented and spoken about is re-framed. Rather than describing 'deficits' or 'impairments' when compared to neurotypical neurology, a young person's preferences, experiences and interests are explored and described within each area. A person's experiences can be explored from the perspective of what is comfortable, natural or intuitive for them, and what is not. Discovering the circumstances within which the young person thrives or best engages can give rich information about their neurology. It is important to explore both strengths and abilities in each area as well as what is challenging so that a complete and detailed understanding can be established.

When using existing criteria from a neuro-affirmative perspective, the approach taken is collaborative, exploratory and respectful. Chapter 15 outlines in further detail how collaboration is undertaken with young people at different ages and stages of development. With younger children, the process involves learning about their experiences of the world through their preferences in relation to play, how they communicate and how they appear to regulate their sensory system. Older children and young people may be able to share their own insights into their experience of the world, again through various communication methods (spoken and non-spoken) and through their interests and preferences. Those who know a young person well (i.e., their parents / caregivers, teachers, other professionals etc.) may also be able to add to a young person's own insights about their experiences.

Although it is possible to work neurodiversity affirmatively with current criteria through a process of re-framing the criteria, this is not an ideal process. This is a process of working with an existing flawed framework, and trying to make it more respectful and neurodiversity affirmative. Rather than re-framing an unsuitable, pathologising set of criteria, what is really needed is a new set of criteria that are developed from a neurodiversity affirmative framework from the beginning. Neurodiversity affirmative criteria that reflect Autistic identity would remove all pathologising language describing Autistic experiences, it would encompass Autistic strengths and abilities as well as differences experienced and it would be informed by Autistic culture.

13.4 Conclusion

In this chapter, we discussed the benefits and limitations of best practice guidelines, looking then specifically at a selection of guidelines in relation to Autistic identification. We also examined how we can use these guidelines to inform a neurodiversity affirmative identification piece with children. We will next look in depth at some of the main assessment tools currently in use in relation to assessing for Autistic neurology.

CHAPTER 14

A Neurodiversity Affirmative Perspective on Autistic Neurology Assessment Tools

14.1 Introduction

Advocates of the Neurodiversity Paradigm critique mainstream Autistic assessment tools for children on several fronts. They argue that these tools often rely on a deficit-based approach, pathologise neurological differences, and prioritise a normative agenda rather than considering the perspectives and experiences of Autistic people (Leadbitter et al., 2021; Yu & Sterponi, 2023). Advocates emphasise the need to shift the focus of assessment from individual skills to interactional experiences and to recognise and value social communicative competencies that may be dismissed as pathologies (Acevedo & Nusbaum, 2020). The Neurodiversity Paradigm calls for a re-framing of effectiveness in interventions, measurement of Autistic prioritised outcomes, and partnerships with Autistic people in research and practice (Rutherford & Johnston, 2023). As described in Chapter 5, it also challenges the notion of being Autistic as a disorder that needs to be fixed or cured, advocating instead for acceptance and support of Autistic individuals' differences (Richman, 2020).

In this chapter, we take a broad look at current assessment tools and the significant issues with them. We also look at screening tools, questionnaires that we have found helpful to the identification process and a possible pathway forward in relation to assessment tools in this area.

14.2 Issues with Current Assessment Tools

14.2.1 Pathologising Autistic Neurology: A Missed Neurodiversity Perspective in Traditional Assessment Tools

The Neurodiversity Paradigm, which is a perspective that advocates for the acceptance of neurological variations as standard and the beneficial aspects of human diversity, posits that Autistic neurology should be viewed as a variant of neural development rather than a disorder that requires correction or remediation (Chapman, 2021). However, it is worth noting that many of the prevalent assessment tools used to evaluate Autistic neurology indirectly treat it as a pathology, thereby deviating from the expected 'norm' (Kapp et al., 2019). These assessment tools primarily focus on the identification of 'deficits' and 'impairments', thereby perpetuating a model that pathologises Autistic neurology and directly contradicting the neurodiversity standpoint, which advocates for an approach that emphasises individuals' strengths and abilities. Most of the assessment tools currently available are measures of how much a person fails at being neurotypical, as opposed to how much their experiences align with Autistic experiences and how much they thrive as an Autistic. As Woods and Estes (2023) highlight, most questionnaires, observational tools and interview questions focus on 'problems' to determine if a person is Autistic or not, and they miss a comprehensive overview of what it means to be Autistic.

14.2.2 The Issue of Rigid Assessment Tools

Multiple evaluation instruments designed for the study of Autistic neurology employ strict standards that lack the necessary adaptability. This inflexibility fails to adequately encompass the full range of Autistic behaviours, especially among those who do not conform to traditional Autistic stereotypes. Consequently, certain groups, such as Autistic people who were assigned female at birth, gender divergent individuals, and those from diverse cultural backgrounds, often face either under recognition or misidentification, primarily due to a bias towards the typical presentations observed in white males (Begeer et al., 2009; Cruz et al., 2024). There exists a limited conceptualisation of who Autistic people are, i.e., an incorrect assumption that those who are Autistic are typically male and white (Botha et al., 2020) which has contributed to under-identification in other minority groups, including people of colour (Tromans et al., 2021) and women (Hull et al., 2020). Please see Section 10.5 for further discussion on intersectionality.

14.2.3 Discrepancies in the Interpretation of Results

The potential interpretation discrepancies in the results obtained from conventional Autistic neurology assessment tools can be attributed to the reliance on the examiner's knowledge and expertise. This heavy reliance on the examiner's understanding of Autistic experiences can often lead to inconsistencies in how the results are interpreted. These discrepancies, as highlighted by Gotham et al. (2015), can be problematic as they introduce a level of subjectivity into the process, potentially undermining the validity and reliability of the assessment. Furthermore, the presence of normative bias issues further complicates the interpretation of results. The examiner's personal biases and preconceived notions regarding Autistic neurology can inadvertently influence their interpretation, resulting in an inaccurate representation of the person being assessed. Therefore, it is crucial to address these interpretation discrepancies and normative bias issues to ensure a more objective and comprehensive understanding of the results obtained from Autistic neurology assessment tools.

Bishop and Lord (2023), two co-authors of the ADOS-2, discussed the intended role for standardised tools in the exploration of Autistic identity. They highlighted that the apparent requirement for certain tools to be used in an identification process has resulted in a large number of professionals being technically trained in the use of specific instruments, but without the broader training in assessment and in understanding Autistic experiences. Bishop and Lord (2023) stated that there are a large number of clinicians who have technical training in the use of specific tools, but who lack understanding and experience of other neurotypes, and the possibility of differential explanations for apparent Autistic experiences. They emphasise the importance of professional ethics codes which state that professionals must work within their competency, including only making identifications they are trained to make (Bishop & Lord, 2023). Where there is a lack of clinical expertise in Autistic experiences and co-occurring conditions, no tool or combination of tools will make up for this (Bishop & Lord, 2023). This needs to be carefully considered in terms of whether such 'gold standard' tools are being used appropriately and the strong likelihood that the outcome is invalid and unreliable if administered by a clinician without the necessary experience.

14.2.4 Limited Scope of Assessment Tools

Predominantly, the evaluation tools designed to assess Autistic neurology tend to prioritise the assessment of communication and social interaction skills, typically viewing them through a neurotypical lens. However, this approach of assessing these skills, where neurotypical styles of communication serve as the gold standard and any deviation from that is considered inferior, poses significant problems and deviates from the principles of scientific objectivity. It fails to acknowledge the importance of other crucial aspects such as sensory perceptual differences, the distinctive developmental trajectory of Autistic children and young people, their cognitive styles like monotropism, self-regulatory actions such as stimming, the role of the environment in shaping their experiences, Autistic-specific communication styles, as well as their unique interests and talents. By solely focusing on communication and social interaction, we overlook the rich tapestry of experiences and abilities that Autistic children and young people possess, thus limiting our understanding of their true potential and the diversity within the Autistic community (American Psychiatric Association, 2022).

14.2.5 Constraints in Age and Cognitive Level Adaptability

Traditional assessment tools used for evaluating Autistic neurology often face challenges when it comes to adapting to various age groups and cognitive abilities, as noted by Bal et al. (2016). These limitations hinder the effective utilisation of these tools, particularly with very young children or individuals who are non-speaking. Furthermore, individuals with co-occurring intellectual disabilities or speech apraxia also face difficulties in utilising these assessment tools. As a result, the current applicability of these traditional assessment methods is compromised, necessitating the development of more adaptable and inclusive alternatives.

Bishop and Lord (2023), who co-developed (amongst others) the ADOS-2, highlight that many standardised assessment tools were not standardised with a range of different populations. As a result, clinicians in the field need to explore and establish ways to hold on to best practice processes for identifying Autistic neurology, which includes comprehensive methods for collecting information, while also being able to be flexible. This is especially the case when working with populations that were either excluded from or under-represented in the validation samples for any particular instrument (Bishop & Lord, 2023).

14.2.6 Overlooked Personal Experiences

Most conventional methods of assessment heavily rely on behavioural observations and third-party reporting, often neglecting to give due consideration to the subjective experiences of Autistic individuals (Milton, 2012). This prevailing approach may inadvertently hinder the tools' ability to fully comprehend and adequately represent the personal, lived experiences of Autistic children.

The common practice of utilising traditional assessment tools, which are widely employed to evaluate individuals for Autistic neurology, predominantly revolves around behavioural observations and the reliance on others to report on their behalf. However, these tools often fail to acknowledge the significance of incorporating the subjective experiences of a child into the assessment process. By solely focusing on external observations and depending on third-party reporting, these assessment methods may inadvertently undermine their potential to genuinely grasp and aptly capture the unique and personal lived experiences of Autistic children. Consequently, there exists a pressing need to devise assessment methods that not only consider behavioural aspects but also prioritise the subjective experiences and perspectives of Autistic people, thereby facilitating a more comprehensive and holistic understanding of their distinct challenges and strengths.

14.2.7 'Test Scores' as Barriers to Accessing Services

It is increasingly becoming common practice that a young person's score on an assessment tool, or indeed whether particular standardised tools have been used at all, is being used by services to determine access to their service. This is hugely problematic and unethical, and requiring the use of specific tools, without exception, is discriminatory and damaging (Bishop & Lord, 2023). Bishop and Lord (2023) highlight the problems associated with using standardised instruments as 'gatekeepers' for access to services, where young people must reach a certain score in order to be given access. They emphasise that such thresholds will never be capable of yielding perfect sensitivity or specificity values, and there will always be Autistic young people who don't reach a formal 'threshold' or score on a standardised measure (Bishop & Lord, 2023). Bishop and Lord (2023) also describe how standardised measures were designed to ensure that relevant information is available in making clinical decisions, and that such measures were never meant to be used to determine access to services, or as standalone tools.

It is apparent that many services have evolved to focus too much on scores on certain tools, and too little on what is gained from the actual administration and clinical reasoning involved in the use of such tools (Bishop & Lord, 2023). Using standardised tools in isolation goes against best practice processes (Bishop & Lord, 2023) and is much more likely to yield an incorrect and unreliable outcome. Prioritising and emphasising the identification process itself will better serve Autistic young people and their families and will give a more reliable outcome. Individual clinicians have a responsibility to ensure that they are appropriately using any tool they choose to use, and it is inappropriate, unethical and discriminatory for services to force clinicians to behave unethically or to practice outside of their scope (Bishop & Lord, 2023). Bishop and Lord (2023) point out that it is clinical judgement, rather than tools per se, that should be used in the 'assessment' process.

14.3 Screening Tools

There is no single measure that will identify all children who are likely to be Autistic (Wieckowski et al., 2023) and due to the complexity of 'screening', it is likely to be impossible to adequately screen very young children, i.e., those aged 18–24 months (Sturner et al., 2017; Toh et al., 2017). The heterogeneity of Autistic experiences also makes accurate screening very challenging (Lee et al., 2023). Screening tools can sometimes be helpful in identifying the possibility that a young person may be Autistic, but they need to be used with a high level of caution. Screening tools can yield high levels of incorrect results and are also poor at detecting possible Autistic neurology within those with sensory differences and / or intellectual disabilities (de Vaan et al., 2016). They are also not definitive and a person's 'rating' on a screening tool can change over time, which highlights the need to view 'screening' as a dynamic and continuous process (Sturner et al., 2022) rather than a one-off occurrence.

When a clinician considers that a young person may be Autistic, and they wish to take this further to establish whether further formal exploration and possible identification is warranted, using a screening tool is often the first step in the process. This is often the first formal introduction a young person and their parents / caregivers may have to Autistic experiences, and the way that this is presented will set the tone for how Autistic neurology is understood. The lens a screening tool takes and the language used within it contribute to the foundational understanding parents / caregivers and young people may gain of Autistic neurology. If the lens and the language are deficit-focused and pathologising, this communicates to a young person and their family that being Autistic is an impairment and something that is undesirable. Using a formal screening tool with a family therefore needs to be carefully considered in terms of what it may represent to that family, and if it is deficit-focused, then it is not going to be helpful in cultivating a positive Autistic identity in Autistic young people.

Below is further exploration of a sample of screening measures that are commonly used. This is not intended to be an exhaustive list, and other screening measures are available. It is advised that a critical appraisal of any screening measure is adopted before use, in relation to its suitability as a neuro-affirmative measure.

14.3.1 The Modified Checklist for Autism in Toddlers, Revised (M-CHAT-R)

The M-CHAT-R (Robins et al., 1999) is a 20-item questionnaire for parents and / or caregivers about their child's behaviour. The M-CHAT-R is intended for children aged between 16 and 30 months, and relies on parental observations of their child's experiences of the world. While the M-CHAT-R has been shown to have statistically acceptable reliability, sensitivity and specificity (Robins et al., 2014), there has been considerable variability in the methods used to examine its psychometric properties (Yuen et al., 2018). Furthermore, the assessment of contextual factors, e.g., the rigor of false-negative case identification strategies, has been limited (Wieckowski et al., 2023). There is, therefore, a lack of consensus about the screening properties of the M-CHAT-R (Wieckowski et al., 2023). A recent study examining the psychometric properties of the M-CHAT-R indicated that the M-CHAT-R frequently resulted in false positives and false negatives, with just over half (57.7%) who scored positively on the M-CHAT-R going on to be identified as Autistic, and almost a quarter of those who scored negatively proceeding to be identified as Autistic (Aishworiya et al., 2023). This highlights how the M-CHAT-R is a screening tool with limitations, and clinical judgement and a more comprehensive exploration of Autistic identity are needed.

14.3.2 The Social Communication Questionnaire (SCQ)

The SCQ (Rutter, Bailey et al., 2003) is a 40-item rating scale completed by parents and / or caregivers about a young person's reciprocal social interaction, language / communication, and behaviours. The SCQ is standardised for children aged 4 years and above and has been widely used in clinical settings to support decision-making in relation to referrals. However, studies examining the validity of the SCQ have yielded mixed results (Lee et al., 2023), with low sensitivity, specificity and utility within certain clinical settings having been found by many studies (e.g., Corsello et al., 2007; Hollocks et al., 2019). In a review of the literature, Lee et al. (2023) concluded that individual differences amongst young people, e.g., cognitive ability, language ability, co-occurring conditions and differences in behaviour appear to impact the effectiveness of the SCQ. Lee et al. (2023) also noted that the referral source and parental / caregiver understanding of Autistic experiences also impact on the outcome of the SCQ.

14.3.3 The Social Responsiveness Scale, 2nd Edition (SRS-2)

The SRS-2 (Constantino & Gruber, 2012) is a 65-item rating scale which measures social characteristics associated with autism in both children and adults. There is also an abbreviated version of the SRS-2 available which is a 16-item measure (Sturm et al., 2017). Multiple raters who have known the person for at least one month can complete the scale, and the adult version also has a self-report form. For children and young people, the SRS-2 is an observation-based measure and relies on third-party observations of a person's experiences of the world (Bruni, 2014). Although the SRS-2 has been shown to have acceptable psychometric properties (Moody et al., 2017), many items on the SRS-2 have been shown to be vulnerable to non-autistic related factors (Frazier et al., 2014; Sturm et al., 2017), including ADHD (Constantino & Gruber, 2012; Reiersen et al., 2007). Those with common co-occurring conditions have been shown to not score as high on the SRS-2 as those without (Constantino & Frazier, 2013), and those who receive high SRS-2 scores may include those who are Autistic and those who struggle with behavioural differences (Hus et al., 2013). The influence of several different factors, including behavioural differences, age, expressive language and cognitive level needs to be considered when using the SRS-2 (Hus et al., 2013).

14.4 Assessment Tools

The primary focus of a comprehensive process of exploring Autistic identity is to accurately identify whether a young person is Autistic or not. Further goals of carrying out a detailed exploration also include identifying the possibility of co-occurring conditions, exploring and uncovering strengths, and identifying areas for support. A range of different 'assessment tools' have been designed with the goal of aiding exploration of Autistic identity. The original intent of developing assessment tools was to formalise the procedures through which clinicians and researchers gather information about Autistic experiences (Bishop & Lord, 2023), however the context within which Autistic experiences are 'assessed' using standardised instruments will drastically impact the information obtained (Lord et al., 1999). Children and young people behave differently, depending on the context they are in (Bishop & Lord, 2023), and therefore the reliability of the information gathered via the use of a standardised instrument needs to be considered when using them as part of an exploration process.

The use of standardised assessment tools in the exploration of Autistic identity has evolved over time, and they have become synonymous with what is considered the so-called 'gold standard' in the identification of autism. However, many researchers are now stressing the over-reliance on such instruments in clinical practice and in research (Freudenstein et al., 2020). Bishop and Lord (2023) highlight the negative outcome of misidentification resulting from the inappropriate use of standardised instruments, and that this has been repeatedly emphasised by clinicians, researchers and Autistic people and their families as being a major challenge in this field currently. Assessment tools tend to lack transparency, do not recognise context, do not consider emotion, fail to recognise differences in interpretation and also foster power imbalances within a process (Timimi et al., 2019). Best practice guidelines do not state that standardised tools must be used (see Chapter 13 for further discussion of best practice guidelines), but that they can be used to support the information-gathering process if needed. In line with best practice guidelines, and with a neurodiversity affirmative process, a bespoke and flexible approach to information gathering that is structured and clear is needed.

Below is further exploration of a sample of assessment tools that are commonly used. This is not intended to be an exhaustive list, and other assessment tools are available. It is advised that a critical appraisal of any tool is adopted before use, in relation to its suitability as a neuro-affirmative measure.

14.4.1 Autism Diagnostic Interview-Revised (ADI-R)

The ADI-R (Lord et al., 1994) is a structured interview designed to be administered by an experienced clinician. It consists of 93 items or interview questions posed to a parent or caregiver, which evaluate a person's current and historical experiences across different domains associated with Autistic experiences. The ADI-R takes approximately 1.5–2.5 hours to administer and can be used with both children and adults.

The ADI-R was originally devised in accordance with DSM-IV-TR and ICD-10 criteria. It has shown variability in terms of sensitivity and specificity (Lebersfeld et al., 2021) and it has been suggested that it is most accurate when used in research studies as opposed to in clinical practice (Yu et al., 2024). As a standardised instrument, the ADI-R has several issues. Notwithstanding the deficit-based language contained within it, one of the biggest issues the ADI-R faces is retrospective recall bias, which increases the older the person is that the ADI-R is focused on. Information gathered via the ADI-R may also be impacted by the inaccurate memory of parents and / or caregivers, particularly if a parent / caregiver did not notice any differences in a child's experiences when they were younger (Havdahl et al., 2017). Information about a person's early developmental history and experiences may play a lesser role in an identification process than their current experiences, particularly for older adolescents (Kamp-Becker et al., 2021). This issue is evident in the low agreement that has been found between Autistic identification based on the ADI-R (thus with a focus on early life experiences) and that based on the ADOS, particularly as children get older or if they don't present typically (Le Couteur et al., 2008). Kamp-Becker et al. (2021) highlighted that instruments that are based on what is understood about Autistic experiences in childhood are likely to not be as sensitive to experiences relative to identification in older people.

14.4.2 Autism Diagnostic Observation Schedule, 2nd Edition (ADOS-2)

The ADOS-2 (Lord, Rutter et al., 2012; Lord, Luyster et al., 2012) is a tool designed to assess characteristics of Autistic experiences through a series of activities. It is designed to be administered by trained clinicians, and aims to provide an opportunity for characteristics to be observed by others in a consistent manner. The ADOS-2 is a lifespan tool that can be used from the age of 12 months up until adulthood, and takes 30–60 minutes to administer.

It has not been validated for use with deaf or blind people, or those with intellectual disabilities or motor differences, i.e., those who use a wheelchair (Lord, Rutter et al., 2012; Lord, Luyster et al., 2012; Bishop & Lord, 2023). The ADOS-2 has several different modules, with the appropriate module being selected by the clinician based on a person's language ability and age.

There are several limitations of the ADOS-2, many of which have been outlined by the authors themselves. The first issue is that the time to administer the ADOS-2 is a very short period within which to observe certain behaviours or experiences, many of which are challenging to elicit in such a short session (Bishop & Lord, 2023). These include, for example, sensory interests and a person's experience of friendships and relationships. Related to this point is that the tool itself is an observational tool, which therefore relies on a rater's observations of another person to determine the presence or absence of Autistic experiences. This fails to recognise the importance of inner experiences and the fact that these can differ significantly from outwardly observable experiences, which may be explained by masking or by the fact that assessment tools rely on stereotypical expectations of what an Autistic person might 'look like' (Pearson & Rose, 2021). Indeed, several studies have shown a difference between the self-reported internal characteristics experienced by Autistic people and how the same person appears to others (as assessed using tools such as the ADOS-2) (Lai et al., 2017; Lai, Lombardo et al., 2019). Pearson and Rose (2021) suggest that the reason for this dissonance lies with how a person is conceptualised and operationalised by the measurement tool, and that such tools have been developed based on non-autistic ideas of what appropriate social behaviour looks like. Therefore, judging how Autistic a person appears to be based on how well they are able to perform non-autistic behaviours doesn't make sense (Pearson & Rose, 2021) and it needs to be acknowledged that Autistic people present in many different ways. Standardised measures, such as the ADOS-2, are limited in their capacity to capture this (Pearson & Rose, 2021).

The authors of the ADOS-2 have themselves highlighted the limitations of the ADOS-2 in detecting Autistic people in all instances, and in failing to identify some Autistic people (Bishop & Lord, 2023). When the ADOS was initially developed, during the standardisation process it was administered by clinicians with extensive training in autism. This is reflected in the validity data, which were collected by experienced and research-reliable examiners, and which show high levels of sensitivity and specificity (Bishop & Lord, 2023). However, when the ADOS-2 is administered in regular clinical practice, it is often not being administered by those with adequate training and knowledge of Autistic experiences and in co-occurring conditions, which limits its reliability. Furthermore, according to Bishop and Lord (2023), the thresholds of the ADOS-2 are not capable of yielding perfect sensitivity and specificity, even when administered by experienced clinicians. The ADOS-2 will always miss some people or suggest that others are Autistic when they are not and something else (e.g., a psychiatric or medical explanation) may better explain their experiences (Elias & Lord, 2022; Klaiman et al., 2024). The likelihood of misidentification using the ADOS-2 was also highlighted by Freudenstein et al. (2020) who sought to compare the classification of autism using the ADOS-2 and the DSM-5 among 8–10-year-olds. They found significant disparity between the ADOS-2 classification and DSM-5 identification of autism, and found that age, additional 'diagnoses' and over-reliance on observation may bias the ADOS-2 classification. Similar to the ADI-R, research has shown that the ADOS-2 shows higher levels of accuracy within research contexts than within clinical practice (Lebersfeld et al., 2021).

Understanding of Autistic neurology has progressed significantly since the ADOS-2 was developed, and there are many aspects of Autistic experiences that are either not reflected in the ADOS-2 or that are understood through a pathologising lens. The ADOS-2 has been criticised for the deficit-focused language it uses, its portrayal of Autistic experiences through a medical model lens, and for the processes involved in its administration that leave the person feeling as though they have been manipulated (Timimi et al., 2019). The ADOS-2 does not align with a neurodiversity affirmative approach or with the preferences of the Autistic community (Curnow et al., 2023).

14.4.3 Childhood Autism Rating Scale-2 (CARS-2)

The CARS-2 (Schopler et al., 2010) is a rating scale for clinicians that consists of 15 items that cover a range of different areas, including social, emotional, adaptive, communication and cognitive functioning. Ratings are based on a clinician's observations of a child across different settings. The CARS-2 was originally developed based on the DSM-III. Its sensitivity and specificity have been shown to be mixed, with acceptable levels in some studies (e.g., Dawkins et al., 2016), but with reduced specificity shown in others (e.g., Moon et al., 2019).

From a neuro-affirmative perspective, there are two main issues with the CARS-2. The first issue is that the CARS-2 is based primarily on a clinician's observations of another person, and ignores the inner experience of that person, which may differ from what is observable on the outside. This is an issue that is shared with most assessment tools currently available. The other issue is the pathologising language that permeates the entire measure. The CARS-2 uses terminology such as 'symptoms', 'impairments', 'abnormal', 'strange', 'bizarre', 'peculiar' etc., which set a child up to be pathologised and also go against the narrative of a positive self-identity.

14.4.4 Monteiro Interview Guidelines for Diagnosing the Autism Spectrum 2nd Edition (MIGDAS-2)

The MIGDAS-2 (Monteiro & Stegall, 2018) is a strengths- and sensory-based schedule that is designed to gather and organise information needed to explore Autistic identity. The MIGDAS-2 can be used with all age ranges and takes approximately 60–90 minutes to administer. It provides a system for gathering distinctive examples of Autistic experiences through the use of sensory materials and encouraging discussion of areas of high interest to the person. The process invites a person to share their worldview through an entry point of preferred topics and sensory materials, and is designed to be adapted to each individual person. The MIGDAS-2 allows for the integration of multiple sources of information, and it facilitates the exploration of co-occurring conditions. The aim of the process is to support children, adolescents and adults to create an individualised understanding of their Autistic neurology. It can be administered both remotely and in-person.

Very little research exists in relation to the clinical use of the MIGDAS-2. The exploratory, supposedly strengths-based, narrative approach that it takes is aligned with a neurodiversity affirmative approach to exploring Autistic identity, and it is an improvement on tools which came before it. However, the language of 'disorder' and 'diagnosis' is still utilised. In addition, the framing of differences is often from the lens of neurotypical ways of being as the 'gold standard'. For example, in looking at template reports provided with the MIGDAS-2, a strength is noted to be a range of facial expressions that are easily recognisable, while speech is described as having an 'excessive' quantity when talking about a preferred topic of interest. This framing is not aligned with a neuro-affirmative approach. Further research in relation to Autistic young people's and adults' experiences of the MIGDAS-2 is needed.

14.5 Helpful Questionnaires

There are a number of questionnaires relating to Autistic experiences that are helpful to include in the exploration of Autistic identity. It must be stressed that these questionnaires assist in the exploration process, and are not definitive in terms of any outcome.

14.5.1 Monotropism Questionnaire (MQ)

The MQ (Garau, Woods et al., 2023) is a self-report measure exploring a monotropic cognitive style amongst those aged over 16 years. The MQ aims to capture different aspects of monotropic cognition, including a person's interests, routines, attention focus and social interactions. Early research indicators suggest that the MQ has good psychometric properties and that both Autistic and ADHD neurotypes were associated with higher mean monotropism scores (Garau, Murray et al., 2023). Further research is required in relation to this questionnaire across different groups.

14.5.2 Camouflaging Autistic Traits Questionnaire (CAT-Q)

The CAT-Q (Hull et al., 2019) is a 25-item measure of social camouflaging behaviours (i.e., strategies to compensate for or mask Autistic characteristics during social interactions). It is a self-report measure, designed for use with those aged over 16 years. The CAT-Q measures camouflaging generally as well as three sub-categories of camouflaging, including compensation (i.e., strategies used to actively compensate for difficulties experienced in social situations), masking (i.e., strategies used to hide Autistic traits and to portray a non-autistic experience), and assimilation (i.e., strategies used to try to fit in with others socially). The CAT-Q has been found to be a valid and reliable self-report measure of social camouflaging behaviours across both research and clinical settings (Hull et al., 2019; Lundin Remnélius & Bölte, 2023).

14.5.3 Survey of Autistic Strengths, Skills and Interests (SASSI)

The SASSI (Woods & Estes, 2023) is a set of questions that can be integrated into an identification process to explore and identify common Autistic strengths. With versions available for use with adults and with children, it is a recently developed tool which taps into Autistic strengths and experiences, including a strong sense of social justice, Autistic communication styles, connecting with neurodivergent others, interests, hyperfocus, systems, routines, physical movement, sensory, play, cognition and connecting with animals. Although this tool requires further research and development, it is a welcome measure that provides an opportunity to highlight strengths-based information within an identification process. This serves to counter the stigmatising messages within society about Autistic people, which are also harmfully promoted by other assessment tools and questionnaires.

14.5.4 First-Hand Account of Experience of Pathologising Assessment Tools

Below is a first-hand account from a young person who attended a pathologising assessment process.

CHILD'S VOICE

EMMA, AGE 17

- Before you went for your assessment, do you remember how you were feeling about it?

  I was hopeful and kind of excited. I like learning more about myself.

- Was there anything the service you went to did to make it easier for you to go to meet with them?

  NO. We went to a community centre that was noisy and full of children, in a small room that was right to next to the community centre coffee shop. They moved me halfway through into a bigger room away from the noise but then there were children banging on the metal industrial shutters on floor to ceiling windows. I had very little privacy.

- Were you given any information about what to expect during the process? If you were given information, did it help? If you weren't given any information, would it have helped if you did have information on what to expect?

No, if I was given the information I would not have gone, and saved money and time.

- What happened when you met the person who did your assessment with you? Did they explain who they were or what would happen? Did you talk with them, or do activities or both?

They did not introduce themselves. My mam had to get them to introduce themselves. I felt like a product on a conveyor belt. They went straight into the actual assessment, as in they didn't ask me anything beforehand.

- What activities did you do as part of your assessment?

The frogs flying on lily pad, they asked me to pretend to brush my teeth which was odd. I don't know how that relates to autism. I had to make up a story with little trinkets.

I don't remember all of it because I feel like I've repressed it.

- How did it feel doing the activities you did? Were they comfortable? Were they enjoyable? Did you learn anything about yourself by doing them?

I felt infantilised. I was told that this was the adult assessment and I still felt like I was being treated like a 5-year-old.

- How did you learn about the outcome of the assessment? Did the person who did your assessment explain anything to you about it?

NO. They told me what to do but that was it.

- How did you feel when you learned about the outcome of your assessment?

Devastated. They told me I wasn't Autistic, and she said to my mam 'she doesn't look Autistic'. That's crazy to hear from a medical professional. They told my parents and not me directly. It felt like everything I had known about myself was just a lie.

I looked at the email, held back tears and proceeded to cry for five hours straight.

- Did you feel as though you learned anything about yourself in your assessment?

  It felt like everything I had known about myself was a lie. I quickly pieced together that the doctor is not the be all and end all.

- Did you feel as though you were included in your assessment piece?

  No. It was very impersonal. They just did the stuff, no asking me about my life.

- What did you think about your report? Is it helpful? Does it explain you?

  At first I thought, 'Oh my god this is it', then I realised it's not me and it doesn't tell me who I am. There were a lot of recommendations for my sensory issues but there were no questions to me about this and my mam mentioned it in passing as she was leaving the parent meeting. The report was clearly cut and pasted as someone else's name was in it.

- For any other child who is coming for the type of assessment you had, how would you describe to them what they should expect?

  Don't have high expectations, don't expect a lot from them. It needs to be more personal and they need to ask you what are you doing, how are you experiencing things, what's daily life like for you. Think critically about it. If it feels silly it probably is. Don't be afraid to ask questions.

- Do you think there would have been a better way to do the assessment you had?

  No I genuinely believe this needs to be replaced with something entirely different.

Reflection Point

If you experience discomfort when reflecting on previous, or current, deficit-based approaches to identification, we urge you to remember that we do things for good reasons – knowledge changes, we did the best that we could with what we knew at the time. Sitting with the discomfort may help you find your good reason for shifting your practice.

See the box below for an occupational therapist's perspective on the use of standardised assessment measures.

PERSPECTIVES OF AN OT: STANDARDISED ASSESSMENT TOOLS

KATIE KERLEY

I know for me, assessment used to be a standardised process – especially when using standardised assessment tools. But over time with experience and reflection, I have realised that this 'one-size-fits-all' approach doesn't necessarily work, and often does not suit our Neurodivergent clients. I know over time, I and many other neurodiversity affirmative clinicians have moved away from standardised assessment, or at least moved away from only or primarily using standardised assessment tools. I always feel no human can be fairly represented in only numerical data, and we are in a privileged position to get to explore so much more with our clients than just what a standardised assessment tool will tell us. We also have to wonder if standardised neurodiversity affirmative assessment tools actually exist. Some occupational therapy assessment tools can be neurodiversity affirmative, but many may require you to adapt the language and wording. Some examples of this are sensory processing assessments in which sensory experiences are categorised as 'dysfunction' or as 'moderate', 'severe' 'typical' as opposed to just being identified as they are. I have also, over the years, moved away from using a lot of these tools in their standardised form. For example, I feel confident enough in my clinical reasoning, my understanding of sensory processing and my ability to explore this with a person to not rely on standardised assessments or to use some standardised questionnaires as the basis for a semi-structured interview.

With younger children and young people who don't flourish with interviews, I can get this information through play and observations.

I personally like some of the MOHO (Model of Human Occupation) assessments that allow a person to self-identify areas of their life in which they think they struggle and then to further identify whether this is important to them or not, the idea being that if that they are not important then we don't need to pursue them. This is true in the OSA (Occupational Self Assessment) and the COSA (Child Occupational Self Assessment).

My personal opinion is that most people who can read an assessment manual or who watch assessment manual training videos can administer a standardised assessment, but this is not where our skillset lies or where we see a whole person for who they are. The X factor that clinicians bring to assessment is our clinical reasoning skills, our ability to explore a person's life experiences and to make a bigger picture with the information we get.

I think it's important we focus on evidence-based practice yes, but more so than that we need to incorporate life experience. There is a move towards lived experience-informed practice.

This is the narrative and story of the individual so anecdotes do matter here. I often find that we get into 'flow' so much better when the process is less formal, and our clients feel comfortable and even a little relaxed (if possible). We can adapt both the environment and the process, and it is important that we do. It is ok to adapt assessment tools to suit your client's comfort levels. The end result is based on your clinical reasoning and your client's lived experience. Standardised assessment tools are one way to get information but not the only way, and often not the best way.

14.6 The Pathway Forward

Traditional assessment tools often do not meet the necessary standards when viewed through the lens of neurodiversity. There are several crucial areas in which these tools fall short including that they are pathologising and deficit-focused, making it imperative for the field to prioritise the development and implementation of assessment and identification tools that align with neurodiversity principles. In the absence of a fully neurodiversity affirmative standardised assessment tool, it is possible within current best practice guidelines to complete an exploration of Autistic identity without using a standardised measure. When developing neurodiversity affirmative assessment tools, these new tools should focus on highlighting the unique strengths of individuals, encompass a wider spectrum of Autistic presentations across diverse demographics, and incorporate the personal experiences of Autistic people by utilising various communication methods. It is crucial that as our understanding of Autistic neurology deepens, our assessment tools also progress in order to accurately capture the diverse experiences and strengths of Autistic people.

14.7 Conclusion

Advocates of the Neurodiversity Paradigm critique mainstream Autistic assessment tools for children on several fronts, arguing that these tools often rely on a deficit-based approach, pathologise neurological differences, and prioritise a normative agenda rather than considering the perspectives and experiences of Autistic people. In this chapter, we took a broad look at the current assessment tools in use, and the significant issues with them. We also looked at screening tools, questionnaires that we have found helpful to the identification process and a possible pathway forward. In the next chapter we will outline the practical steps to conducting an identification process in a neuro-affirmative way.

CHAPTER 15

Conducting the Identification Process

15.1 Introduction

In this chapter, we will bring you through the steps of conducting a neurodiversity affirmative child autism identification process that meets best practice standards. This includes preparing for the process, selecting tests / questionnaires and working with other informants, creating a safe space, gathering information about the child's inner experiences and gathering wider information such as medical and mental health history, trauma experiences and gender identity. Support is given on how to map this information onto a newly framed neurodiversity affirmative diagnostic criteria, as is helping the child and their family make sense of their Autistic experiences. Also covered in this chapter is how to support children who do not want to attend, the involvement of a multi-disciplinary team, the utility of cognitive and other assessments, and how to write high-quality, supportive reports and documentation.

15.2 Preparing for the Process

Prior to undertaking an exploratory process with a young person and their family, it is essential for both the clinician(s) and the family to prepare. The absolute core aspect of any piece of work is collaboration, and the collaborative approach begins with the preparation as this will be different for every child and family and must be tailored to suit their needs specifically. It cannot be a 'one-size-fits-all' approach as each family will have their own communication preferences and needs and will process information in different ways (see Section 10.2 in relation to power and process issues). Upon embarking on a piece together, the clinician has the advantage of knowing what to expect during the process, but it must be considered that the family and specifically the young person do not have this knowledge and they do not know what to expect, which can lead to significant anxiety ahead of a collaborative piece beginning.

The range of emotions experienced by a family prior to an exploration piece is vast and varied, and multiple feelings can be present simultaneously. Often, there may have been a significant waiting time for the piece to begin, and when it finally arrives there can be feelings of relief and hope for parents / caregivers particularly. Alongside these feelings, there can also be significant fear and worry that the outcome of the piece will not align with what they know of their child, or for many young people who may have requested the piece themselves, that the outcome will not align with how they know themselves.

Parents / caregivers can feel deeply concerned about how their young person will cope with the process of undergoing an assessment piece, and it can be hugely stressful for young people to meet with new people during the process. Often a young person can be managing mental health challenges, or there may have been significant challenges in relation to school or accessing education and there is therefore a high level of stress before entering the process. Clinicians need to be cognisant of the multitude of emotions a young person and their family may be experiencing before beginning the piece, and they need to consider how best to support the family in navigating the experience.

CHILD'S VOICE

HANNAH, AGE 9

- How were you feeling when you first learned you were going to come to meet us?

  Nervous. I wanted to know what type of brain I had but was worried about what type of brain it would be.

- Was there anything we did that made it easier for you to come to meet us?

  Not really.

- What did you enjoy when you had your session with us?

  I liked answering all the questions and I liked talking about my things. I liked playing games – that made it easier to be there.

- Was there anything you did not enjoy about your session?

  Just the long journey. It might be better if I there was a beanbag or peanut ball for kids if they need a break.

- How did you feel when you learned that you are Autistic?

  I understand my brain, instead of thinking I'm really worried and I don't know what to do, I know it's just my autism and I'm not going crazy.

- Was there anything we did that helped you when you first learned this?

  I liked how she said it. It was easier on the computer.

- What did you think about your report or letter that we sent you?

  I really liked it. I liked that they added all the things I like to it. It made me feel really special.

- For any other child who is coming to meet with us, how would you describe to them what they should expect when they meet us?

  People are kind and you will learn all about your brain. They will ask questions about you and play fun games.

- What would you say to any other child who is worried about coming to meet with us?

  Don't worry, people are really kind.

Embarking on a neurodiversity affirmative exploration of identity with a young person and their family means collaboration from the outset. The young person and their parents / caregivers need to be given information about the process and consulted on what their requirements are in accessing the process during the course of the piece (see Chapter 12 on 'Making the Identification Process

Accessible' for further considerations in relation to families accessing the process). It is important for families to be aware that the key component of the piece is that all involved will work together to make sense of a young person's experiences, and that young people, their families and the clinicians involved are all equal partners in the process. Collaborating in relation to preparation for the piece not only ensures better access for families and a more comfortable process for young people, it also sets the tone from the outset that an equal, collaborative partnership is a core component of the entire piece.

As professionals, our role in an identification process includes the following:

1. Create a safe space for a young person to explore their experience of the world.

2. Acknowledge their experience as valid.

3. Support the young person in making sense of their experiences.

4. Support the young person to have a better understanding of themselves and their experience of the world.

5. Support the young person to develop their own narrative (see Chapter 4 for further discussion of narratives that are created in relation to being Autistic).

CHILD'S VOICE

A, AGE 10

- How were you feeling when you first learned you were going to come to meet us?

  I was feeling nervous.

- Was there anything we did that made it easier for you to come to meet us?

  Having a picture of the room helped.

- What did you enjoy when you had your session with us?

  I enjoyed the fidgets and playing Uno.

- Was there anything you did not enjoy about your session?

  No.

- How did you feel when you learned that you are Autistic?

  I felt like a bit sad but then I said I am the same me.

- Was there anything we did that helped you when you first learned this?

  Explaining it in a way that made sense like the different bears.

- For any other child who is coming to meet with us, how would you describe to them what they should expect when they meet us?

  They are really nice and don't be worried.

- What would you say to any other child who is worried about coming to meet with us?

  They are nice.

15.3 Selecting Tests / Questionnaires and Working with Other Informants

The process of undertaking a neuro-affirmative assessment involves a detailed process of gathering information about a young person's experiences of the world. There are many ways to gather this information, with the most important information coming from the child and young person themselves as to how they experience different aspects of the world. This information may be in what they communicate through their actions and interactions during play, or it may be in their direct communication (spoken or unspoken) about their experiences when asked.

In gathering information, there are a number of different options available to clinicians, with some being more reliable and informative than others. Reliable and informative information can come from multiple sources and is not just the information that is gathered via standardised instruments. It is important to be aware of testimonial justice and that information coming from professionals isn't any more 'valid' by virtue that it comes from a professional than information coming from parents / caregivers or young people. Young people can and do experience different environments in different ways, and therefore the information provided from different sources may differ but be equally valid. There is a significant lack of standardised instruments that are neurodiversity affirmative, particularly for young people (see Chapter 14 for further analysis of current available assessment tools and the problems with their use), and there is much misinformation that standardised tools must be used in an assessment process for it to be valid. This is categorically not the case, and over-reliance on standardised measures often results in a completely inaccurate outcome. Clinicians also need to be aware of potential power imbalances in the information being gathered, with certain 'voices' sometimes being given more weight than others, e.g., information from teachers is sometimes given more power than information from parents / caregivers. Young people often can experience different environments in different ways, and clinicians need to be careful not to dismiss information based on the information being different to descriptions of children in other settings.

The tools and instruments that currently exist are primarily designed to supposedly help clinicians to gather information about a young person's experiences. However, as outlined in Chapter 14 of this book, there are currently no assessment tools available that are fully neuro-affirmative, and sole reliance on tools that exist currently will give rise to limited information as they typically focus on outward presentation. Furthermore, existing tools such as the ADOS-2 have been reported to induce shame, humiliation and frustration for adults and leave them feeling patronised (Lockwood, 2023; see also https://wrongplanet.net/forums/viewtopic.php?t=385368). In a service evaluation of an autism assessment team in the UK, Thresher (2019) found that young people who had experienced an ADOS-2 as part of their assessment reported some of the activities as being challenging, and that the ADOS-2 activities contributed to them experiencing a degree of stress, worry and anxiety. In exploring whether a young person is Autistic, the aim is to learn as much as possible about a young person's inner experience of the world, and existing tools do not assist with this aim as they focus on what is outwardly observable. The best way to learn about a person's inner experience is to move away from existing tools – across all age ranges – and to focus on learning as much as possible about the inner experience of the young person by joining them in their experience. Be curious, immerse yourself in their interests, learn about the circumstances within which they thrive, find out about what leads them to feeling overwhelmed, join them in their play activities, and ultimately share in their experience of the world.

The way in which inner experiences are learned about will likely differ across different ages, but the same principles of collaboration, respect, creating a safe space, and supporting a person to develop their own narrative apply to all processes and all ages. With very young children, who may not yet have developed insight into their experiences or who may not be able yet to articulate their experiences, as well as non-speaking children, the emphasis is on what can be learned about their experience of the world through their play, their interests and how they communicate. Be careful, however, not to always assume that younger children who use spoken language cannot articulate their experience and ensure that the option to provide information about their experiences is always given. It is important also not to assume that non-speaking children are unable to convey their experiences – many articulate their experiences through body language, play, music, art etc. There will also be important information to gather from those who know them best – the people who care for them and who spend the most time with them. Older children and adolescents can often express their own experiences of the world, and again those who know and care for them can support them in articulating and expressing their experience.

> When gathering information about a young person's inner experience of the world, it is essential to remember that the most important and most valid information comes from the young person themselves. This may be in what they tell you about, it may be in their writing or drawing, it may be in their play or it may be in their actions or body movements. Other informants can provide supplemental information, but unless this information is coming from a parent or caregiver, then it is not as reliable as the information gathered directly from the young person. Information from a parent or caregiver can help to make sense of what a young person is communicating, but it can sometimes also differ from the information gathered from a young person (e.g., Nordahl-Hansen et al., 2014). This can be due to double empathy issues, where perhaps a parent is not Autistic themselves, or is masking; or it can be a lack of knowledge about Autistic experiences. It is also important to reflect on the weight that is placed on different sources of information during an exploration process, particularly when information differs from different sources.

Further exploration is required in situations where, for example, a parent or caregiver appears to be 'over-stating' a young person's needs, or where a young person is masking significantly, and parents or caregivers are unaware of their true inner experiences. Exploring these scenarios collaboratively and respectfully can allow for a consensus on the best understanding of a young person's neurology to be reached.

Reflection Point

The process of undertaking an 'assessment' with a young person and their family should reflect a therapeutic process. Although the word 'assessment' is used, this incorrectly implies that the clinician(s) will be making judgements about the young person exclusively and that the other parties (young people and their parents / caregivers) are on the periphery of the process. This is not the case with a neurodiversity affirmative piece. The process is one of collaborative discovery and of exploring identity. All involved share in the responsibility and in the process of making connections, seeking understanding and arriving at a shared understanding of a young person's experience of the world. For clinicians who are more familiar with 'traditional assessment' approaches, this requires a significant shift in thinking and understanding and a different approach moving forward. This may require some reflection and consideration on how this can be achieved and on the experiences of a young person and their family in the process.

15.4 Steps in a Neuro-Affirmative Process of Exploring Autistic Neurology with Children and Adolescents

Within a neurodiversity affirmative process, there are two distinct processes occurring at the same time. One aspect of the process is the technical aspect of ascertaining whether a person's experiences align with current criteria. The other aspect relates to the process of supporting a person to explore their sense of identity and how they understand themselves and their experience of the world. This exploration of identity is a broad process and is one that continues long beyond the technical piece of examining criteria. It is essential for clinicians to hold in their minds the importance of a person's narrative and their own sense of identity. When supporting a person to explore whether they are Autistic or not, the shift in identity for older children can be very significant for some, and for younger children, learning about their identity is significantly formative to their sense of self. Our role in this as clinicians is crucial, and it extends far beyond the technical examination of criteria being met. The words we use, the approach we take, the understanding and support that we offer, and the sense of connection to similar others that we can open up all have a huge impact on cultivating a positive sense of Autistic identity for a young person (see Chapter 4 and narrative accounts of a neurodiversity affirmative process from children and young people captured earlier in this book).

When embarking on a neurodiversity affirmative process with a young person and their family, there are a number of key steps to undertake. The core principles of collaboration, respect, transparency, flexibility and support are the foundations of the process and should be maintained throughout. With these principles in mind, the following steps may need to be adjusted and tailored to meet the needs of the person. These steps are:

1. Create a safe space within which to explore a child's inner experiences of the world.

2. Gather information collaboratively about a child's inner experiences.

3. Gather information about a child's medical history, mental health history, and their experience of significant life events or trauma events.

4. Map the information gathered onto current criteria re-framed to a neurodiversity affirmative perspective.

5. Support a child / adolescent and their family to make sense of their experiences.

15.4.1 Create a Safe Space

Creating a safe space for a young person and their family to explore their neurology within is essential to a neurodiversity affirmative process. This space is not only the physical space that they may come into but is also the emotional space provided by clinicians. Exploring neurology requires vulnerability, openness, transparency and trust, and it can be a very significant challenge for children, young people and their families to feel secure and comfortable in the physical and emotional space provided. Detailed information on how to create a safe environmental space is outlined in Chapters 11 and 12 of this book.

Creating a safe emotional space is equally as important as creating a safe physical space. The process of exploring neurology has major implications for a person in terms of shifting their sense of identity, and this can only be done within a space that is psychologically safe. Reflective practice is a key component to creating a safe psychological space for children and young people to explore their identity. Within reflective practice, clinicians should reflect on and unpack any ableism (both internalised and externalised) along with connecting and listening to the Autistic community in terms of their experiences of 'assessment' pieces.

CHILD'S VOICE

AARON, AGE 15

- How were you feeling when you first learned you were going to come to meet us?

  A bit nervous.

- Was there anything we did that made it easier for you to come to meet us?

  Talking about the interests that I had.

- What did you enjoy when you had your session with us?

  Talking. I also enjoyed telling you about the flags and countries.

- Was there anything you did not enjoy about your session?

  I enjoyed everything, nothing was bad in my opinion. I felt relaxed.

- How did you feel when you learned that you are Autistic?

  I didn't think much about it. I just wanted to know. Everything made sense about the way that I am.

- Was there anything we did that helped you when you first learned this?

  The letter you sent.

- What did you think about your report or letter that we sent you?

  I agreed with it. Everything made sense.

- For any other young person who is coming to meet us, how would you describe to them what they should expect when they meet us?

  They are going to give you lots of questions and try to ask about your interests and know more about it. You will expect relaxation and lots of fidget toys. Very quiet and understanding.

- What would you say to any other young person who is coming to meet with us?

  Don't be nervous, it's not the end of the world. They will try lots of stuff to make you less nervous and more calm.

Many young people and their families may have had negative experiences within healthcare settings prior to undertaking an exploration of Autistic neurology. There can be a variety of reasons for this, including being misunderstood, environments not being accessible etc. (see Chapter 12 for further discussion of the barriers in accessing healthcare and accessibility considerations). Determining what is a safe space needs to be carefully considered with each individual we meet with as professionals, and the definition of a safe space will be different for each person. The decision about what is a safe space is not for professionals to determine, although our role in creating a safe space is significant. When establishing a safe space, professionals need to employ a trauma-informed approach and also to consider how to meet various communication needs. A safe space needs to ensure that all communication methods are honoured and supported.

15.4.2 Gather Information About Inner Experiences

The core aspect of a neuro-affirmative assessment process with a child or young person relates to gathering information. As discussed previously in this chapter, the core information being gathered comes from the young person themselves – their own research into Autistic neurology, their own insight into their experiences, or what they communicate within their play, actions or body movements. Information should be gathered respectfully and collaboratively. The questions asked and how the answers are interpreted should be within a neurodiversity affirmative framework and with neurodiversity affirming language.

15.4.2.1 Preliminary Information Gathering

Prior to meeting with a young person and their family to begin the process of exploring their neurology, it can be helpful to gather preliminary information about a young person and what has prompted the exploration piece. This may include information from referral agents, but most importantly this should be information from the young person and their family. Within the process of an exploration piece there is much information to gather, and having a 'sense' of a person's experiences prior to commencing can be very helpful in our role of supporting a person to develop their own narrative.

When gathering preliminary information, information is most often sought from parents or caregivers. This information can give a detailed overview of a child's birth and medical history, early development, educational history and mental health history. Parents and caregivers can also offer wider information in relation to strengths and abilities, experience of communication, play preferences, friendships, passions / interests, sensory experiences, experience of change and transitions and regulation experiences. It is important that young people also have the option to offer this preliminary information if they would like to. Preliminary information can be gathered either via non-spoken methods (e.g., by writing or completing intake forms) or via spoken methods (e.g., via voice recordings). Gathering preliminary information from both the young person and their caregivers allows for the process to begin and removes some of the pressure of having to 'explain' everything when meeting in-person.

15.4.2.2 Session with Parents / Caregivers

Gathering information from parents and / or caregivers is an essential component within the process, and even though the most important information comes from the young person themselves, it is advised that the parent / caregiver session happens first for a number of reasons. Meeting with parents / caregivers first is advised to ensure consent and to provide information that may help to support a young person through the process. It is also an opportunity to ascertain the family's understanding of Autistic experiences and to begin having neuro-affirmative conversations about Autistic neurology. For young people of all ages, meeting with parents / caregivers first gives space to ascertain what a child's understanding of the process is and whether or not they know what is being explored is whether they are Autistic or not. Many parents / caregivers are unsure about whether or not to inform their young person about the nature of the piece. Some young people already know what the piece is about, and many may have even requested it or instigated it. Meeting with parents / caregivers first gives space for these conversations and allows for a plan of support to be implemented if needed.

Meeting with parents / caregivers prior to meeting with a young person allows for the gathering of rich and detailed information about a child's development and their apparent experiences of the world. Prior to meeting with parents / caregivers, consideration needs to be given to their communication needs and styles, and how this part of the process can be accessible to them (see Chapter 12 for further discussion in relation to accessibility). Most often, there are many questions to ask and many experiences to explore, and it is advised to offer parents / caregivers the option of having a list of the questions they will be asked in advance. Knowing what they will be asked in advance allows parents to reflect on their child's development and early years, and it also means that if another parent or caregiver cannot attend the session then they will have an opportunity to contribute to the information being gathered if they wish to. Providing the questions in advance and also giving space and time for reflection means that the information being gathered will be much more rich and detailed than if questions are asked spontaneously with no opportunity for reflection. Parents / caregivers should also be offered different options for supplying the information, with both written and spoken methods (or a combination of both) being made available.

Along with gathering information from parents / caregivers about the core areas within the criteria, information also needs to be gathered about experiences outside of 'criteria areas'. These experiences include (but are not limited to): Autistic communication, Autistic joy, a sense of justice and fairness, creativity, empathy and compassion, hyperfocus and masking. Gathering wider information to include the above supports the cultivation of a positive sense of Autistic identity as the process of exploring and discussing the full range of Autistic experiences allows a young person to develop their narrative and their Autistic identity.

15.4.2.3 Session with Young Person

Following the gathering of preliminary information from a young person and their family, and also following an initial meeting with parents / caregivers, the next step in a neurodiversity affirmative process is to meet with a young person themselves. Prior to undertaking this step, it is vital to be aware that it can often be an exceptionally challenging experience for a young person to come into an unfamiliar space and to meet with unfamiliar people. It is essential to remove as much uncertainty as possible in relation to this meeting and to create a safe space for a young person to come into. Providing information in advance about what to expect during the session is essential (see Chapter 12 for further detail on how to make the process accessible). Photographs and / or a video of the space that a young person will come into are extremely helpful to most in understanding what the room will look like and what it contains. Similarly, photographs and / or videos of all clinicians they will meet helps to take away the uncertainty of who they will meet with.

For all young people, having the option to bring something that is a comfort to them is very important. Familiar items offer comfort and also certainty in an unfamiliar space. Some children bring favourite teddies or toys, while others bring sensory items or preferred snacks. Bringing something with them also allows for an opportunity to share their interests and passions, and exploring these together can be a joyful and validating experience for all. Seeing the detail and creativity in artwork or learning about a niche aspect of a particular topic provides clinicians with rich information about a person's experience of the world and is most likely to be a comfortable and enjoyable experience for a young person.

For very young children (preschool age), the emphasis of the session is on the child's experience of play and exploration. Having toys or items available for play and activity for a child to explore is helpful, but there should be no agenda or set of activities to complete. A child may also bring their own favourite toys or objects, and again very rich information can be learned about a child's inner experience through sharing in their play and activities. This session should be led by a child and there should be no pre-determined structure to the session. Learning about a child's experience of the world through their play and their interests means joining in with their activities (if they are comfortable with being joined) and playing in the way that they are playing. It means paying attention to what they notice and sharing in the joy they glean from an action or activity. A child's choices and communication should always be respected, and no toy or object should ever be removed or made unavailable (unless there is a safety reason for doing so). For some children, entering an unfamiliar space can be very overwhelming, and they may need a little time without the presence of an unfamiliar person to acclimatise to the setting. It can be helpful for clinicians to leave the space for a short time to give this adjustment time where needed.

Having a range of toys and activities available for children to explore if they wish is helpful. It is advised to have a range of the following available:

- Toys for sensory play (e.g., fidgets, textured toys, toys that light up or make sounds etc.).

- Toys that allow for precise and detailed play (e.g., toy figures that can be sorted or arranged into different categories, toy animals that can be arranged etc.).

- Toys that have a repeated aspect to them (e.g., cars being pushed down a track over and over).

- Open-ended toys (i.e., toys that are not specific in their purpose and can be used for anything).

- Materials for arts and crafts.

- Toys for pretend play (e.g., dolls, toy figures, role play costumes etc.).

- Toys that require or result in an action (e.g., pop-up toys, cars that can be wound up to move, toys that fly in the air when wound up, bubbles etc.).

- Construction toys (e.g., Lego™, bricks, shape sorters etc.).

- Different types of books (e.g., fact-based books, story books etc.).

- Board games, card games.

For adolescents, the emphasis again is on creating a safe space and reducing as much uncertainty as possible. With the advent of social media, many adolescents have engaged in a lot of research prior to engaging in formal exploration of their identity, and many are aware of Autistic experiences and feel as though their experiences of the world align. It is important to acknowledge and validate their experiences and to engage with them in a way that allows for learning about and sharing in their experiences. For adolescents, there can be a high level of stress in relation to what they will be asked about during their session. Giving the option of seeing in advance the types of questions that will be asked can be very helpful in reducing stress regarding the session (see Appendix 3 for a sample of the types of questions / areas that are helpful to explore). Many young people choose to write down their information in advance of a session, and this could be explored during the session. For those that are non-speaking, they may communicate information about their experiences in other ways. Whether a young person uses spoken or non-spoken communication, it is important that they know that all of the room is available to them when they are present. This means that they may choose to engage with some of the toys or items in the room if they wish, and they may choose to sit or stand where they wish in the room, or to move about if they need to.

For children who are older than preschoolers but younger than adolescents, usually a combination of play and activities while exploring their experiences through conversation (if they use spoken language), written methods or artwork is most comfortable and helpful to the process. Children of all ages can be incredibly insightful in relation to their own experiences of the world, and they are most likely to share their insights when the environment facilitates them to do so and when they feel safe, comfortable and that their experiences will be treated with care.

It is important that even though there may be spoken conversation about their experiences, this doesn't have to be an 'interview-style' session and should be more informal and exploratory. Let the young person know in advance of the session (and give a reminder at the beginning of a session) about the following to make the experience more comfortable for them:

- They can choose whether they would like to come into the room alone or if they would like to have someone familiar with them.

- They are welcome to sit wherever they like – on the floor, on the table, on a chair, on a swing etc.

- They can move about the room as much as they like.

- Anything in the room is available to them and they are welcome to bring their own items if they wish.

- Eye contact is not expected (ensure to reduce yours too if you naturally make eye contact with others and particularly if you know eye contact is uncomfortable for the young person).

- They do not have to talk about anything that they don't feel comfortable talking about.

- They do not have to talk at all, if they would prefer to write about their experiences (have paper and pencils available for use).

- This session is not the only opportunity to share information. Something may be remembered after a session and can be sent on to the clinician for inclusion in the piece.

See the box below for speech and language advice on assessments with children who use communication methods other than the spoken word.

PERSPECTIVES OF AN SLT: CONSIDERATIONS FOR CONDUCTING AN ASSESSMENT OF A CHILD / YOUNG PERSON WHO CANNOT RELY ON SPEECH ALONE TO BE HEARD OR UNDERSTOOD

ELAINE MCGREEVY

The temporal, bodily and stylistic characteristics of communication need to be respected and facilitated in an AAC-mediated interaction. For those who used aided AAC, direct eye contact is often difficult, and turn taking is slowed down significantly. Silence not only allows for processing and formulating messages, it also has communicative power itself.

Some basic etiquette for clinicians to remember:

- Respect the person's AAC device and any other aid.

- Do not touch the AAC device without gaining consent first. Even if the child / young person cannot clearly answer, always ask first and wait.

- Do not lean on a young person's wheelchair.

- Allow considerable time for the young person to construct a message and wait for them to finish their message and play it before responding.

- If the young child is exploring their device and their message is unclear, acknowledge that you heard them. Encourage them to try again or show you in another way if you don't understand.

Prior contact with the family will help the clinician prepare alternative modes for a young person who may not be able to speak during the assessment. As a rule, pen and paper or markers and colouring pencils should be available as a way for the child or young person to give information, and some may use drawing as a way to regulate. The therapist may need to significantly adjust their question types to allow yes / no / don't know responses. Consider making available a communication board with key self-advocacy messages in text, symbols, or photos, e.g., 'I need a break', 'I don't want to', 'I don't know', 'I need a different way to tell you', 'I'm tired / thirsty', 'I want to go home / to the toilet'.

The clinician may need to provide a questionnaire format of questions relevant to their experiences when exploring situational non-speaking. The table below (developed by Elaine McGreevy) is an example of a communication assessment that the young person can complete with a parent or the clinician.
Yes No Sometimes Don't know

I can use mouth words to say what I need at home.
I can use mouth words to talk about something I like at home.
I can use mouth words when I am angry at home.
I can use mouth words when I am upset at home.

I can use mouth words when I am excited at home.

I can use mouth words when I am tired at home.

I can use mouth words when I am sick at home.

I can use mouth words to talk to friends in online games.

I can use mouth words when I'm upset or angry in online games.

Sometimes, I can talk but I don't want to talk so I stay quiet.

I know what I want to say in my head, but the words don't come out of my mouth.

I know what I want to say but I am too tired to say it.

I know what I want to say but I can't be bothered to say it.

I can't speak with mouth words because there are no words in my mind at the time.

When my brain is thinking too much, I can't get my mouth words to work.

When it's been too noisy or too many people, my mouth words stop working.

When the words won't come out, I feel like my lips are shut tight.

When the words won't come out, I feel tight in my throat.

When the words won't come out, I feel uncomfortable feelings in my body.

When exploring a young person's experiences of the world, the areas being explored include the areas within the criteria and also Autistic experiences that are outside of the criteria. As mentioned above, these include (but are not limited to): Autistic communication, Autistic joy, a sense of justice and fairness, creativity, empathy and compassion, hyperfocus and masking. Exploring these areas with a young person allows for opportunities to acknowledge and validate their experiences, and to begin the process of making connections within their experiences to Autistic ways of being and cultivating a positive sense of Autistic identity.

When gathering any information from or about a young person in terms of their communication, interaction, friendships / relationships, interests, sensory experiences and how they process information, the emphasis in each area being considered should always be on the following:

- What is their preference in this area?

- What is comfortable for them?

- What is their interest?

- What are their strengths in this area?

- What is uncomfortable for them in this area?

Throughout the process, consideration needs to be given to whether a young person's experiences align with Autistic experiences or another neurotype.

15.4.3 Gather Wider Information about the Young Person

When supporting a young person to explore whether or not they may be Autistic, it is not only important to gather information about their Autistic experiences, but also to gather information about their wider experiences. This is important in helping to explore whether there is a different explanation for their experiences elsewhere, and also in differentiating Autistic experiences that may be there from other experiences. When considering wider information, it is important to gather information about a young person's medical history, mental health history and trauma history. See the box below on taking an experience-sensitive approach to assessment.

PERSPECTIVES OF AN SLT: AN EXPERIENCE-SENSITIVE APPROACH TO ASSESSMENT

ELAINE MCGREEVY

An experience-sensitive approach (Pavlopoulou, 2021) enables the practitioner to shift their lens and practice from neuro-disorder to a neuro inclusive, humanistic framework of healthcare. The approach 'promotes a sense of agency and identifies strengths, barriers and needs to support well-being and to create opportunities for the person to flourish authentically, living their best life, according to their own norms'. (McGreevy et al., 2024). The humanising lifeworld framework, first proposed by Todres et al. (2009), underpins the experience-sensitive framework of healthcare and places individuals at the centre of care by considering how support can uphold the key aspects of what it means to be human, as outlined by the eight dimensions of care. Considering the SLT assessment in the context of an autism assessment, Table 15.1 below describes examples of the practical application of a dimensions lifeworld framework discussed in McGreevy et al. (2024) which enable an experience-sensitive approach.

Table 15.1: Practical applications of the dimensions of a lifeworld framework in SLT / autism assessment

Dimensions of a Lifeworld Framework	Practices
Insiderness	• Cultivate emotional safety and a collaborative approach. • Facilitate the child / young person to express their own experiences and share their interests. • Follow their lead. • Use multi-modal communication and honour all forms of spoken and non-spoken communication. • Avoid using reductionist and deficit tools and associated deficit language to describe challenges. • De-emphasise the use of standard assessments and standard deviations when evidencing support needs. • Post-identification, collaborate with the individual to facilitate their self-discovery of their neurodivergence and include family to promote shared understanding.
Agency	• Gain consent / assent for each step of the assessment. • Create the possibility for the child / young person to make choices and take decisions on how they can comfortably occupy the therapy space. • Avoid rushing the child / young person to allow time to develop connection so the child or young person feels cared for. • Avoid power-over, coercive strategies such as the use of rewards. • Ensure that the voice of the child / young person is heard, both directly and through others who know them well, and amplify their voice in reports and recommendations for further support. This includes ethically listening to non-spoken forms of communication which support self-advocacy and expression of preferences.

Uniqueness	<ul><li>Autistic children / young people are unique and should be seen as individuals with many identities. Affirm Autistic communication and processing styles.</li><li>Validate Autistic play.</li><li>Avoid 'cut and paste' template reports and support plans.</li><li>Provide an affirming post-identification letter to the child / young person.</li><li>Co-construct a communication passport or one-page profile of needs and accommodations.</li><li>Support the young person's self-understanding.</li><li>Use culturally sensitive practices and use interpreters as needed.</li><li>Information should represent the individual's cultural and social identity.</li></ul>
Sense-making	<ul><li>Sense-making involves a motivation to find meaning and significance in things, places, events and experiences. The child or young person is viewed as the story maker of their own life.</li><li>Consider how Autistic ways of play help with sense-making and learning about the world.</li><li>Seek the individual's perspectives on their school, community and families.</li><li>Honour stimming.</li><li>Use neurodivergent affirming language and language that honours gender and cultural identity.</li></ul>
Personal journey	<ul><li>Support the child / family as they journey through the discovery of the child's neurocognitive profile.</li><li>Provide clarity around time frames, involved professionals and steps in the process of assessment.</li><li>Proactively facilitate each child's / young person's personal journey planning by identifying strengths, interests and passions.</li><li>Co-create plans that meet needs and self-identified goals by ensuring the child / young person makes choices and expresses preferences.</li><li>Use information gathered to inform supporters at times of transition.</li><li>Provide clear information and an agreed plan for next steps.</li></ul>
Sense of place	<ul><li>Autistic children / young people should feel welcome and safe in the therapy room and in their everyday environments. They should be encouraged to bring support objects and have anchoring people accompany them.</li><li>Ensure sensory comfort as a means to empowerment and creating acceptance in environments.</li><li>Learn from the child / young person about what supports they need to feel a sense of belonging and inclusion at school and home.</li><li>Provide visual communication supports to create a sense of predictability and safety.</li></ul>

cont.

Dimensions of a Lifeworld Framework	Practices
Embodiment	• Avoid making assumptions or value judgements. • Presume competence – all children / young people with communication disabilities have something to express, even if others do not yet understand their communication. • Provide AAC without gatekeeping. • Validate Autistic body language and non-spoken communication. • Explore and describe Autistic ways of languaging, playing and sensing without defaulting to a deficit / disorder narrative. • Consider using energy accounting and monotropism to enable participation in the session.
Togetherness	• Set up a communication space that fosters meaningful connection and curiosity where the therapist and child / young person can take time to get to know each other. • Consistency, transparency and practice of 'power-with' strategies ensure that the child / young person / parent / carer can feel safe and this helps build trust with the practitioner. • Validate the child / young person so they can express worries / fears, argue, protest / reject, ask for help, as well as share fun and intimate moments. • Signpost the child / family to safe, neurodivergent sources of information and peer support.

15.4.3.1 Medical History

In terms of medical history, it is important to gather information about a person's experience of medical illnesses, injuries and potential genetic / chromosomal differences for a number of reasons. First, there may potentially be a different explanation for their 'Autistic experiences' in their medical history. Second, it may be the case that they have co-occurring medical conditions alongside being Autistic and they may require support and adjustments in accessing healthcare.

There is a growing body of research that highlights the barriers for Autistic people in accessing healthcare (Doherty et al., 2022) and Autistic young people with any of the below medical conditions or with any other medical history will require advocacy and support in relation to the adjustments they require to access the healthcare they need. Exploring a young person's medical history is important in understanding their overall experience of the world and in supporting them to access the care they need.

Research has shown that Autistic people experience an increased level of co-occurring medical conditions compared to the general population. These can contribute to a worsening of social communication and behaviour, lower quality of life, higher morbidity and premature mortality (Sala et al., 2020). Research also suggests there is greater diversity in brain development in Autistic people compared to non-autistic people. For example, research (albeit relying mainly on Autistic male children) has indicated that there are structural and connectivity differences in the brains of Autistic people, such as diversity in cortical thickness, hippocampal volumes, with the amount of cerebrospinal fluid, grey matter volume and developmental trajectories of neurobiological processes often lasting longer into adulthood and being less fixed (Braden et al., 2017; McAlonan, 2004; Raznahan et al., 2010).

There are a number of medical conditions that frequently co-occur with Autistic neurology. These include Ehlers-Danlos syndrome / hypermobility (see www.sedsconnective.org/), epilepsy, POTS (postural orthostatic tachycardia syndrome), gastrointestinal conditions (e.g., constipation, diarrhoea, abdominal pain, irritable bowel syndrome), asthma, allergies, migraines, insomnia, and fibromyalgia. For example, Holingue et al. (2023) explain that gastrointestinal symptoms are common amongst Autistic children, although estimated prevalence rates vary due to the diversity of Autistic experience and difficulties with accurate and reliable measurement of gastrointestinal symptoms. Similarly, a systemic review by Leader et al. (2022) found that gastrointestinal symptoms are common in Autistic children, young people and adults, pointing out that these can result in irritability, withdrawn behaviour, anxiety and sleep difficulties.

Epilepsy (a condition of the central nervous system) is common in the Autistic population. Epileptic seizures are thought to be caused by abnormalities in brain activity. A systemic review by Liu et al. (2021) found that epilepsy is more prevalent in the Autistic population than in the general population, and that there are higher rates of epilepsy among Autistic adults than Autistic children. Liu et al. (2021) reported that 1 in 10 Autistic individuals has epilepsy and that epilepsy increases with age, gender (increasing for females) and co-occurring intellectual disability.

Ehlers-Danos syndrome (EDS) and hypermobility syndrome (hEDS) also occurs in Autistic people at higher rates than in non-autistic people. These can affect proprioception, resulting in such symptoms as increased fatigue and pain. Kindgren et al. (2021) found that EDS and hEDS co-occurred at a higher rate in Autistic children and those who are ADHD compared to neurotypical peers, reporting three times the expected rate of hEDS and EDS in ADHD children, and an estimated twice the expected rate in Autistic children. Many girls did not seek medical care until after puberty, and boys were diagnosed with hEDS and EDS on average two years earlier (peak age for males was 5 to 9, compared to 15 to 19 for girls). In a national Swedish population-based study looking at EDS and hEDS in those with different neurodivergencies and psychiatric conditions, Cederlöf et al. (2016) found that Autistic individuals and individuals with bipolar affective disorder, ADHD and schizophrenia had an increased risk ratio of having co-occurring EDS and hypermobility syndrome.

15.4.3.2 Mental Health History

Across all areas of mental health, higher rates of mental ill-health are experienced by Autistic people in comparison to neurotypical people. For many Autistic people, their mental health challenges often begin in childhood or adolescence, and often mental ill-health may be the first indicator that a person is Autistic as they unknowingly struggle to navigate neurotypical environments. A young person who is unaware that they are Autistic will most likely do the best that they can to navigate a neurotypical world, which can impact significantly on their mental health in terms of higher levels of anxiety, lower mood, higher levels of overwhelm, and a higher likelihood of shutdowns and meltdowns as they struggle to cope. Many Autistic young people experience eating disorders and OCD. The level of unidentified Autistic neurology among those who experience eating disorders is at such a high rate that it is advised that consideration should be given for all young people experiencing an eating disorder to whether or not they may be Autistic.

Similar to the barriers in accessing physical healthcare for Autistic people, the same barriers in accessing mental healthcare also unfortunately exist. Autistic adults have also shared their experiences of being 'misdiagnosed' as adolescents and their Autistic neurology being missed (see Autistic Science Person, 2022). Many have also shared their experiences of negative experiences of mental health support, and feeling invalidated, unheard and isolated (Brede et al., 2022). Working with children and young people, there is an opportunity to impact change in terms of their mental health experience at a younger age, and hopefully to better support their mental health going forward into adulthood. This is achieved by supporting young people to understand their neurology, their identity, their mental health experiences and how each of these things are interwoven. Exploring mental health experiences also opens up access to support and understanding. For a young person, it is best in terms of their mental health and their sense of self if they can access support to help both with understanding their Autistic identity and with their mental health within the one service. However, unfortunately this often is not possible, and it can be challenging for Autistic young people to access mental health support that also understands their Autistic neurology.

15.4.3.3 Experience of Significant Life Events Including Trauma Experiences

It is clear that there are higher levels of trauma exposure and higher rates of PTSD amongst the Autistic population than amongst the general population (Koenen et al., 2017; Reuben et al., 2021). As a result of there being such a high prevalence rate of trauma amongst the Autistic community (see Section 9.3 for further details about the intersection between Autistic neurology and trauma experiences), it is essential that an exploration of Autistic experiences being undertaken with a young person also includes an exploration of potential trauma experiences. This is important for two reasons. First, it is essential to learn about trauma experiences in order to differentiate between Autistic experiences and trauma experiences. Second, it is vital that following the piece of exploration in relation to Autistic identity, if trauma experiences have been identified, children and young people have access to trauma support that also understands their Autistic neurology.

In gathering information about significant life events and potential trauma, a trauma-informed process means that there is awareness that for some, communicating about their trauma experiences may be re-traumatising. Gathering information about trauma experiences needs to be carried out carefully, gently and safely. For most young people, this may begin with those who know them well who can provide information about whether it is likely that they have been exposed to potentially traumatic experiences, bearing in mind that the person providing the information may have co-experienced the traumatic event and may also need support in relation to this. Depending on the age and the situation for the young person, this may also involve their own reflections on their trauma experiences, but it doesn't have to in order to arrive at a conclusion on whether they are Autistic or not. This is because it is possible to understand whether a person who has experienced trauma in their lives is Autistic or not by focusing on their Autistic experiences rather than their trauma experiences, if this is re-traumatising or potentially re-traumatising for them.

When trying to disentangle trauma experiences from Autistic experiences with children and young people, there are a number of areas to consider:

- Consider the timeline of events for the young person. If their trauma experiences stem from particular events, explore whether their Autistic experiences pre-date their trauma experiences.

- Consider the nature of early play and friendships throughout their life. Young people who have experienced trauma but who are not Autistic may have an interest in connecting with their neurotypical peers and their play preferences will be more aligned with neurotypical play than with Autistic play. Autistic children and young people who have experienced trauma will most likely gravitate towards friendships and connections that are typical of Autistic or neurodivergent friendships or connections, or they may prefer to play or spend time alone rather than with others.

- Consider the nature of hand and body movements. Young people who have experienced trauma but who are not Autistic are likely to move their hands and bodies in similar ways to Autistic children, e.g., they may rock their bodies etc. This is typically in an effort to soothe their distress or in response to a trauma trigger. Autistic young people will also move their hands and bodies to regulate any distress they experience, but they are also likely to move their hands and bodies to express joy, excitement, and to support their concentration or focus.

- Consider the use of language and speaking. Autistic young people often enjoy using language in different ways to their neurotypical peers. They may enjoy a whimsical use of language, they might like to play with language and words and develop new words, or they may enjoy words in different languages or accents. Autistic young people may be very direct and honest in their communication style, and they may prefer a monologuing conversational style over back-and-forth conversation. All of these aspects of language use are aligned with Autistic neurology and are different to neurotypical use of language and communication.

- Consider routines and how a young person manages change. Young people who are not Autistic but who have experienced trauma may have particular routines or ways that they need to do things, and these are typically related to avoiding a trigger of their trauma or a trauma memory. Autistic young people may also have particular ways of doing things that might be related to avoiding distress, but they will also have routines that reduce the amount of processing or uncertainty in their environment, and that are unrelated to trauma experiences.

- Consider interests and passions. Autistic young people are more likely than their neurotypical counterparts to have the capacity to hyperfocus on their interests. They are more likely to have a strong ability to acquire deep knowledge about their interests and their interests are likely to be more specialist than their neurotypical counterparts. Young people who are not Autistic are much less likely to have abilities relating to hyperfocus, and may find their attention and concentration is negatively impacted when they are experiencing a trauma response.

- Consider sensory experiences. Young people who are not Autistic but who have experienced trauma may have sensory experiences that they find challenging to tolerate and that are typically related to their trauma experience. There may be a particular smell, sound or element of touch that triggers a trauma memory, and that the young person therefore tries to avoid. Autistic young people will also have sensory experiences that they are unable to tolerate, but they are also more likely to have sensory experiences that they seek and that are necessary in order to regulate their system.

- Consider what triggers overwhelm. For neurotypical young people who have experienced trauma, the most likely trigger for their sense of overwhelm is the memory of their trauma experience being triggered. It can also be the case for Autistic young people that a trauma memory will trigger their overwhelm, however there are more likely to be other factors that trigger their overwhelm also. Sensory aspects of the environment, experiences of masking, over-exposure to social events that are stressful and unpredictability or uncertainty are more likely to trigger overwhelm for Autistic young people than their neurotypical peers.

- Consider the presence of Autistic strengths and abilities. An Autistic young person is more likely to have a profile of Autistic strengths and abilities than a neurotypical young person, regardless of their trauma experiences. Autistic strengths and abilities include (but are not limited to): hyperfocus, deep passions and interests, specialist knowledge in relation to interests, curiosity, creativity, a strong sense of justice / fairness, being analytical and methodical in their approach to tasks, having a strong ability to notice and attend to detail etc. These strengths and abilities are typically unrelated to trauma experiences.

By focusing on the presence of Autistic experiences rather than the nature of trauma experiences (which may be re-traumatising during a relatively short process), it is possible to determine collaboratively whether a young person is also Autistic alongside their trauma experiences. The process of exploring the differentiation between Autistic and trauma experience needs to be trauma-informed.

A trauma-informed process includes the following elements:

1. Routinely ask parents and caregivers about the possibility that a young person has experienced trauma in their lives.

2. Be mindful that previous experiences within health services may have been traumatising for a young person and their family. They may have felt unheard, been misunderstood, or experienced difficult dynamics. They may have experienced trauma from having to be in an unfamiliar and / or unpredictable environment when accessing healthcare settings. Their trauma from these experiences may have the potential to be re-triggered by engaging in the current process.

3. Be aware of power dynamics within the piece. For healthcare professionals, even if they don't seek power within the interaction, it is there. It is important to work to share power within the dynamic.

4. Understand the challenges experienced by many in talking about trauma experiences, particularly if their time within the process is

short-lived and the clinician won't be involved in the post-assessment support piece. Within a short piece, there hasn't been scope to develop deep trust and psychological safety, and it may be psychologically unsafe for a young person (or their parents / caregivers) to communicate in-depth in relation to their trauma experiences.

5. Consider the possibility of Autistic neurology and trauma co-occurring. All too often, young people and their families are told that it cannot be determined whether they are Autistic or not as they have experienced trauma and their experiences are likely because of their trauma. This happens without consideration being given to the presence of Autistic experiences that cannot be explained by trauma experiences.

6. Be aware that trauma support for those who have experienced trauma in their lives will be required following the process. If the young person is Autistic, this support will need to be tailored for them using an Autistic framework.

15.4.3.4 Gender Identity

As outlined in Section 10.4 of this book, there is a high rate of gender variance amongst Autistic people. Many young people who along with their families seek to explore their Autistic neurology are also exploring their gender identity or already identify as a gender different to that which was assigned at their birth. For clinicians, it is essential to understand the intersectionality between neurodivergence and gender identity, as ableism and pathologising Autistic identity create barriers for young people in exploring their gender identity.

In creating a safe space for young people that is both neuro- and gender-affirming, the following should be carried out within the process:

1. Clinicians need to be aware of the high overlap between Autistic neurology and gender variance.

2. Use gender-affirming language throughout the piece – whether a young person is openly exploring their gender or not.

3. Ask about preferred pronouns and their preferred name. Ensure preferred pronouns and names are used.

4. Check what name and pronouns are to be used in documentation.

5. Do not assume that all stress is associated with gender variance or mental health. Consider the likelihood of stress being associated with being Autistic and trying to navigate neurotypical environments.

6. Engage with the LGBTQIA+ Autistic community.

15.4.4 Mapping Information

When the process of gathering information about a young person's experiences of the world has concluded, the next step in the process is to map this information onto current best practice criteria. As discussed earlier in this book, current classification systems are not neuro-affirmative in their description of Autistic experiences, and they also exclude many Autistic experiences from their outline (see Chapter 13 for further evaluation of current classification systems). Nevertheless, despite the problems associated with the classification systems, they must be used as part of a best practice process.

Reflection Point

When gathering and mapping information as part of the process of assessment, while the main areas outlined within the international criteria need to be considered, the way in which these areas are considered needs to be interpreted differently. When thinking about Autistic experiences, the areas within the criteria are broadly useful to explore collaboratively with a young person, but the language used to describe those experiences is problematic, deficit-focused and inappropriate within a neurodiversity affirmative framework.

Rather than framing a person's experiences as 'impaired' or 'deficient' when compared to the majority neurotype, it is important to explore a young person's experiences from the perspective of what their preferences are in each area, what works well for them and is comfortable for them, how they thrive or best engage in each area, and what are their strengths and abilities in each area. Alongside exploring these aspects, it is also important to learn about a young person's needs and what they find uncomfortable in each area, what are the challenges that have arisen for them, and what does not work well for them. In exploring all of the above, it can then be considered whether or not a young person's experiences align with Autistic experiences or the experiences of another neurotype.

See Appendix 1 for examples of many aspects of current criteria re-framed within a neuro-affirmative framework.

During the process of gathering information and mapping this information onto re-framed criteria, it is important to ensure that this process is collaborative with a young person and their family, and that it is respectful to their experiences. Everyone involved in the process has the option to contribute to the mapping process and documented information should be reviewed and subject to change by a young person (where possible) and their parents / caregivers prior to being finalised. The process should be centred around the 'voice' of the young person and should reflect their actual inner experiences where they can articulate these, or the most accurate estimation of their inner experiences based on their communication through their actions. All of a young person's experiences should be documented and added to the relevant section of the criteria (see Appendices 4 and 5 for samples of mapping documents that are aligned with DSM-5-TR and ICD-11 criteria).

15.4.5 Making Sense of Experiences

Following the collaborative process of gathering and mapping information about a young person's experiences, the next step in the process is to make sense of the experiences. This has traditionally been known as a 'feedback' session, but this term is problematic for a couple of reasons. First, it implies that this session is the first time that the outcome may be discussed. Within a neurodiversity affirmative process, this should not be the case. The process should feel like a sense of shared understanding is being arrived at and that everything is converging towards the outcome. There should be conversations along the way as experiences are being explored to establish whether a particular experience aligns with Autistic experiences or whether they align with the experience of a different neurotype, so that an overall picture is being built and arrived at. It shouldn't be the case that there is a 'surprise' ending that hasn't been explored prior to the outcome session. The second reason that the term 'feedback' is problematic is that it implies that the conversation is one-way, from a clinician to a young person and their parent / caregiver. Again, this is not what a neuro-affirmative process should be. It is not the role of the clinician to 'decide' on another person's neurotype without any input or involvement of the other person. This should be a conclusion that is reached collaboratively, and the clinician's role is to support the young person to make sense of their experiences and support them in developing their narrative and identity.

The outcome session is a collaborative and exploratory session and is the culmination of a process of 'discovery' about a young person's experiences of the world. The session might begin with the clinician re-sharing their thoughts and understandings of a young person's experiences and whether (having mapped the information gathered collaboratively) their experiences overall align with the experiences of Autistic children and young people. A conversation then usually ensues in relation to whether this continues to make sense to the young person in how they know themselves and the parent / caregiver in how they know their young person. Through discussion and collaboration, there is then an opportunity to establish where thinking converges and where there may be differences in thinking. If the understanding of the outcome is not shared, i.e., if the clinician believes a young person is Autistic and the young person and / or parents / caregivers do not, or vice versa, then it is important that the process proceeds in relation to re-examining the information gathered and further considering whether any key information is missing. It may also be the case that further exploration of Autistic experiences and how they align or don't align with a young person's experiences may need to take place. This process should continue until a shared understanding is arrived at.

In approaching the outcome session, parents / caregivers often query whether their young person should attend the outcome session. It is always the case that a young person is very welcome to attend the outcome session if they would like to. This is about them and their neurology, and they should be part of the discussion and conversation. If a young person is going to attend, it is important that their communication needs are met within the session and that they have access to their preferred method of communication. Many young people choose to be at the session but state that they do not wish to speak. It is important that they are aware that they may communicate if they wish and that they do not have to if they don't wish to.

Learning about their neurotype is a powerful and important experience for most young people. It may be the first time that they have had an opportunity to understand themselves and their experience of the world. Being excluded from this can be detrimental to their narrative, but being involved in it can support the cultivation of their positive sense of identity.

Where possible, it is helpful to offer different options for the outcome session in terms of whether it happens remotely, in the young person's own home or in the clinic setting. Offering a choice of these options to a young person and their parents / caregivers empowers them to decide what would be most comfortable for them in discussions about the process they have undertaken. Being at home (whether the session happens there or happens remotely) offers the option for the young person and their family to control their environment and to maintain their physical comfort. It also means that they are in their familiar and comfortable surroundings immediately following the session, which would be beneficial to most. Ultimately, the decision on where to hold the session should be shared and with different options available.

15.5 Supporting Children and Young People Who Do Not Wish to Attend

For most children and young people and their parents / caregivers, undertaking the process of exploring their neurotype is a very welcome venture of validation and understanding. For some, however, they find the opportunity exceptionally overwhelming and challenging. Some young people express that they do not wish to 'be Autistic' and that they do not wish to explore their experience of the world, even though it may be clear to those around them that their experience of the world is different to the neurotypical majority. It may be the case that the young person has a limited understanding of the Autistic neurotype, or maybe their peer group have incorrectly made assertions about Autistic ways of being through their own lack of knowledge or guidance.

In supporting all young people where the possibility that they may be Autistic has been raised, it is important to maintain respect and collaboration regardless of whether they are open to exploring their neurology or not. For those who are reluctant to engage in the process or who have expressed that they do not wish to engage in it, creating a safe space where they can explore their fears and reluctance prior to engaging in any further process is a helpful approach. It often takes time to establish trust and safety in order to support a young person with exploring their fears, but this can be a key support in progressing with supporting their understanding of their identity. On occasion, the process of exploring their reluctance might be better undertaken in the home environment via parents / caregivers with support from afar from professionals, as perhaps the prospect of meeting any professional for any reason is overwhelming.

For some young people who are reluctant to engage in a process of exploring their neurology, a more helpful place to begin the process might be in offering support with their needs rather than a process to understand where their needs come from. Often, the needs of young people centre around their sensory regulation or their mental health. Offering therapeutic support in relation to these areas that is informed by a neurodiversity affirmative framework can be a gentler introduction to the process of exploring their neurology, while also offering support with their needs.

15.6 Involvement of Multi-Disciplinary Team Professionals

Current best practice guidelines broadly agree that there should be a range of different professionals involved in the process of exploring Autistic identity. The NICE guidelines (UK) state that the core group of professionals who should be involved in the process are a paediatrician and / or child and adolescent psychiatrist, a speech and language therapist, and a psychologist. The SIGN guidelines (Scotland) state that the process should involve a 'multi-disciplinary team', but do not specify the disciplines that should be involved. The Australian best practice guidelines specify that the lead practitioner in carrying out this piece should either be a medical practitioner (either in the field of community child health, general paediatrics, psychiatry or neurology; or who has at least six years of relevant experience in terms of working with Autistic young people), or a psychologist (clinical, educational / developmental or neuropsychologist). At least one additional practitioner should be included, who can be another medical practitioner with the relevant experience as specified above, an occupational therapist, a psychologist or a speech pathologist.

In practice, it is essential that all practitioners working as part of a team have a deep understanding of neuro-affirmative practice. In our experience, the most beneficial core group of practitioners to be involved in the process include a psychologist or psychiatrist, a speech and language therapist and an occupational therapist. Not only are the core areas of work for these disciplines (i.e., mental health, communication, regulation and occupation) central in identifying Autistic experiences, these are also the disciplines that are likely to be required following the piece in terms of support. These disciplines can therefore give tailored input during the process that provides the foundation for support following the piece. Other practitioners are also helpful, and the practitioners that provide the most helpful support will of course be bespoke to the child / young person in terms of their needs.

15.7 Cognitive and Other Assessments

There is a general consensus amongst best practice guidelines across the world that within a best practice process, consideration needs to be given to alternative explanations for a child's experience of the world, and also to co-occurring conditions. None of the current best practice guidelines specify that any particular assessments outside of the core exploration of Autistic identity need to take place as standard as part of a 'diagnostic process', but they all clearly state that they may be needed and should be considered in terms of each child's individual needs.

The NICE guidelines (UK) recommend that differential explanations are considered along with the possibility of co-occurring conditions. The guidelines advise that consideration should be given to whether specific additional assessments are needed in terms of language, intellectual disability, developmental coordination disorder, mental health and ADHD; without any particular additional assessment being specified.

Australian best practice guidelines state that it is good practice to obtain information from a recently completed Assessment of Functioning and Medical Evaluation for the purpose of informing the outcome of the exploration piece. The guidelines state that other sources of information (e.g., allied health practitioner reports, school reports and information provided formally and informally by others) should also be considered within the core piece. They don't, however, state that any additional assessments should be undertaken as part of a core process.

The SIGN guidelines (Scotland) state that a cognitive assessment will not assist in identifying whether a child is Autistic or not but may be helpful in establishing a profile of strengths and areas of need and in whether a child has a co-occurring intellectual disability. The SIGN guidelines state that occupational therapy and physiotherapy assessments should be considered where relevant, along with biomedical investigations, and that all Autistic children should have an evaluation of their communication skills with a speech and language therapist. They also state that Autistic children may also have additional developmental differences, medical needs and emotional support needs and may need access to a range of therapeutic assessments and supports following their initial piece exploring their Autistic neurology.

In Ireland, the PSI (2022) guidelines state that consideration should be given to alternative explanations for a child's presentation, including 'differential diagnosis and psychosocial influences'. The guidelines state that 'Consideration should be given to other conditions as relevant, including mental health, intellectual disability, stress and / or trauma, motor disorders, sensory impairments, behavioural issues, neurological conditions, and genetic conditions' (p. 18).

USA guidelines vary according to state, and are therefore not explored in full within this book. Clinicians seeking information about the addition of cognitive assessments to their autism identification process should seek out individual state guidelines.

In practice, cognitive assessments are broadly speaking unnecessary in establishing whether a young person is Autistic or not. Most often, it can be determined clearly without undertaking other formal assessments whether a young person's experiences align with Autistic experiences and whether or not it is likely that there may be other aspects to consider. This is with the exception of a circumstance where it is unclear whether a young person's experiences of the world may be linked to their level of cognitive ability, and it isn't clear that their experiences are related to Autistic ways of being. Most often, however, a cognitive assessment provides information about strengths and needs in terms of learning, and it also allows for additional time to be spent with a young person, which may be helpful in learning about their experiences of the world. However, it also must be considered that additional assessments can be very stressful for many young people as they occur in unfamiliar settings and they have standardised components which may be challenging for many to engage in. It is absolutely better practice for cognitive assessments to be considered only as necessary, and not to be necessary as standard within an exploration process.

In terms of other assessments, e.g., assessments of communication, sensory experiences, motor skills, mental health etc., information from previous assessments carried out can be exceptionally helpful in learning about a young person's development and experiences over time. Where these are available, they need to be considered, however it should always be the case that a young person's and their parent's / caregiver's feedback should be sought as to whether they felt previous assessments were a reliable or valid assessment of their experiences at that time or not.

15.8 Reports and Other Documentation

When considering reports and other documentation following an exploration piece with a young person and their family, the same principles of respect and collaboration that were central to the exploration piece still apply. Documentation that will be required should be discussed with young people (where possible) and their parents / caregivers and should be finalised collaboratively. Reports need to be respectful of gender identity, and be written using the correct pronouns. In collaboration with a young person and their caregivers, where gender identity is still being explored, it can be helpful to offer the option of issuing two sets of documentation – one set in the young person's legal name and one set in the name that they use. This allows for flexibility in the future in terms of gender identity, while also giving access to supports at the current time.

For most young people, a detailed report is required in order for them to access services, educational supports and state supports. Alongside a detailed report, the following documentation is also helpful and often necessary:

- A short letter stating that a young person has undergone an assessment process, and that the outcome is that they are Autistic. This letter is important as it can be used as 'proof' or 'evidence' where a young person or their parents / caregivers do not wish to submit their detailed report.

- For younger children, a version of the report that is just for them and that explains the concepts in the main report in a way that they can understand. This is an important document as it supports the cultivation of a positive Autistic identity, and also it ensures that a young person has a good understanding of what was learned during the process of the piece and what it means.

- For older children and adolescents who have the capacity to read and understand their main report, a separate letter explaining the piece that was undertaken, their Autistic identity and the next steps is helpful in finalising the piece.

- Many young people may be eligible to apply for state benefits. Letters supporting their application can be helpful and should be provided.

CHILD'S VOICE

ERIN, AGE 10

- Was there anything we did that made it easier for you to come to meet us?

  Nice messages to my Mum about me and looking forward to talking about Harry Potter.

- What did you enjoy when you had your session with us?

  Talking about Harry Potter, and playing with the fidget toys. I liked the quietness.

- Was there anything you did not enjoy about your session?

  Getting lost on the way to the office and Mum was stressed out.

- How did you feel when you learned that you are Autistic?

  I felt fine.

- Was there anything we did that helped you when you first learned this?

  Being given time to tell people when I wanted to.

- What did you think about your report or letter that we sent you?

  Fine, it makes me know that I am Autistic. I liked to hear it all.

- For any other child who is coming to meet with us, how would you describe to them what they should expect when they meet us?

> A 45-minute long session that is not scary.

- What would you say to any other child who is worried about coming to meet with us?

> You might be nervous to meet new people and not want to go but it is not bad as they are kind and happy.

15.8.1 Main Report

When writing the main report following an exploratory piece with a young person and their family, it is important to co-write the report and to collaborate when considering the recommendations from the piece. There are some helpful guides to writing neurodiversity affirmative reports (e.g., Day et al., 2024). The report needs to foster a positive Autistic identity, and the language within it should be validating, affirmative and non-judgemental. It is important that the report reflects a young person's strengths and abilities as much as it needs to outline what they need support with. Goals should be co-created and bespoke to the young person and their specific needs. Young people should have input into what the recommendations are, specifically in terms of what is important to them and what would feel comfortable to them. The report also needs to signpost a young person and their family to how they can connect with the Autistic community, as well as promoting self-advocacy and autonomy.

> ### Reflection Point
>
> The report that is written upon concluding the piece is going to last forever. It is essential for those writing the report to consider whether they feel comfortable with the young person reading it now or in the future, and whether it supports the young person to feel empowered in the future. Clinicians need to reflect on whether the report has acknowledged a young person's strengths as well as their support needs, and how they would feel if the report was being written about them or a person they care about.

Reports should not be pathologising or traumatising for a young person or their family to read. They should not include any normative or curative goals and should not have any recommendations relating to compliance-based behavioural interventions or neurotypical-only social skills training. Using compliance-based behavioural interventions teaches children to ignore their needs and to comply with others' wishes. They promote masking and do not support autonomy and self-advocacy. They increase a young person's vulnerability. Similarly, neurotypical-only social skills training is problematic as it teaches Autistic children to behave in neurotypical ways, which invalidates their neurology and experience of the world and it promotes masking. There are many excellent Autistic-led social skills resources that promote a strong Autistic identity while supporting children and young people to navigate the neurotypical social world, e.g., Konnect by Ausome Training, Neurobears etc.

> It is essential that all reports are flexible and reflect that a young person's needs will change over time and will need to be re-considered. This review does not have to happen formally but should be advocated for within the report in terms of the adults in a child's life understanding that their strengths and needs will change. Supports offered should reflect this, and should always be accessed or implemented in collaboration with a young person and their family.

15.8.2 Short Letter Stating the Outcome

There can be many reasons why a young person or their family do not wish to submit their full detailed report to a service or support they are trying to access. It may be that the report contains sensitive information that they do not wish to share, or it may be the case that the report was written a long time ago and doesn't reflect their current needs. It is also the case that there are many supports and services that can be accessed, e.g., assistance when travelling through an airport, without the need to share detailed information. To this end, it is very helpful to provide a short letter of just a few lines which states that a young person has undergone an exploratory process in line with best practice criteria, and that the outcome is that they are Autistic.

15.8.3 Report for Younger Children

Younger children can of course read their main report, but depending on their age and ability they may not have the capacity to read and / or understand this document until they are older. Given that the piece is about them, it is essential that at the outcome stage they have a document that helps them to understand the piece that was undertaken, what was learned about them, what their strengths are, what their needs are and what the outcome is. If they are Autistic, then explaining what this means and how it was learned about them is crucial. Having a version of their main report that is just for them is a powerful and empowering experience for most young children. It supports their development of a positive Autistic identity, and it is respectful to their needs.

15.8.4 Letter for Older Children and Adolescents

Just like younger children, older children and adolescents can read their main report and are more likely to have capacity to understand it. However, for them, even though they can read and understand their main report, it is very helpful to the cultivation of their Autistic identity to have a letter that affirms their Autistic identity and that explains about neurodiversity. This letter can also emphasise their strengths and abilities as well as the adjustments that they may need and their rights to those adjustments.

15.8.5 Letters in Support of State Benefits Applications / Educational Support

As stated above, depending on the country they live in, many Autistic young people may be eligible to apply for specific supports from their government / state. At the time of writing, state systems are generally pathologising in their view of Autistic ways of being, and the application process for welfare supports is often lengthy, detailed and deficit-focused. It is important to prepare families for the likelihood that the state body application process will not be neurodiversity affirmative. They will also need to know that there may need to be particularly pathologising wording in terms of any letter in support of an application. Informing families that the letter will be very different to their young person's neurodiversity affirmative report and that the letter does not reflect the whole view of their young person's experience of the world is essential.

In different jurisdictions it is important to be aware that there are different systems in terms of supports that young Autistic people can access. In many areas, these systems are not neuro-affirmative, and it is likely that in order to access different supports particular wording, recommendations or statements need to be made. Often, these need to be framed from a deficit perspective in order to satisfy the requirements of the service gatekeepers. Clinicians need to be aware of local requirements in their own particular area, and of the balance that is required in terms of fostering a positive Autistic identity and the need to access supports.

15.9 Conclusion

In this chapter we explained how clinicians can undertake a neurodiversity affirmative autism identification process with children of all ages and varying communication preferences, using the core aspects of collaboration, respect, transparency and flexibility. To do this necessitates professionals creating a safe space to explore a child's inner experience, gathering information collaboratively about their inner experience, gathering other vital information, mapping the relevant information onto a re-framed criteria document, and finally supporting the child and their family to make sense of their experiences. In the next chapter, we provide comprehensive practical advice around post-identification support.

CHAPTER 16

Post-Identification Support Recommendations

16.1 Introduction

This chapter offers a comprehensive guide for supporting Autistic young people following identification of Autistic identity, including clinical-, school- and home-based recommendations. The information and resources presented aim to help clinicians to support parents / caregivers and educators in better understanding and supporting the needs of Autistic young people. By implementing the recommendations and resources provided, we aim to foster a more inclusive and supportive environment for Autistic young people to thrive.

First and foremost, we recommend that the young person connect with their Autistic peers. The importance of building a community with people who share similar neurological experiences can't be overstated. The young person will discover that their communication style and way of experiencing and existing in the world are no longer seen as atypical or deficient, unlike what they might likely experience when spending most of their time with non-autistic peers. They will gain from being around like-minded peers who accept them, which, in turn, will help them to learn to accept themselves. For older children and young people who have adapted to mask their true selves, this will offer an opportunity to discover that it can be safe to be more authentically themselves. This is a vital step in developing their self-advocacy skills and enhancing their self-esteem with a positive Autistic identity.

Next, we strongly recommend that family members deepen their understanding of Autistic culture, ways of being and interpreting the world (see Chapter 6). It's likely that one or both parents, as well as multiple extended family members, will recognise many of their own neurodivergent traits when they learn more contemporary understandings of Autistic neurology, particularly when they become aware of Autistic-led 'insider' research as opposed to the older theories which were dominated by non-autistic people, and this is to be welcomed. Teachers, therapists and all others involved with the young person should ideally be educated on the progressive understanding of neurodiversity and Autistic neurology. The goal is to foster a culture of acceptance and understanding, while recognising the multi-dimensional, dynamic and temporally fluid challenges that accompany being Autistic in a predominantly neurotypical world (see Chapman, 2023).

16.2 Within a Neuro-Affirming Framework, Is Support Needed?

Prior to discussing clinical-, school- and home-based recommendations, it is important to reflect on what we mean when we discuss support from a neurodiversity-informed perspective. If a neuro-affirming approach to neurodivergence, specifically Autistic neurodivergence, is to appreciate that Autistic people are not deficient in any way but simply part of the natural variety of people, then does it follow that support is actually needed?

What do we mean by support?

Support is a process of providing assistance and resources to a person in order to help them adapt to their challenges, achieve their goals and improve their quality of life. Support can be provided in various settings and domains, such as education, healthcare, employment or social relationships. However, support can also have negative impacts on Autistic young people, such as infantilising, controlling or isolating them, or depriving them of their rights and choices.

The Autistic young person should always be at the centre of any support considerations. Their needs and rights should be prioritised. Historically, support recommendations adopted a deficit model, focused on changing the child to fit the environment, rather than adapting the environment to fit the child. Within a neurodiversity affirming framework, our primary focus is to uphold the young person's right to authenticity, ensuring they can remain true to themselves rather than attempting to teach them to conform to conventional, neuro-normative concepts of well-being.

In a world that has been designed primarily for non-autistic people, we argue that support to live an authentic empowered life must focus on adapting the environment, not the young person. Keeping our support focus rooted in Beardon's (2020) Autism + Environment = Outcome model, we can empower families and young people to flourish.

Support, therefore, should be provided with caution and care, and always with the following principles in mind:

- Support should be provided with the consent and involvement of the Autistic young person, and their parents / caregivers. They should be informed about the options, benefits and risks of the support, and their views and preferences should be respected and valued.

- Support should be provided by professionals, peers or mentors who are ideally Autistic themselves, or at least have cultural competence, knowledge and training on the neurodiversity affirming approach, and who adopt a respectful and empathetic attitude towards Autistic young people. This is in line with Damian Milton's (2012) double empathy theory (see Section 6.10). By having support provided by those who share the same neurology, Autistic young people may find it easier to relate, communicate and feel understood, leading to more effective and meaningful support (Milton, 2012). Coercive or aversive techniques should never be employed, instead using positive and collaborative approaches to facilitate the learning and development of Autistic young people.

- Support should be provided using strategies and interventions that are appropriate and effective for Autistic young people, and that enhance their strengths and interests, as well as recognising and validating their challenges and needs. They should avoid using one-size-fits-all or standardised programmes, and instead use individualised and flexible plans that suit the Autistic young person's personality, communication preferences and pace.

- Support should ideally be provided in a context that is comfortable and familiar for the Autistic young person, and that maximises the opportunities and resources that they have. They should be given enough autonomy, freedom and dignity to make their own decisions and mistakes, and be supported to use their preferred modes of communication and expression.

- Support should be provided for the benefit and empowerment of the Autistic young person, and never for the convenience of others. Support goals should be decided in collaboration with the young person themselves, taking into account their unique sensory needs and social communication style.

- For Autistic young people with additional learning disabilities who may require assistance from parents / caregivers in expressing their preferences, it is essential to ensure that the parents / caregivers are well-informed about the neurodiversity affirming approach and can effectively advocate in collaboration with the young person. Parents / caregivers should involve the young person in the decision-making process to the fullest extent possible and respect their autonomy. For those with profound and multiple learning disabilities (or other complex needs) a multi-agency approach with any medical professionals will need to be in place. It is essential to validate the parents / caregivers' voice and deep understanding of their child. They will be best placed to understand the more nuanced ways their child communicates their preferences and engagement levels. Guardians' opinions will be invaluable in providing information for professionals so a suitable plan can be formed that honours the importance of feeling safe, creating a sense of belonging with the young person's parents / caregivers and the world around them.

- Greatest care should be taken to always seek to embrace the young person's authentic self rather than change their essential way of being.

- Support outcomes should be evaluated based on the Autistic young person's satisfaction, happiness and well-being, as determined by themselves, and not by the expectations or standards of others. For those with learning disabilities, this may involve using alternative methods of communication to gauge their contentment and progress.

- Ensure parents / caregivers are validated and that neuro-affirming parenting styles are supported.

- As highlighted by McGreevy et al. (2024), an experience-sensitive approach is essential, taking into account the unique perspectives and experiences of Autistic children and young people. This approach emphasises the importance of humanising care, being with people, creating a sense of togetherness, valuing insiderness, helping people make sense of their personal journey, promoting agency and celebrating uniqueness so we can adapt support accordingly.

16.3 Educational and School-Based Recommendations

Anxiety-based school avoidance, and indeed just a general unhappiness and overwhelm in a traditional school environment that does not match their neurology or meet their needs, is very common for Autistic young people. As clinicians, it is our role to make recommendations in reports that target education in order to advocate for schools to change practices in order to support their Autistic students better. In fact, unhappiness in school and a lack of adequate support there is frequently one of the main drivers for parents / caregivers wanting to explore an Autistic identity for their child.

In these recommendations, we draw upon our professional experience with schools and families, as well as lived experience as parents of Autistic young people, and the invaluable work of organisations like The Autistic Girls Network, which provides support and resources for Autistic girls and women; Square Pegs, which advocates for children with school-based anxiety; and Not Fine in School, which supports families of children who experience barriers in attending school. These organisations offer unique insights and expertise that inform our guidance in relation to education.

The recommendations provided here can and should be adapted for individual young people, although many can be applied universally:

1. **Language**

   All school staff need to be educated in using the identity-first and respectful language chosen by the Autistic community. The language appropriate to use changes over time and so it is important staff know that they need to keep continuously up to date in this area by listening to Autistic people.

2. **Learning about neurodiversity in schools**

   It is vitally important that learning about neurodiversity and neurodivergence is part of the general curriculum for all children in school and this should be recommended in reports. Currently available and recommended is the LEANS programme (for children 8–11) which is a free curriculum (developed in the UK) introducing pupils to the concept of neurodiversity, and helping them explore how it impacts experiences at school.

3. Presenting differently at home and school

All children are unique and have a range of needs, but the needs of neurodivergent children are often misunderstood for a variety of reasons. One common issue is the disparity between a young person's presentation at school and at home. When parents / caregivers inform teachers of the struggles their children face, teachers may respond with, 'they seem fine in school' as they often don't see beyond the young person's masking behaviours. Therefore, it is vital that education staff are educated about this disparity and why it occurs. They need to know that this difference in presentation is in fact very common and why, and it is our job as clinicians to ensure that this information is provided clearly and authoritatively. Otherwise, this disconnect can lead to a breakdown in the relationship between the school and the home environment, resulting in the young person not receiving the support they need. In many cases, guardians' concerns may be dismissed, and in the worst-case scenario, safeguarding concerns may be raised, questioning parenting skills (Murphy, 2021; also see Chapter 10). These situations can further strain the relationship between the school and the family, making it difficult for the student to receive the appropriate support and understanding they need to thrive.

4. Home / school communication

A variety of ways for parents / caregivers to communicate with the school need to be provided, in ways that suit both the parents / caregivers and teachers to ensure success. This will greatly help build relationships and help bridge the empathy gap. This is especially relevant for secondary school-age children, where there is often less guardian face-to-face communication, and alternative methods will likely be needed to establish and maintain a positive home–school relationship (Honeybourne, 2018). A strong home–school relationship is important for all students; however, it can become particularly crucial for Autistic students at key transitional points such as starting school, and changing year groups or school settings. Increased communication between home and school is vital during these times.

5. Homework

In our experience as clinicians undertaking both assessment and therapeutic work, the issue of homework for both young people and parents / caregivers is an area that can cause the most distress and disruption to the daily life and well-being of the family. This area is also in our experience something that teachers and schools are extremely reluctant to be flexible about, or provide the necessary disability accommodations needed.

The negative impact of homework for Autistic and otherwise neurodivergent children cannot be over-stated. Resentment, dysregulation, overthinking and dread related to homework are all common and impact not only on the Autistic child and their parent but also their siblings, who after school, instead of experiencing a happy relaxed home environment and a calm guardian, are surrounded by daily homework 'battles' and overwhelmed family members.

As stated previously, the sensory impact of the busy, loud school environment cannot be overestimated for Autistic young people. When they come home they quite vitally need down time and quiet time in order to regulate their nervous systems. Allowing this gives them time to recharge and regulate in order to build 'strength' and gain 'spoons' to face the next day in school. And yet instead, they are expected to sit once again and engage in more work that they often find difficult. In our experience, the disability adjustment of allowing no homework can mean the difference between a happy Autistic child going to school and a permanently school-refusing child.

Teachers and schools that are highly resistant to implementing the disability accommodation of no homework could be encouraged to instead provide collaboratively engaging, self-directed after-school tasks that tap into the child's personal interests and need for both autonomy and recharging.

6. Key members of staff

Young people need to have a say in who they feel safe and most comfortable being with in schools. Effective co-regulation will not be able to take place unless there is a sense of shared belonging and a genuine feeling of trust and that the person 'gets them'. Although unfortunately often not possible in practice, ideally offering a choice of a few key members of staff, rather than just allocating someone whom a student may not feel comfortable with, will help to ensure that students have a sense of autonomy and feel safe in their setting (Bagley, 2022, Chapter 11, cited in Morgan & Costello, 2022).

Staff must understand that just because an Autistic student may be able to talk verbally that does not mean it is always in their best interests or manageable for them. Balancing the various sensory and environmental demands of a school setting while simultaneously trying to communicate effectively can be incredibly challenging for an Autistic person. This overwhelming combination of factors often leads to intense sensory overload, which may result in meltdowns or shutdowns. Knowing a key member of staff cares, understands their communication preferences and is there for them can make all the difference to a young person feeling like they are able to even attend school. Having check-in points with a trusted adult can provide space to just have time to breath, co-regulate and navigate potentially difficult lessons to work around any potential triggers and avoid a crisis point.

Scheduling regular check-ins throughout the day or week with a trusted adult can provide an Autistic young person with the necessary space and time to breathe and co-regulate. These check-ins serve as valuable opportunities to focus on the individual's strengths, share moments of joy and success, and create a safe space to navigate potentially difficult situations.

7. Support plans

Having a support plan that is regularly reviewed and (vitally!) developed in conjunction with the young person, parents / caregivers and teachers is a must. However, different countries and jurisdictions will have different rules governing whose responsibility it is to ensure that a school delivers any additional provision that a child needs and how this is implemented and reviewed, and there are often multi-level systems involved. In an idea world, it should also be the responsibility of all staff to ensure that children's needs are met and support plans are implemented and regularly evaluated. It is vital to consider how information is shared across the setting and that documents are not merely tokenistic.

8. Visual timetables

While not all Autistic students think visually, a visual timetable adapted to how they process information may be helpful, and having options for alternative ways of communicating will help Autistic students manage their energy. It is important to note though that timetables can be very stressful for young people with anxiety-based demand avoidance who can see them as a demand. In addition, the timetable needs to be worked out with the child as to what works for them. Many children do not want, for example, a timetable on their desk which differentiates them from their classmates.

9. **Multi-modal assessment**

Assessments in an education environment should have the option of being multi-modal. This may include combinations of spoken and written work, drawings, photos, videos, the use of technology, text-to-speech, reader pens and other devices and forms of communication depending on the young person and subject. A flexible approach and extra time may be needed for this to be used effectively across the day and to ensure consistency of provision and access across all subjects. This could be especially beneficial for those with learning disabilities and non-speaking students with profound and multiple learning disabilities.

10. **Extra time in exams**

To support Autistic young people's neurology, it is essential that they are provided with extra time for exams and alternative arrangements for environmental considerations, such as taking exams in a small, quiet, familiar room instead of a large hall. Additional support, including equipment, scribes, technology and sensory tools, should also be recommended as needed to ensure equitable access to assessment. However, while these should be recommended in every report, the unfortunate reality of the situation is that there can often be wider systemic barriers to these vital things being provided. However, they should still be advocated for strongly.

11. **Educate about masking and burnout**

Many Autistic students mask at school and it is essential for teachers to consider the impact of Autistic masking and ways for students to feel safe in school to reduce the risk of Autistic burnout and other mental health conditions (Pearson & Rose, 2023). It is better to spend time ensuring students feel a sense of safety, agency and autonomy over their learning space and to be able to plan together before events rather than using the same amount of time, or more, trying to crisis manage ineffective preparation when a student's needs have not been met.

12. **School events**

In our experience, it is often a deeply held belief by most school staff that all children should attend all big school events, and typically this comes from a very well-meaning place. However, it is important to give students input and autonomy over how they wish to be involved in school events, especially large group events such as assemblies that may cause additional sensory and social anxiety. Young people generally want to be included, but it is important to consider how their inclusion looks so their needs are met. Autistic young people should not be coerced into joining in roles and events they may feel uncomfortable with, building confidence and resilience is not achieved by young people feeling forced into situations in states of high anxiety. These events will need to be carefully planned with the students, providing adequate time to prepare and supportive cushioning on either side of the event to help them prepare and regulate. This approach ensures that the experiences can be enjoyable in ways that suit their needs, however that may look.

13. Multi-modal and adapted learning opportunities

Learning opportunities in the classroom should ideally be multi-modal and adapted to suit the needs of the young person. If it is possible to work with the teachers on practical ways that they can do this without creating significant amounts of extra work for them this would be very helpful also, as teachers can become overwhelmed at the thought of the additional work involved. Some empathy for teachers in this area goes a long way in terms of getting them on board with trying new ways to teach.

The following can be considered:

- When planning lessons, offering multi-modal learning opportunities by providing written instructions / outlines / notes to accompany any verbal information.

- Breaking down tasks into more manageable chunks or giving extra processing time.

- Providing access to information prior to a lesson, either with their teacher or another familiar member of staff, to help reduce any anxiety over the unknown.

- Ensuring students' physical and sensory needs are met in the classroom (are they happy where they are seated, are they positioned near a door / window / access to the toilet and drinks when needed?).

- Ensuring resources / sensory tools and any AAC are set up as needed for the specific student and lesson content.

- Small-group instruction.

- One-to-one support.

- Writing or text-based communication between teacher and student.

- Opportunities for peer-to-peer support (this can be especially beneficial for those with similar needs and experiences).

14. A total communication approach

If children do not have a means of effectively understanding their teacher and are unable to express themselves in a way that meets their needs, then learning cannot take place and no support can be provided.

A total communication approach (speech / text / pictures / symbols / signing) is therefore recommended for all schools, and across the whole school so that everyone feels and is included (Mueller, 2021); this should not be exclusively for Autistic classrooms or only if there is a child with a communication or learning disability. Using this approach means that everyone benefits from a combination of different ways to access communication (of course including AAC). Access to communication needs to be in place and accessible throughout the day, including break times.

In addition, as Lewis (2009), states, it is valuable to consider that 'listening better includes hearing silence'. We must not try to force students to speak or communicate when they feel unable, we need to be compassionate and understand that their internal world may be very intense and they may need longer to process (Davis et al., 2000). Conversations and work may need to be revisited at a more appropriate time and with advice from a neurodiversity affirming speech and language therapist.

15. Inclusion strategies

Depending on the individual child's profile, it will be crucial to consider different inclusion strategies, such as peer friendship programs where students look out for one another at unstructured times such as lunch. In some circumstances, it may be necessary to watch out for bullying and social isolation and provide additional support. However, it will also be important to check in with the child to make sure that they are not choosing to be alone because they need or want alone time. Peer friendship programmes need to be managed in a neurodiversity affirmative way, with all children being educated about all neurotypes, including being neurotypical and that real friendships are encouraged as opposed to the Autistic child being 'minded' by other well-meaning children.

16. Interest groups

Setting up interest groups (depending on the actual interests / passions of the young people) in schools can be a good way for Autistic children to feel a sense of belonging, share their joy and join in alongside others (Wood, 2019b). It may also be worth considering the benefits of starting a neurodiversity network / peer group for young people to get to know each other. Mixing with other neurodivergent children is vital, one example being the increased options for parallel play which alongside being beneficial is generally a more natural and less demanding way of socialising and a great way of embracing neurodivergent communication and socialisation (Murphy, 2023; Payne, 2022).

17. The school sensory environment

It is vital to consider how the sensory system impacts young Autistic students in school, as this is often one of the main reasons why Autistic young people find school so challenging. As previously mentioned, getting the views from parents / caregivers and the students themselves is imperative as part of this process. See Chapter 11 for a detailed explanation of doing a sensory audit of a clinical environment which can be adapted to be used in a school environment.

Luke Beardon's (2020) work demonstrates the importance of understanding the impact the environment can have on Autistic people in his equation: 'Autism + Environment = Outcome'. If the environment meets children's needs, they will be able to have good educational, personal, social and mental health outcomes.

Environmental and sensory considerations should include a flexible school uniform policy, using a different school alarm or music system for lesson changes, having a more relaxed start or end to the day, or quieter entrance and exit routes for those who prefer to avoid crowds and noise. A student will not be able to learn effectively if the texture of their uniform is causing extreme discomfort or pain, and if each time the alarm goes off, they become dysregulated. Keeping routines and classroom layouts as consistent as possible will benefit most Autistic students, as will being mindful not to change seating arrangements without prior preparation when it can be helped (Beardon, 2022).

18. Teach educators about monotropism

Most Autistic / ADHD people learn monotropically (Garau, 2023; see Sections 6.12 and 7.5). We want people to embrace authentic Autistic ways of being – working with the flow of monotropic processing, not against it, which might end up with someone 'stuck' and in a state of Autistic inertia which could lead to burnout, affecting executive functioning further. Many people are not even aware that inertia can be 'the single biggest problem' (Murray, 2017) arising from being Autistic, creating a life that is 'a lot smaller and less than it should be' (Buckle et al., 2021, p. 17). Having a greater understanding of the impact of sensory processing, monotropism and Autistic inertia will be essential in supporting young people with their education.

Having a narrow curriculum goes against the flow of an Autistic person's organic way of learning. However, a busy school timetable with frequent changes of staff, subject matter, teaching style, changes of room and the different expectations of each lesson can be exhausting for Autistic students and affect them more intensely than others. Dividing attention between multiple cognitive and sensory channels through the day means Autistic children have to constantly break up their natural attention flow and use a lot of energy to realign themselves onto their next task.

Minimising interruptions and distractions so students can easily enter and remain in a productive flow state will be helpful. It will also be helpful to have resources to support states of Autistic inertia which may be magnified by monotropism, and to have visual or auditory reminders to start and end tasks or stay on task (Edgar, 2024; Lawson, 2011; Murray, 2019). These will need to be developed with the young person so they are involved in the process (as described earlier in this chapter) and are happy with the plan. Teachers will need to ensure that the support resources, such as timers and staff, do not end up disrupting the very flow states they were intended to help (Wood, 2019b).

Enabling Autistic students to embrace their natural monotropic way of being may require some creativity on the part of the teacher to weave in more topic-based learning that can be easily adapted to lean into Autistic students' strengths and interests so they can enter a flow state (McDonnell & Milton, 2014; Wood, 2019a, 2019b). The research by Wood (2019b) highlights the wonderful benefits of developing a deeper understanding of monotropism to support Autistic children's extracurricular activities. Setting up interest-led groups in school could help peer relationships and has positively impacted their communication skills. Inclusive interest-led activities alongside like-minded peers will likely be more beneficial than withdrawing a child from a lesson for 1:1 talking therapy (unless that is what the young person wants).

Teachers versed in monotropism theory will understand the importance of providing flexibility and more time between subject changes to allow for a smoother transition between attention tunnels. It takes enormous energy and effort for Autistic people to change tasks and move from one attention tunnel to another; it is important to try and keep a flow state flowing (Rapaport et al., 2023). If there are constant obstacles and barriers to learning throughout the day breaking up flow, it will cause dysregulation and be a very difficult, exhausting environment to navigate. Unexpected changes to routine, and needing to switch tasks frequently without enough time to rest and recover can lead to Autistic burnout (Murray, 2023). It can help having access to movement and sensory tools that Autistic young people feel safe enough to use without fear of being judged by others. Stimming and movement can help with self-regulation and remaining in a flow state to help maintain concentration in a lesson, and can also help with transitioning between different spaces / subjects / activities in school (Murray, 2023).

19. Self-directed learning

Autistic students often learn best through self-directed learning as that meets their monotropic learning style (Fisher, 2023; Wood, 2019a). Self-directed learning allows autonomy over the direction their interests take them. This has shown to not only be a way to learn more effectively in the moment, but also enables students to retain more of what they have learned (Seli et al., 2015). Encourage teachers to include as much self-directed learning as possible in a child's curriculum.

20. Detentions and exclusions

Some schools have rigid detention and exclusion policies that discriminate against neurodivergent neurology. It is worth considering the value and aim of detentions and exclusions for any student but it could be especially harmful for Autistic students if it is caused by executive function or processing issues, e.g., forgetting equipment, being late, being unable to find the class, being slow to get changed, being slow to form a group and other factors that may be impacted upon by unmet needs in the environment. A review of school policies in this area is recommended if needed.

21. Educational placement

For many Autistic children, over time, school environments that do not provide the necessary disability accommodations become too much to bear and are eventually traumatising.

Issues include a lack of understanding of neurodiversity in their peers and teachers, the barriers of an ever-inflexible curriculum and rigid success criteria (Ball, 2003), the ever increased expectations and workload, a tightened curriculum and reduced body autonomy as they are expected to sit at their desks for extended periods (Fisher, Chapter 1, cited in Morgan & Costello, 2022). The rich variety of continuous provision provided in preschool education, including for example the free flow of indoor and outdoor self-directed learning opportunities and different spaces to regulate their sensory systems through various types of play and physical activity, is hindered and often comes to an abrupt end as a child begins primary school, especially in mainstream settings. This puts Autistic children at a greater risk of being in physical, sensory and cognitive dysregulation making it difficult if not impossible to learn. Over time, without the proper support, masking and living in permanent states of dysregulation and constantly wavering between dysregulated states can lead to Autistic burnout and more severe mental health difficulties (Phung et al., 2021), and school will have become a traumatic environment.

Some students may thrive in a mainstream classroom setting with the necessary support and accommodations, while others may require a more specialised environment, such as a dedicated autism class or school. For other young people, even a specialised setting may be too much for them at that particular time. Even with the world's best support staff, the physical school environment may not be the best place for some individuals (Fisher, 2023).

This puts many parents / caregivers in the very difficult position of balancing the need for their child to be educated and their child's mental and physical health.

In an ideal world there would be a range of educational options available to parents / caregivers and young people to meet individual needs. However, in reality (depending on where they live and their individual economic and family circumstances) there are often very few options. Specialised environments for Autistic young people are often scarce and extremely difficult and time-consuming to access. In some regions there may be other options, for example Democratic or Sudbury schools which focus on self-directed learning. Home education or flexible, hybrid or online placements may also be available to some. While many parents / caregivers (who are able to provide it, many aren't) have found that home education was ultimately the only option that kept their child learning and found a supportive network of parents / caregivers to guide them through the process, it is important to be aware that while home education is supported in some jurisdictions, in others it is considered taboo and may even be illegal.

The reality for most families is, that although their child is being traumatised in their educational environment, accessing special, hybrid, home schooling or alternative educational options is more often than not a massively complicated process that is inaccessibly difficult and oftentimes impossible to access.

It is very important for clinicians to be aware of not only the educational options available to a family depending on where they live (e.g., specialised classes and schools, alternative schools, flexible arrangements or home schooling), but also realistically how long the waitlists are, how available the places are, and just how much work the family will need to do even to potentially be in with a chance of accessing such a placement. While it is ultimately individual for every family, trying to fight the systems they are currently in may in the long run be more detrimental than choosing other options (if available). Helping parents / caregivers work this out by providing realistic and up-to-date information is vital.

Families will often need additional documentation advocating for certain educational options (if legal and available) and it is vital this is provided alongside other identification documentation.

If a change of setting is to occur, it will be essential to involve the young person and their family in discussions about any changes in the setting and manage this carefully so the young person feels involved and happy with the alternatives so the change does not negatively impact their mental health. If parents are able to access alternatives such as self-directed home education or hybrid education, it will be essential that they do not try to recreate school at home and that it offers the flexibility and support the child needs and the family can support. See the box below for an educator's view on supporting meaningful connections.

PERSPECTIVES OF AN EDUCATOR: MEANINGFUL CONNECTIONS

HELEN EDGAR (AUTISTIC REALMS)

As a late-identified Autistic person, parent to two neurodivergent children and a teacher with 20 years of experience working in special educational needs settings, I have first-hand experience working with the neurodivergent and disabled community personally and professionally. I can see the consequences of an education system that is currently not meeting the needs of Autistic people. Through my engagement with young people and their families, I feel the harm it is causing to their mental health with many young people unable to attend school due to Autistic burnout. There are enormous systemic issues throughout many countries' education systems making it virtually impossible for many neurodivergent families to access the right kinds of supports or educational placements for their children, leading them to breaking point. There is a massive disconnect between the education and school policy (including prescriptive, rigid curricula) and young people's expansive, fluid needs, which I believe is at the heart of this crisis. Autistic and multiply neurodivergent children need an approach that sways away from the neuro-normative expectations and ideals of how people think students 'should be taught' and the 'best' ways people think they 'should learn'. We must move towards a more flexible, interest-led, strengths-based educational system focusing on differences rather than deficits, that is actually accessible to those who need it.

To achieve this, we need to bridge gaps between professional educators, young people, their families and the neurodivergent community. I believe that by adopting a humanist approach, embodying kindness and compassion, we need to strive towards creating a sense of true belonging in our schools, where all children feel valued and proud of their authentic identities. Young people need to feel safe in their learning environments. They need settings and resources which support them properly, and which nourish their bodies and minds so they are in the best place to engage in learning. These settings need to be actually accessible to those who need them, when they need them. We should work towards igniting curiosity and developing interests and passions so that learning is meaningful and young people are intrinsically motivated. Educators need to be vigilant against imposing neuro-normative ideals, adapting teaching approaches and expectations to their neurodivergent students' needs. For example, providing – within the constraints of having to work within national curricula for those in formal settings that do not foster flexibility in teaching and learning approaches – autonomy over their learning journey and encouraging students to be active participants in all aspects of their lives, however that may look for them individually.

Following a neurodiversity affirmative paradigm enables us to move away from the idea of trying to 'fix children' who are not even broken. I firmly believe an understanding of the theory of monotropism (Murray et al., 2005) will be incredibly beneficial for Autistic / ADHD students, and believe it should be embedded in professional training. Understanding how students' minds and bodies work monotropically will enable educational facilitators to embrace young people's strengths and plan effectively to support their areas of need. A deeper understanding and application of the theory of monotropism will help to enable and maintain a more regulated flow of embodied learning and the potential for greater outcomes. All young people need adults who genuinely care for them and need to feel like they belong and are valued in their community. I don't believe we should aim for our children's needs to be merely 'met'; young people deserve to be able to flourish and become the people they want to be. By committing to the paradigm shift as outlined in this book, I hope it will be the catalyst educators need to re-frame the deficit-based autism narrative still permeating many settings and practices. A starting point in re-storying Autistic experience is thinking carefully about the language and underlying assumptions used in young people's reports and recommendations made, and how these are shared by professionals with families and young people. I hope the positive changes that emerge from this book will radiate outwards so that the systemic barriers facing Autistic young people are reduced and we can celebrate the unique strengths of Autistic young people and support them to thrive.

16.4 Home-Based Support Recommendations

To support families, we recommend gaining a comprehensive understanding of contemporary Autistic theories about Autistic experiences. Learning about how their young person perceives and interacts with the world can help bridge the double empathy gap for allistic parents / caregivers. We suggest providing families with information as outlined in Chapter 6. Additionally, staying up to date by reading first-hand accounts from Autistic people can offer wonderfully insightful perspectives. Encouraging and facilitating opportunities for their young person to spend time and connect with Autistic peers is crucial, as it can provide a sense of belonging, understanding and shared experiences that will be difficult to find in predominantly allistic environments. We highly encourage engaging with books, art and materials that provide the insider's point of view; however, it is critical to remember that each Autistic person's journey is unique and there is no one, singular, universal Autistic experience. When exploring resources, practice critical thinking and be particularly cautious of books and advice that aim to mask Autistic traits or teach a young person how to act as if they were neurotypical. Be alert to the phenomenon of neurodiversity-lite where token gestures towards neuro-affirming language mask the deficit-based approach (Neumeier, 2018). When in doubt, look to the Autistic community for guidance.

We present a brief overview below of our home-based support recommendations. We encourage deeper study on each suggestion and highly recommend seeking out Autistic-led neurodiversity affirming training and resources for further guidance.

16.4.1 Routines and Schedules

It is essential to understand the difference between a routine and a timetable when supporting Autistic individuals. A routine is a set of activities that are regularly followed, providing a sense of structure and familiarity; as such, they can reduce uncertainty and help decrease anxiety. In contrast, a timetable is a specific schedule with set times for each activity. While visual supports such as now / next boards and timers can be very helpful for some Autistic individuals, it is important to recognise that they can also cause anxiety if not used flexibly.

The key to reducing anxiety for many Autistic young people lies in the flexibility around routines. When an Autistic person knows what to expect throughout the day and has enough time to prepare for transitions, they may be able to reduce any anxiety and maintain flow. It is important to keep in mind our understanding of monotropism theory (Murray et al., 2005), which suggests that having more time and flexibility to change attention tunnels, as well as opportunities to regulate between events, can help prevent feelings of overwhelm and manage energy levels. Consistency and predictability within a flexible framework often foster a sense of autonomy.

It is essential to recognise that these strategies must be tailored to the age, cognitive abilities and sensory processing differences of the individual young person. While structure with visual schedules, timers and advance notifications of changes can reduce anxiety for many Autistic young people, there is often a misconception that these tools will reduce anxiety for all Autistic young people.

It is also important to recognise that many neurodivergent young people experience 'time blindness', meaning abstract concepts like time can be challenging for them to use to provide structure. In these cases, linking schedules visually to specific tasks and events can be more helpful than relying solely on time. For example, using images or apps to convey 'first we have breakfast, then we leave for school' might provide more clarity than simply stating '7am breakfast and 7:30am leave for school'. This approach helps bridge the gap between abstract time and concrete activities, making the schedule more understandable and actionable for young people.

▦ PRACTICE POINTS

◇ Meaningful collaboration is essential when supporting Autistic young people. Consider the story of Max, a 15-year-old Autistic young person who struggled with transitions in his daily schedule. Max experienced a deep love of music and often found it deeply challenging to switch off his headphones and transition to the next activity in his daily life. Max's family, with guidance from his support team, recognised the need to co-create a more personalised approach to help him navigate his day.

◇ Through open communication and active listening, they gained valuable insights into Max's perspective. Max, an AAC user, shared that he found comfort in certain songs that helped him feel more relaxed and focused while other songs helped him feel more energised and excited.

◇ Based on this information and the advice from Max's support team, the family worked together to create a customised schedule anchored by

Max's love of music. They developed a visual schedule using musical notes and symbols to represent different activities and with Max's lead, they incorporated a playlist of Max's favourite songs to help him transition more easily between tasks.

◊ Max's lead in the co-creation of his schedule was crucial. He selected the songs for his playlist and matched each one to the relevant activity and helped design the symbols used in his schedule. This collaborative approach not only resulted in a more effective support tool but also empowered Max to take an active role in shaping his daily routine.

◊ The impact of this collaboration was significant. With his personalised schedule, Max reported experiencing greatly reduced anxiety during transitions. His parents found a greater appreciation for his passion for music and Max was able to have ample time to transition his focus of attention from one activity to the next. His sense of autonomy and self-advocacy also improved as his perspective was valued throughout the process.

◊ This example demonstrates the power of meaningful collaboration in supporting Autistic young people. By actively involving Max in the process of developing his schedule, his family created a tailored approach bespoke to his individual needs and preferences, respecting his passions. This approach not only enhanced family harmony and met Max's needs, but it also helped to cultivate a positive sense of agency and empowerment for Max. Moreover, this collaborative process provided his family with a valuable framework for future decision-making, ensuring that Max's voice and unique perspective remain central in all aspects of his life.

It is imperative to respect the deep engagement Autistic people have with their passions. Special interests (SPINs) are often a wellspring of enjoyment, comfort and learning. They provide opportunities for the young person to gain knowledge and skills in areas they are passionate about. Forcing a child to suppress or hide their SPINs to conform to neurotypical standards can be deeply damaging and is strongly discouraged (e.g., Long, 2024; Wood, 2019b).

Thoughtful consideration will have to be given to providing ample opportunity for the young person to engage in their interests on an ongoing daily basis, while balancing their other needs such as hygiene, education, meals and exercise. Autistic people can find their interests so deeply satisfying and sustaining, they may easily enter a flow state while engaged with them (see Rapaport et al., 2023; Thompson-Hodgetts et al., 2023). Transitioning into other activities or thoughts may be deeply challenging, and emotionally or even physically painful. Understanding the concept of monotropism, as discussed in earlier chapters, will help you comprehend the intensity of focus and the significance of engagement with SPINs.

Making a 'sensory toolbox' with items like fidget toys, noise-cancelling headphones, weighted blankets, and other calming or engaging materials can help an Autistic young person self-regulate their emotions and senses. It is helpful to regularly check in with the child to see what specific items help them feel focused and relaxed. Providing access to both stimulating and soothing tools lets the young person choose what they need in the moment.

Many Autistic young people will require emotional regulation and co-regulation strategies that align with their unique neurology. While traditional methods such as deep breathing exercises, mindfulness techniques and progressive muscle relaxation can offer concrete ways for Autistic children to manage feelings of overwhelm or anxiety, it's essential to recognise that these approaches will not suit everyone. For instance, engaging in physical stillness, which is often a prerequisite for these techniques, can be particularly challenging and far from relaxing for many neurodivergent children. Recognising the impact of each individual's experiences of alexithymia and interoception will be vitally important considerations also (see earlier chapters).

It's essential therefore to explore alternative forms of emotional regulation that may better resonate with their sensory and cognitive styles. Activities such as music, dancing, yoga, art, martial arts, climbing, bouncing or building with Lego™ could provide more suitable and enjoyable ways for Autistic young people to calm and centre themselves. Always ensure that the young person's interests are never weaponised or used inappropriately (e.g., rewards / punishments as part of a Positive Behaviour Support programme) as this can be detrimental to a young person's mental health (Rapaport et al., 2023).

Ultimately, understanding and respecting each young person's unique methods of finding comfort, calm and joy is vital. By gaining a deeper understanding of the ways the individual young person finds comfort, excitement and happiness, we ensure that emotional regulation strategies are not only accessible but also meaningful and beneficial to the young person's overall well-being and autonomy.

Autistic young people often require more solitude as compared to non-autistic children. This solitude can recharge their social battery as well as act as a preventative measure against the risk of burnout (Phung et al., 2021). This requirement highlights the importance of ensuring Autistic children have enough alone time (as determined by them) after social situations, such as school or clubs or teen hangouts with friends, to relax and decompress. Social environments can be loud and noisy, filled with uncertainty and unexpected behaviours – Autistic teens may have been masking or camouflaging and consciously trying to work out all the billions of micro moments of social cues and expectations they may feel pressured into (Pearson & Rose, 2023). These environments can be overwhelming, and providing uninterrupted time for solitude (or alongside a trusted adult if this is their preference) and / or engagement with their SPINs, if desired by the young person, is crucial.

Forced socialisation when an Autistic young person needs and wants solitude can greatly increase anxiety and lead to overload. It's essential to recognise and respect the young person's need for quiet time, allowing them the space to process their experiences and recharge in their own way. This solitude should not be misinterpreted as isolation or anti-social or depressive behaviour. Instead, it should be viewed as a necessary period of recovery and self-care that supports their mental and emotional well-being.

If so desired, collaboratively incorporating regular, scheduled periods of downtime (such as daily, after school and one weekend day) into the young person's daily routine can help them manage their internal resources more effectively. This approach ensures that the young person will know there will be a time reserved for them to unwind, where no demands will be made. This can help foster a sense of control of their environment and create a sense of belonging and safety. It is essential that young people feel comfortable advocating for themselves when they reach the stage of understanding their need for personal time, knowing that they won't be judged and that others will understand them (McGreevy, 2024). Providing education to family members, educators and peers about the importance of this personal time can foster a more conducive environment for the young person and help to build their capacity to manage their own internal resources and advocate for themselves as they grow.

Personal time allows Autistic individuals to engage in SPINs, stims and other sensory regulations that relax and interest them, which can be essential for their emotional and cognitive development. These activities should be encouraged and respected as part of their individual needs for recovery and personal growth. See below for a deep dive from an OT's perspective on meaningful occupation.

PERSPECTIVES OF AN OT: MEANINGFUL OCCUPATION

KATIE KERLEY

Occupational therapists bring a unique and important skillset to the multi-disciplinary team and are experts at exploring lived experience for our clients and especially at exploring meaningful occupation. What brings value, joy and purpose to people's lives? How do they live their everyday lives in a way that is right for them as an individual? This is where we can shine.

The Association of Occupational Therapists of Ireland (2024) uses the term occupation to describe 'all the things we do to take care of ourselves and others; to socialise and have fun; to work and learn; and to participate and contribute to our community and society'. Basically, if humans do it, it's an occupation.

The World Federation of Occupational Therapists (2019) states that engagement in occupations is not only a right, but also a need.

Meaningful occupations are things that take up a person's time that are purposeful, relevant to their individual needs and desires and that fit into the context of their lives. OTs believe that this is fundamental to physical and mental well-being and to quality of life.

Occupational therapy is heavily built on occupational science – which is a field of academics that studies the nature of human occupation and how it connects to well-being.

Another important component of occupational therapy is occupational justice.

This is a concept that emerged in occupational therapy in the 1990s and it stems from social justice.

Wilcock and Townsend (2009) talk about the fact that having access and opportunities to have basic needs met, to have equal life opportunities to meet goals and work towards one's potential, to have access to meaningful occupation in a way that is right for each person, is occupational justice and a human right. Occupational justice means that people are enabled to engage in occupations that have value to them. This is more fragile and challenging for people who are marginalised.

Occupational therapists have an ethical and moral duty to ensure that our clients get to engage in occupations that are meaningful to them. We do not get to decide what is meaningful to a person. This is diverse and unique to each individual. Historically, Autistic people have been encouraged or forced to meet neuro-normative standards and to engage in neurotypical occupations or not supported to engage autistically or in their own self-determined occupations. This denies an Autistic person the right to their own individuality and autonomy and does not support them to have a life that is right for them.

I absolutely always explore meaningful occupation in whatever form that may be. I always explore the context a person exists in – their physical, social, cultural and institutional environments. I almost always explore sensory processing experiences. I sometimes explore executive function experiences.

Our responsibility is to enable people to be their most real and authentic selves through the medium of occupations and activities that provide joy, purpose or value to them. This may look different for Autistic people than for a neurotypical. It is so important that we let people guide us through what is meaningful for them and not the other way round.

16.4.2 Screentime

Recent research has begun to challenge the conventional wisdom surrounding screentime and its impact on child development (Menezes et al., 2023). While excessive screentime has been associated with potential risks, it is necessary to consider the unique relationship that neurodivergent children may have with screens and digital technologies.

For many Autistic young people, screens can serve as a valuable tool for learning, communication, self-expression and self-regulation. Engaging with digital media can provide a sense of control, predictability and comfort that may be difficult to find in other aspects of their lives. Additionally, screens can offer opportunities for social connection, particularly with other Autistic peers who may share similar interests and experiences.

When considering screentime for Autistic children, it is essential to approach the topic with understanding and flexibility. Rather than imposing strict limits or banning screens altogether, we recommend working with young people to develop gentle transition strategies that respect their needs and interests. This may include providing clear, visual schedules for screentime, using timers or other preferred cues to signal upcoming transitions (see section 16.4.1 above on routines and schedules), ensuring to respect the young person's attentional focus and avoid 'ripping' their attention away prematurely (see monotropism).

It's also essential to consider the content and purpose of the young person's screentime. Engaging with educational apps, creative software or online communities that foster the young person's passions and skills can be highly beneficial. Parents / caregivers should be mindful of the historical context of moral panics surrounding new technologies, such as the concern over excessive book reading in the past, and approach screentime with a balanced, flexible perspective.

We strongly encourage parents / caregivers to join their Autistic children and young people in screentime activities wherever possible. By engaging with digital media alongside their children, parents / caregivers can gain valuable insights into their children's interests, skills and challenges. This shared experience can also provide opportunities for bonding, communication and learning. Parents / caregivers can help model healthy screen habits, discuss the content being consumed, and help young people navigate any difficulties they may encounter. Collaborative screentime can be a powerful tool to help strengthen family relationships.

Another critical aspect to consider is the role of interoception and alexithymia in Autistic young people's experiences with screens. Interoception refers to the ability to sense and interpret internal bodily signals while alexithymia describes the ability to identify and express emotions. Many Autistic young people may experience differences in these areas which can impact on their ability to notice and regulate their physical and emotional needs.

Working with a neuro-affirming occupational therapist can be an invaluable strategy in supporting Autistic young people to navigate the balance between their screen-based interests and their physical needs for movement, eating, toileting and self-regulation. OTs can help young people develop strategies for recognising and responding to their body's signals, even when engrossed in screen-based activities.

By approaching screentime with empathy, flexibility and a focus on the individual young person's needs and interests, families can support Autistic young people in harnessing the potential benefits of digital media while promoting overall well-being and development.

16.4.3 Stimming

As discussed in earlier chapters, stimming is a valuable and common trait of many Autistic people. It serves a variety of functions. Research has shown that stimming can help regulate emotions, manage sensory input and alleviate stress and anxiety (Kapp et al., 2019). Engaging in repetitive movements or behaviours can provide a sense of calm and help people cope with overwhelming situations. Moreover, stimming can facilitate self-expression, communication and the processing of complex emotions. Recognising and supporting a person's need to stim, rather than attempting to suppress or eliminate it, is essential for promoting overall well-being and mental health (McCormack et al., 2023; Orsini & Smith, 2010). Families need to be supported in understanding the value of stimming and referred to an occupational therapist for support if a stim is harmful for the individual, as creative satisfactory substitutes will need to be identified in these cases.

16.4.4 Competing Family Needs

It is necessary to recognise that within a family, there may often be what can be termed 'competing needs' that require fluid management and accommodation. This is especially true in families where multiple members, including parents, may be Autistic, given the strong hereditary likelihood (Sandin et al., 2017). For example, one Autistic family member may have a strong need for quiet environments while another may seek out and find comfort in louder more stimulating sounds. Supporting everyone's needs while finding a balance that works for the family unit is key. This could involve designated quiet spaces and times, using noise-cancelling headphones, or finding compromises that meet everyone's needs to some degree. This is another opportunity for collaboration and open discussion with empathy and flexibility, and is an ongoing process for families to navigate together. It provides a space for empowerment and an opportunity for family members to advocate for each other's needs (O'Donnell-Killen & Zadurian, 2023).

16.4.5 Mealtimes and Food Considerations

Mealtimes and food can be significant challenges for Autistic people and their families, often requiring a complete re-imagining of traditional expectations. Research with neuro-affirming families highlights the importance of adapting mealtime expectations to accommodate the diverse needs of Autistic family members (O'Donnell-Killen & Zadurian, 2023). For example, the common expectation that everyone should sit together and eat at the same time may be unrealistic for some families due to sensory processing differences such as misophonia, where the sounds of others eating cannot be tolerated. Some Autistic individuals may need to move around while eating, such as bouncing on a ball or pacing, to regulate sensory needs. The smell of food preparation can be overwhelming for some. Additionally, food sensitivities related to texture, taste and smell should be carefully considered and respected, moving away from labelling individuals as 'picky eaters'.

As described in Chapter 2, many Autistic young people (and adults) have a need for 'safe foods', foods that will provide a consistent experience (e.g., the same brand of cracker). This need will often intersect with a routine (e.g., eating the crackers sitting in the chair facing the window, while watching their favourite cartoon on their tablet). The understanding and recognition of these needs may vary depending on the region and clinical perspective. In some areas, these needs are more commonly understood as a potential indicator of avoidant / restrictive food intake disorder (ARFID), while in others, there is a growing recognition that these needs may be a common aspect of Autistic sensory processing differences (Nimbley et al., 2023). It's essential for practitioners to consider both possibilities and to be aware of the potential for diagnostic overshadowing, where co-occurring conditions such as ARFID or other eating disorders may be overlooked if a young person is identified as Autistic. This can lead to difficulties in obtaining appropriate support and treatment for these conditions. Clinicians must remain vigilant and consider the possibility of co-occurring conditions while also being mindful of the differences in understanding and interpretation of these needs. It's imperative for parents / caregivers to be aware of these needs and for clinicians to stay up to date on this rapidly changing area. Embracing flexibility and finding creative solutions that work for each individual and family is key to promoting positive mealtime experiences.

16.5 Pervasive Drive for Autonomy and Low-Demand Parenting

Pathological demand avoidance (PDA) is a term used to describe a profile characterised by a pervasive need for autonomy and resistance to everyday demands. Many neurodivergent individuals and advocates (along with these authors) prefer the term 'pervasive desire for autonomy', as it re-frames the experience in a more empowering and positive light. While there is ongoing debate about the validity of PDA as a 'diagnosis', it's essential to recognise that many Autistic individuals and their families strongly identify with this profile and find it helpful in understanding their experiences. Regardless of the terminology used, creating a low-demand environment is a key strategy for supporting Autistic young people (and adults) with this profile (McDonnell & Milton, 2014). This involves minimising pressure and expectations, prioritising autonomy – providing age-appropriate choices and flexibility whenever possible, and respecting the young person's need for autonomy and control over their own life. By adopting a low-demand approach as also advocated for by Greene (1998), families and professionals can help reduce anxiety and stress, promote self-determination, and foster more positive relationships and outcomes for Autistic individuals who experience a strong need for autonomy. In a recent study on neuro-affirming parenting, O'Donnell-Killen and Zadurian (2023) reported that many participants shared how embracing a low-demand, neuro-affirming approach to parenting their Autistic children led to life-changing improvements for their family. This approach enhanced their children's well-being, autonomy and empowerment while strengthening relationships within the family, as they shifted from constantly working against their child to collaborating with them.

As an Autistic child gets older, it is helpful for families to proactively learn about accommodations and supports available at school, college and in the workplace. These will differ from region to region. Planning helps smooth major life transitions and may help to prevent gaps in services. It will also be helpful for families to engage in open communication with the young person about upcoming life transitions. It will be important to validate concerns and accommodate preferences while providing reassurance and support. Families may wish to visit new settings in advance and make the transition as gradual as possible, helping the young person familiarise themselves with the environment. This can greatly reduce uncertainty and promote a smoother transition.

16.6 Clinical Recommendations

When providing clinical support for Autistic young people and their families, it is essential to adhere to the same principles outlined in both the home-based support recommendations section above, and Chapters 6, 10 and 12. This includes ensuring that all practices are neurodiversity affirmative, goals are co-created with the young person and family, and interventions never aim to mask or suppress the young person's authentic self. The primary focus should be on adapting the environment and supporting the child to foster a positive Autistic self-identity. It is important to note that first-wave and second-wave behavioural therapies, such as Applied Behaviour Analysis, Positive Behaviour Support, and any compliance-based interventions, are strongly contra-indicated (see Chapter 6). Cognitive behavioural therapy may be helpful, in some contexts, for some Autistic people, but only if adapted to account for Autistic processing differences, employed with cultural humility and extreme care to avoid epistemic injustice, and within a neuro-affirming framework. The impact of interoception and alexithymia cannot be underestimated and should be carefully considered in any therapeutic approach (see Chapter 6).

When needed, professionals should refer Autistic young people to other specialised services, such as:

1. Occupational therapy (OT): OT is vital for supporting Autistic children with sensory regulation, understanding processing differences and support with daily activities.

2. Speech and language therapy (SLT): SLT can help with communication challenges, understanding gestalt language processing and other differences in communication. Augmentative and alternative communication should be explored in all circumstances where a young person struggles to express their thoughts orally.

3. Physical health: Consideration should be given to co-occurring physical conditions commonly associated with Autistic individuals such as hypermobility, Ehlers-Danlos syndrome and gastrointestinal issues.

4. Mental health services: Autistic young people may benefit from support in managing co-occurring conditions such as anxiety or depression and also OCD. However, providers must use neuro-affirming approaches and avoid any deficit-based interventions that aim to make a child appear less Autistic.

When working with Autistic young people and their families, clinicians should:

- Adopt identity-first language as the default (Kenny et al., 2015) but honour personal preferences. Familiarise themselves with Autistic theories and concepts, such as the double empathy problem and monotropism, sensory experiences, the impact of Autistic masking, energy accounting / management (described below).

- Assess for any co-occurring conditions and provide appropriate support.

- Use neurodivergent-friendly communication strategies.

- Discuss puberty, sexuality, gender identity and relationships in concrete, clear terms without assuming a neurotypical developmental trajectory.

- Ensure that the young person sets their own goals whenever possible, rather than imposing neuro-normative or guardian / teacher goals. If the young person seeks to self-impose a neuro-normative goal, work with them to unpack internalised ableism prior to goal setting.

- Include the young person's passions and interests in goal setting while never weaponising them.

- Educate family members about Autistic experiences and provide neurodiversity affirmative support.

- Consider neurodiversity affirmative family therapy to help with family dynamics and communication.

- Be aware of competing needs within a family and work with siblings and parents / caregivers to find solutions that validate challenges while nurturing strengths.

- Provide support for Autistic young people and their families with co-occurring learning disabilities and profound and multiple learning disabilities.

By following these recommendations, clinicians can provide effective, neuro-affirmative support that promotes the well-being and autonomy of Autistic young people and their families.

ENERGY ACCOUNTING AND SPOON MANAGEMENT

Energy accounting and spoon management are essential strategies for Autistic children and adults to maintain their well-being. Spoon management, as conceived by Christine Miserandino (2017) through her metaphor Spoon Theory, helps us understand and manage energy levels effectively. The concept was initially designed to be applied to the chronic illness community and has been shown to be highly relevant for other populations, including the Autistic community. In essence, each activity, from social interactions to daily tasks, requires a certain number of 'spoons' or units of energy.

Energy accounting, a concept introduced by Autistic psychologist Maja Toudal, builds on this idea by re-imagining energy use like a bank account, where energy deposits and withdrawals can be tracked. This helps prioritise essential activities, plan for rest and avoid burnout. Young people should be supported in identifying energy-draining as well as energy-giving activities. Once identified, they can be encouraged to promote their self-care and advocate for necessary accommodations, ensuring a balanced and sustainable approach to daily living.

In a practical sense, energy accounting may look like this: list the tasks that generally give energy (deposits) and take energy (withdrawals). Reflect on a week's activities, noting where energy has been gained and where it has been taken away. See how you can help a young person budget their energy so they are balancing tasks that drain and tasks that replenish energy throughout the day and week. It's important to remember that energy needs fluctuate, and energy-giving and -draining activities are fluid too, depending on context and time. Each person will have individual experiences with this. Some will start the day with several units of energy, or spoons, while others may have less. Break down tasks into steps: waking up, getting out of bed, brushing teeth, showering, entering a noisy, smelly kitchen and having breakfast, getting dressed, and taking the trip to school. Look throughout the day to see what costs and what gives energy. Aim to learn how to budget energy effectively.

By incorporating energy accounting and spoon management into their daily lives, Autistic young people can develop a greater understanding of their own needs and limitations. This self-awareness can help them make informed decisions about how to allocate their energy, prioritise self-care and communicate their needs to others.

See the box below for post-identification support recommendations from an occupational therapy perspective.

PERSPECTIVES OF AN OT: POST-IDENTIFICATION SUPPORT

KATIE KERLEY

The role of occupational therapy in post-identification support is quite unique.

We are experts at helping people explore ways in which their lives may be most satisfying to them.

Our main skillset is to focus on meaningful occupation. But we can also focus on the foundations for meaningful occupation; that is, the things that underpin the ability to engage in your life in the right way for you.

OTs can have specific knowledge and training in these relevant areas:

• Sensory processing and how this may differ for neurodivergent people.

• Executive function and how this may differ for neurodivergent people.

• Environmental adaptations to support engagement.

• Motor coordination and muscle tone.

• How to adapt tasks and demands to make life easier.

• Lifestyle design.

• Emotional regulation.

- Interoception and self-care.

- Eating as an occupation.

We are in a strong position to advocate for supports, accommodations and environmental adaptations for our clients across other environments, like home, school, leisure environments etc.

All of us allied health professionals engage in CPD (continuing professional development) but not a lot of CPD available to us is neurodiversity affirmative. Some of this we need to discard altogether, but a lot just involves us using our skills flexibly, blending approaches to suit our client's individual needs and desires, and modifying what we do. No approach will be neuro-affirmative unless you are.

Occupational therapy focuses on meaningful occupation – things you do that have meaning or value to you. These things can range from mundane everyday tasks like brushing your teeth or getting dressed, to work or study, eating, cooking, paying bills to what you do for fun or to relax. Literally anything that occupies your time! If humans do it, it is an occupation.

We are person-centred, which means that we approach each person as an individual. You, as a unique human being, get to decide what is meaningful and important to you and it is up to us to help you experience this in an accessible way.

An aspect that is sometimes overlooked is that only an individual can determine what is meaningful to them. We don't get to determine this for other people – where this has been overlooked has been in the context of Autistic occupation. Often Autistic people are told, either by society or professionals interacting with us, that our way of being needs to be altered, that we need to change to fit in with the world. This really isn't true. Healthy and positive Autistic lifestyles cannot be determined by non-autistics.

Occupational therapy for Autistic people needs to support and enable us to live our lives Autistically. This is true across all the lifespan.

We also have an ethical duty to our clients to ensure that occupational justice occurs – to ensure that our clients get to engage in occupations that are meaningful to them. Our responsibility is to enable people to be their most real and authentic selves through the medium of occupations and activities that provide joy, purpose or value to them. I think a helpful distinction for me is that it is my job to enable people to do things, not to get them to do things.

Another thing that was part of my evolution was the realisation that autonomy and independence are not the same thing. Sometimes people say that OT is all about independence and function, but it's not. It's about meaning, self-determination and living a fulfilling life. I have come to realise that humans are not independent creatures, rather we are interdependent. No man is an island and all that. None of us exists in a vacuum and we are all standing on the shoulders of giants. Where this has really manifested in my practice is how I set goals for my clients. I no longer say, 'this person will do this task independently', but 'this person will be able to this in this context and with these supports'. See the difference? We all need supports to different extents and it's absurd to think that we should expect people to not need them.

Side note: neuro-normative goals will not serve neurodivergent clients. This is something I am guilty of in my past – setting goals based on what is considered typical rather than what is meaningful to this person. I read past goal documents I wrote for clients and shudder. Now, we co-create goals, especially with teens and young people who are finding their way in the world and have plenty to say about this. We talk about it together, what would make their life better for them, not for the people around them. Goals are not targeted towards making a child appear more neurotypical (this is associated with poor mental health and sense of identity). We also focus on self-advocacy, agency and self-determination.

This has been so rewarding for me too, and has opened up a whole world of diverse goals and desires. Some examples are: a client who wanted to be able to go into a shop and buy herself an ice cream without feeling crippling anxiety and the agony of being perceived; a client who wanted to be able to make dinner for himself and his mum without needing support; a client who wanted to self-advocate in medical appointments; a client who wanted to go on a school trip abroad so that they could plan for more travel in the next few years, knowing that they had already done so successfully. Being perceived is about being seen, noticed, or having the fact that you exist observed by others. This is usually out of our control once we are around other people, and it can be an uncomfortable experience when you are acutely aware of it.

Something that I find really interesting and really endorses our role in neurodiversity affirmative practice is that if you look at many of the conceptual models used in occupational therapy, neuro-affirmative practice really fits into these frameworks. I personally like the MOHO (Model of Human Occupation) as it blends volition, habituation and performance capacity (sometimes referred to as the will, the drill and the skill) and places these in the context of a person's life. These conceptual frameworks allow us to see people as complex beings and to explore the environments in which they exist.

16.7 Conclusion

In this chapter, we have presented some of our recommendations for supporting Autistic children and youth in various settings and domains, based on the latest research and best practices. We have also shared some insights and perspectives from our own experience as a neurodiverse team of clinicians and parents of Autistic young people. Our aim was to provide a neurodiversity-affirming support guide that respects the autonomy, dignity and identity of Autistic young people and that promotes their well-being, inclusion and empowerment.

We hope this chapter will inspire and inform professionals, parents / caregivers and allies who work with or support Autistic young people and contribute to a more positive and respectful understanding of neurodivergence. This chapter can be a springboard to open up ideas and further conversations; our lists and recommendations are not exhaustive but will provide a solid foundation for many Autistic young people and settings. It is also our deepest hope that this chapter will empower Autistic young people and encourage them to embrace their Autistic identity.

CHAPTER 17

Conclusion

It is our hope with this book that professionals will have gained the confidence and knowledge to transition to undertaking identification work with Autistic children through a neurodiversity affirmative framework, using the core aspects of collaboration, respect, transparency and flexibility.

We have sought at all times to provide an account of Autistic experience from the inside, with an approach which conceptualises being Autistic as a different neurology, unlike the medical model and deficit-based approaches that many professionals will be familiar with. We encourage readers to continue examining how they know what they (think they) know about Autistic experience, where this knowledge came from, what may have influenced that knowledge (e.g., whose voices were heard and whose were ignored), and how they will continue to explore Autistic experience within a neuro-affirmative approach.

Identification work, sensory audits, reports, additional documentation and support recommendations that respect the autonomy, dignity and identity of Autistic young people and that promote their well-being, inclusion and empowerment are all vital and explained. It is our deepest hope that professionals through their work will support the Autistic children they work with to embrace, self-advocate and celebrate their authentic Autistic selves.

Undertaking the practicalities of the identification work outlined in this book necessitates clinicians creating a safe space to explore a child's inner experience, gathering information collaboratively about their inner experience, gathering other vital information, mapping the relevant information onto a re-framed criteria document, and finally supporting the child and their family to make sense of their experiences. However, more important than any practical advice is the shift in thinking required to become truly neurodiversity affirmative.

Surrounded by rigid systems, it is easy to become paralysed in a position of 'we've always done it this way' and feel overwhelmed at how to introduce different ways of working clinically when the systems surrounding us appear to provide little flexibility. Making a change in how we approach our thinking about Autistic experience and stepping outside familiar ways of conducting an identification piece can launch us back to the perhaps floundering feelings we experienced as trainee practitioners or when we started learning how to conduct the typical, deficit-based autism 'assessment'. This can feel intensely uncomfortable, and changing established methods or practices is not easy. If you experienced discomfort when reflecting on previous, or current, deficit-based practice, we urge you to sit with this discomfort, which may help you find your good reason for the shift.

This shift can, of course, be challenging when we work in systems that are inherently deficit-based. There will be resistance – but our job is to find which doors give, and push on those. Changes can be incremental. Even an avalanche starts somewhere with a single snowflake. Each time in a team meeting you suggest a clinician use 'Autistic' rather than 'ASD' or 'ASC' or 'having autism', you are making a difference, advocating for the Autistic voice and for change.

Moving towards neurodiversity affirmative practice is a process of ever-becoming: you will never arrive. Seek to always learn from the Autistic community in general, and the Autistic children and young people with whom you work. The way in which you work, and the environment that you provide to support the child and young person's engagement in the process, will have a profound impact on their lives moving forward and how they relate to their Autistic identity. Show yourself compassion as you unlearn, re-learn and ever move forwards. Learning is an ever-looping process of becoming: it is not linear. Welcome this.

CHILD'S VOICE

ERICA, AGE 16

- How were you feeling when you first learned you were going to come to meet us?

  I was very happy and excited to finally be seeing someone about an autism assessment. I was a bit nervous though since it was a new environment and I didn't know what to expect.

- Was there anything we did that made it easier for you to come to meet us?

  Sending photos of the building and room I was going to be in and also sending photos of who I was going to meet and their names.

- What did you enjoy when you had your session with us?

  It was nice that you had a bucket of fidgets that I could use. You also told me that I didn't need to make eye contact and it was fine to look out the window the entire time.

- Was there anything you did not enjoy about your session?

  No, everything was great.

- Did it help you understand yourself better?

  It helped confirm what I already thought about myself.

- Was there anything we did that helped you understand yourself better?

  You just confirmed my suspicions.

- What did you think about your report or letter that we sent you?

  I was very happy about it. Reading it made me feel seen and like there was someone who understands me a bit more.

- For any other young person who is coming to meet with us, how would you describe to them what they should expect when they meet us?

  Expect very kind and patient people. You won't feel pressured during the session.

- What would you say to any other young person who is worried about coming to meet with us?

  It's less scary than you think. You can worry but after you'll be confused as to why you were worrying.

Appendices

Appendix 1: An Outline of Many Aspects of Current Criteria Re-Framed Within a Neuro-Affirmative Framework

(Reprinted from Hartman et al., 2023.)

Deficit-focused statements or aspects of current classification systems	Re-framed from neuro-affirmative perspective
Persistent deficits.	*Consider how a person's experiences may change across their lifespan.*
Deficits in social communication and interaction, abnormal social interaction, failure to engage in normal interaction etc.	*Experience of social-emotional reciprocity, e.g., social approach, conversation styles, sharing of interests / emotions / affect, initiating and responding to social interactions.* Within this area, consider a child or young person's communication and interaction preferences. What works best for them in terms of how they communicate with others? What do they like to communicate about? How do they experience neurotypical expectations for communicating and interacting, e.g., 'small talk', conversations, etc.? Do they engage in an Autistic communication style (clear, direct, and honest communication) and find neurotypical communication styles confusing (e.g., sarcasm, not saying things directly so as not to appear rude etc.)? How do their experiences in these areas relate to 'masking' (depending on age, they may not be consciously aware of this)?

Deficits in non-verbal communication, poor use of communication, abnormalities in non-verbal communication, deficits in understanding non-verbal communication, a lack of non-verbal communication.	*Experience of non-spoken communication, e.g., eye contact / body language / gestures / facial expressions.* Within this area, consider a child or young person's experience of non-spoken communication with others. Are they comfortable or uncomfortable with it? Do they appear confused by it? How do they experience eye contact? Do they find it more comfortable or easier to communicate if eye contact is not expected (e.g., when driving in a car with someone or walking alongside them)? Is body language clear or confusing? Is masking a role here for them (i.e., are they masking discomfort in relation to eye contact because others have taught them they must make it)?
Deficits in friendships and relationships, impairments in adapting to a situation, problems with sharing play and making friends, no interest in peers.	*Experience of friendships and relationships.* Within this area, consider whether a child or young person has friendships or not, and whether they are interested in having friends. Are they comfortable with their friends – would they like more or fewer? Do they spend time alone? Would they prefer to spend time alone? Do they have Autistic friendships (sporadic or irregular contact, engage in things side-by-side, etc.) or neurotypical friendships? Do they have pets? Do they find it easier to be around animals rather than people?
Restricted or repetitive behaviours.	*Calming, alerting, and / or balancing movements / activities; task engagement preferences; interests; and sensory experiences.*
Repetitive or stereotyped movements, speech, or play of objects. Atypical or unusual movements.	*Particular or repeated hand or body movements, use of objects, or vocalisations / use of speech that a person may find balancing or self-regulating.* Within this area, consider whether a child or young person does anything with their hands or body that they find calming or energising. Do they make any sounds or noises that they enjoy or find calming or alerting? Do they do anything with objects that they find balancing (either calming or energising)? Did they do any of these things in the past? Consider why a child or young person might do these things – is it only for comfort or also to express positive emotions?
Persistence in wanting things to stay the same, inflexibility, ritualised behaviour, rigidity, lack of adaptability, excessive adherence to rules.	*Preference or need for routines and specific ways of doing things; response to change and transitions; preference and / or need for familiarity.* Within this area, consider a child or young person's experience of change, both planned and unexpected. Do they prefer familiar surroundings? How do they manage transitions? How do they experience new surroundings? Do they thrive within structure or a routine? Do they have particular preferences for how they arrange their belongings? Or how their food is prepared? How do they experience it when other people do things differently to them? How do they experience uncertainty? Are they more comfortable if things are predictable? Do they have a strong sense of social justice?

cont.

Deficit-focused statements or aspects of current classification systems	Re-framed from neuro-affirmative perspective
Interests that are restricted or fixed, abnormal focus.	*Particular interests or passions for particular topics or activities.* Within this area, it is important to explore what a child or young person's interests are. What are they passionate about? Are there particular things they have been interested in for a long time, or do they 'cycle' through interests? How do they like to engage with their interests? Do they engage with interests via multiple modalities (e.g., reading about them, watching programmes, talking about them, listening to podcasts, etc.)? Do they experience hyperfocus? Does hyperfocus interfere with self-care tasks such as feeding themselves or remembering to move or use the bathroom? Are they able to sustain their attention on their interests for long periods?
Hyper-response or hypo-response to, excessive, persistent or unusual interest in sensory information.	*Hyper- and / or hypo-reactivity to sensory input or interest in sensory aspects of the environment, seeking out certain sensory pleasures.* Within this area, it is important to explore how a child or young person experiences sensory aspects of their environment – what they find difficult to tolerate and what they seek out more of or enjoy. Explore their experiences within all eight senses – visual (sight), gustatory (taste), tactile (touch), auditory (hearing), olfactory (smell), vestibular (balance), proprioception (movement), and interoception (internal communication between sense and emotional states) which refers to recognising signals within the body such as hunger, thirst, pain and needing to use the toilet.
Social awareness, inappropriate social behaviour.	*Experience of masking.* Within this area, explore the child or young person's experience of masking their Autistic experiences. Do they put effort into appearing to be like others? Do they engage in particular movements in private? Have they put a lot of effort into trying to make sense of the behaviour of others, i.e., by researching or role playing? Do they prepare scripts in advance of interactions? Depending on their age, a child or young person's experience of masking may be entirely unconscious.
Understanding the emotional states and thoughts of others.	*Experience of emotion, empathy, and compassion.* Within this area, consider a child or young person's experiences of emotion. Are they able to identify and understand their own emotions? Do they experience alexithymia? What is their experience of others' emotions? Do they experience others' emotions intensely? How do they understand others' behaviour within different contexts?

Ability to share interests with others.	*Experience of sharing experiences of the world with others.*
	Within this area, consider the child or young person's preferences in relation to how they engage with others about their experiences of the world. Do they seek to share experiences with others? Are they content to engage with experiences in their own way and / or without others' involvement? How did / do they like to play? What toys or objects do they like to play with and what do they like to do with them? Do they like to play by themselves or with another person or people? If they like to play with others, what games do they enjoy?
Onset of symptoms occurs in the early developmental period.	Within each of the areas above, if a young person is over the age of 4 years, explore with them and their parents / caregivers their experiences in each area when they were under the age of 4 years.
	Note: Current classification systems allow for there to only be noticeable characteristics of Autistic experiences at a later stage in life when neurotypical social demands might exceed a child or young person's capacity to manage.
Autism symptoms give rise to impairment in various aspects of a person's life, or there is a functional impact on the person.	Consider the support needs a child or young person has. Explore with them and their parents / caregivers the adjustments and supports they require across different areas of their life. Consider also that some children and young people may be accessing environments that are adjusted to suit their neurology (i.e., perhaps they are growing up within a neurodivergent family, they might be home schooled or attending a child-led learning setting). For these children and young people, there may be no observable 'impairment' or 'functional impact' as the environments they are in suit their neurology. However, consider what their needs would be if they were placed within an environment that does not suit their neurology or if the adjustments they access currently were removed.

Appendix 2: Sensory Audit Checklist

Sensory Audit Checklist					
Space	Date	Conducted by	Autistic Consultant	Status	Notes

Planning Stage

Category	Checklist Item	Status Yes / No)
Consultation	Have you engaged the services of an Autistic Consultant who meets the four criteria outlined in this chapter to assist you in your sensory audit of all your spaces?	☐ Yes ☐ No
Audit Planning	Have you planned your sensory audit to address the entire process, including all spaces involved, e.g., physical spaces, transitional spaces, communication spaces and online spaces?	☐ Yes ☐ No
Audit Flexibility	Has your audit been designed to accommodate future re-evaluation and updates to keep up with ever-changing spaces?	☐ Yes ☐ No
Staff Training	Does your audit involve training for all people who work in your spaces to build awareness and understanding of the distinct perceptual mechanisms, communication and interaction styles of Autistic people?	☐ Yes ☐ No
User Sensory Needs	Does your audit consider the diverse sensory needs of users by providing adaptable sensory inputs that reduce overload and enrich the sensory experience?	☐ Yes ☐ No

Auditory Assessment

Category	Checklist Item	Status (Yes / No)
Awareness and Adaptability	Are users of the space informed about the typical noise levels, changing noise levels at different times or in different areas?	☐ Yes ☐ No
	Can users control ambient noises to suit their needs? (wearing headphones, playing background sound in online environments)	☐ Yes ☐ No
	Are spaces welcoming for auditory stimming without judgement?	☐ Yes ☐ No

	Are tools like remotes for TVs / radios accessible to everyone? With clear instructions on how to use them.	☐ Yes ☐ No
Excessive Noises	Are electrical sounds from devices noticeable to any users? (Computers, fan systems, microwaves.)	☐ Yes ☐ No
	Are the noises from extension cords, fluorescent lighting and aging light bulbs noticeable?	☐ Yes ☐ No
	Can any users hear deterrent devices for rodents, bats or loitering mosquito alarm hums?	☐ Yes ☐ No
Unexpected Noises	Are external noises like conversations, car horns, door closures audible?	☐ Yes ☐ No
	Are noises from online calls, like background noises, a problem? Issues with out of sync audio due to technical / connectivity issues?	☐ Yes ☐ No
	Can plumbing sounds or kitchen noises be heard by any users?	☐ Yes ☐ No
Acoustic Improvements	Have you considered using acoustic panels to reduce noise?	☐ Yes ☐ No
	Have you considered using plants to absorb sounds and enhance calmness?	☐ Yes ☐ No

Visual Assessment

Category	Checklist Item	Status (Yes / No)
Initial Assessment	Have you looked at the celling, floor and straight ahead and out of any openings when assessing spaces?	☐ Yes ☐ No
	Have you assessed the space at different times when there are differing light levels and directions?	☐ Yes ☐ No
Lighting Balance	Is the lighting neither too dim nor too bright, and free from visual flicker and noise?	☐ Yes ☐ No
Lighting Adaptability	Are there options like dimmer switches or adjustable lamps to control light direction and intensity? With clear information on how users can adapt lights best for their needs.	☐ Yes ☐ No
Visual Clutter	Is the amount of visual information balanced, avoiding both overload and under-stimulation, while still remaining adaptable for the diversity of needs of users?	☐ Yes ☐ No
Adaptable Stimuli	Are there adaptable stimuli like controllable lamps or biophilic elements which can be easily be moved and adapted for different sensory balances?	☐ Yes ☐ No

cont.

Visual Assessment

Category	Checklist Item	Status (Yes / No)
Transitional Spaces	Have you considered visual inputs from transitional spaces like corridors and waiting areas?	☐ Yes ☐ No
Artwork	Is the artwork appropriate, avoiding over-stimulation while providing positive visual input?	☐ Yes ☐ No
Navigational Clarity	Are doors and pathways clearly marked and predictable, reducing uncertainty and anxiety? Have you prepared an easily updatable map of your space which is made available to users before they arrive at the space?	☐ Yes ☐ No
External Visual Input	Have you assessed your space for visual stimulus from outside windows, like movement or surprises?	☐ Yes ☐ No
Alternative Lighting Options	Are there provisions for using natural light or non-fluorescent lighting options?	☐ Yes ☐ No
Fluorescent Light Management	If you cannot avoid using fluorescent lights, have measures like using sleeves and covers been adopted to diffuse the light?	☐ Yes ☐ No
Lighting Variety	Are RGB lights (which are capable of producing light in any colour) and daylight lighting used to enhance transitions and mimic natural light?	☐ Yes ☐ No
Visual Integration	Are different areas of the space integrated smoothly using consistent or complementary visual themes? (Considering balance, avoiding primary colours, avoiding blank walls and empty spaces, using moveable plants and pastel colours.)	☐ Yes ☐ No
Furniture Positioning	Is the furniture arranged to support visual comfort and reduce distractions?	☐ Yes ☐ No
Windows	Have window coverings been assessed? Avoiding doily and venetian blinds which can introduce distracting / distressing visual flicker and noise to a space. Opting instead for blackout blinds or unpatented curtains.	☐ Yes ☐ No
Visual Navigation	Are there clear visual signs that indicate areas for movement, quiet spaces or directions which can contribute to a sense of orientation and balance?	☐ Yes ☐ No
Material Spaces	Have the visuals of material space been assessed for balance, being aware that black text on white pages with no imagery or colour can be just as overloading as a document of multiple fonts, colours and images?	☐ Yes ☐ No

User Autonomy and Choice	Do users have choices in how they engage with the environment, like selecting seating or routes?	☐ Yes ☐ No
Integrated Colour Design	Is colour used effectively to navigate and transition through different spaces, enhancing accessibility?	☐ Yes ☐ No

Olfactory Assessment

Category	Checklist Item	Status (Yes / No)
Scented Product Usage	Are scented products like candles, incense, cleaning products, perfumes and air fresheners eliminated or reduced?	☐ Yes ☐ No
	Are cleaning products unscented and natural?	☐ Yes ☐ No
	Is there an option for controlled olfactory input essential oil in an airtight box that people can take out to smell and then easily put away that will not linger in a space?	☐ Yes ☐ No
	Are movable flowers used instead of air fresheners for adaptable scent solutions?	☐ Yes ☐ No
Material Considerations	Are low-toxicity and non-lingering materials used in space design?	☐ Yes ☐ No
Odour Management	Is the space well-ventilated to quickly disperse strong odours? (Human error means even with the best plans, unpredictable odours could occur and need a way to be dispersed.)	☐ Yes ☐ No
	Can windows be opened or ventilation activated when needed?	☐ Yes ☐ No
	Have you considered using plants to absorb smells and reduce odours? (e.g., in transition spaces between designated eating space and other spaces)	☐ Yes ☐ No
Space Specific Design	Is there a designated, well-ventilated area for food consumption?	☐ Yes ☐ No
	Are measures in place to prevent food smells from spreading to other areas?	☐ Yes ☐ No
	Is gum chewing and eating during meetings minimised to reduce odours and noise?	☐ Yes ☐ No
	Are coffee areas and similar scent sources located in designated spaces?	☐ Yes ☐ No

Gustatory Assessment

Category	Checklist Item	Status (Yes / No)
Relevance of Taste Assessment	Is the space used for eating or drinking?	☐ Yes ☐ No
	Are plain and separate food options available?	☐ Yes ☐ No
	Is plain still water readily available?	☐ Yes ☐ No
	Are users allowed to bring their own food and refreshments?	☐ Yes ☐ No

Proprioception and Tactile Assessment

Category	Checklist Item	Status (Yes / No)
Furniture and Seating	Are seating options stable and varied in height, support and movement to suit different users' needs?	☐ Yes ☐ No
	Are there adjustable seating options that allow for different postures and comfort?	☐ Yes ☐ No
	Is there a balance between soft and firm furniture to accommodate diverse proprioceptive needs?	☐ Yes ☐ No
Feedback	Do floor and surface materials provide appropriate tactile feedback? (Considering, carpets, hard floors, transition-signalling texture floors.)	☐ Yes ☐ No
	Are uneven surfaces used moderately and explained clearly to users before entering a space?	☐ Yes ☐ No
Space Arrangement	Is the space organised to allow free movement and access without obstructions?	☐ Yes ☐ No
	Are environmental features like steps, stairs and paths clearly navigable?	☐ Yes ☐ No
	Are door handles and other fixtures suitable for users with fine motor difficulties or hypermobility?	☐ Yes ☐ No
Proprioceptive Tools	Are tools like weighted blankets or wrist weights available for users needing extra proprioceptive input?	☐ Yes ☐ No
Tactile Stimulation	Are there soothing or stimulating tactile materials available based on user preference?	☐ Yes ☐ No
	Is the environment designed to be adaptable to offer a varied balance of tactile stimulation?	☐ Yes ☐ No

Vestibular Assessment

Category	Checklist Item	Status (Yes / No)
Seating and Movement Options	Are dynamic seating options like swivel chairs, beanbags, rocking chairs or floor sitting available to accommodate various vestibular needs?	☐ Yes ☐ No
	Are seating options designed to support different postures and movements?	☐ Yes ☐ No
Navigation and Space Design	Are corridors and waiting areas designed for safe, easy navigation with wide, obstacle-free pathways?	☐ Yes ☐ No
	Is the layout of the space conducive to pacing, walking or stimming without disruption?	☐ Yes ☐ No
Designated Movement Areas	Are there designated movement areas that offer gentle vestibular challenges like soft inclines or balance beams?	☐ Yes ☐ No
	Can these vestibular stimulation areas be easily avoided by those who are hypersensitive to this type of input?	☐ Yes ☐ No
Information and Preparation Spaces	Is detailed easily updateable material provided beforehand explaining the physical layout and types of vestibular related resources available?	☐ Yes ☐ No
	Are users informed about the availability and location of movement areas within the space?	☐ Yes ☐ No
Movement Breaks and Flexibility	Have users been made aware that they can take movement breaks in both physical and online spaces to support vestibular health?	☐ Yes ☐ No
	Is there flexibility to adapt sessions or environments to include unconventional spaces like cars, walks or pools for vestibular input?	☐ Yes ☐ No
Interactive and Virtual Elements	Have you considered virtual reality or other movement-based activities utilised in online spaces to engage vestibular senses for users who would benefit from that?	☐ Yes ☐ No
Space Adaptability	Are spaces adaptable to meet the needs of those requiring frequent vestibular stimulation as well as those who require less vestibular input?	☐ Yes ☐ No
Safety and Accessibility	Are all movement and stimulation areas designed with safety in mind to prevent accidents or discomfort?	☐ Yes ☐ No

Interoceptive Assessment		
Category	**Checklist Item**	**Status (Yes / No)**
Temperature and Climate Control	Is there clear signage on ability and how to adjust temperature settings like opening or closing windows?	☐ Yes ☐ No
	Are users informed about how to adjust the climate to their comfort during meetings?	☐ Yes ☐ No
Hydration and Nutrition	Is drinking water visibly available and easily accessible?	☐ Yes ☐ No
	Are individuals offered water or refreshments during meetings? Are users made aware of this before arriving at a space?	☐ Yes ☐ No
Bathroom Accessibility	Is there clear signage directing to the bathroom with prompts for users?	☐ Yes ☐ No
	Are users informed about bathroom locations and ways to communicate their need for a break at the start of meetings?	☐ Yes ☐ No
Communication and Reminders	Are reminders about appointments and follow-up requirements communicated in multiple formats?	☐ Yes ☐ No

Appendix 3: Questions to Send to Young People in Advance of Their Session to Help Them Prepare and Provide Predictability

(Different communication options for sharing information should be provided.)

Interests

- Tell us about your hobbies and interests.

- Is there anything that you are particularly passionate about or have a strong interest in?

Sensory Experiences

- Tell us about how you experience sensory information – sight, smell, taste, touch, hearing, balance, awareness of your body and body signals.

- Is there anything that you find difficult to tolerate in your senses, or anything that you find really calming?

Communication

- If you could choose, how would you prefer people to communicate with you and how would you like to communicate with them?

- Are you comfortable with people talking to you or would you prefer if people wrote information down?

- Do you prefer texting or messaging?

- Is using the phone ok?

- How do you experience things like 'small talk' – are you comfortable with it or would you prefer not to do it?

- What is it like for you having conversations with others?

- Do you have any particular things you like to have conversations about (any particular interests)?

Non-Spoken Communication

- How do you experience things like eye contact?

- Are you comfortable with it or is it too much?

- How do you find picking up on cues or body language from other people ('reading' others)?

- Do others read your body language well?

Friends and Relationships

- Can you tell us a little about your friends?

- Would you like to have friends / more friends?

- What do you and your friends like to do together?

- Are you more comfortable being by yourself?

Hand / Body Movements and Vocal Sounds:

- Is there anything you do with your hands or body that helps you to feel calm? For example, lots of people tap their fingers, flap their hands, pace up and down or rock / sway their body. Do you do any of these things?

- Do you do anything with your voice that helps you to feel regulated? For example, hum, sing, chant, say particular words, use different accents or languages?

Routines

- Do you have any particular ways you like to do things? For example, when preparing food or organising your belongings at home – do you like to do these things in certain ways?

- How do you find change?

- What is it like for you doing new things or going to new places?

Mental Health

- How is your mental health at the moment?

- Do you experience low mood, anxiety, overwhelm or distress?

- Do you feel as though you need any additional mental health support at the moment?

Gender

- What is your gender identity?

- Do you identify as male, female, non-binary or are you still exploring your gender?

Appendix 4: Neuro-Affirmative Autistic Criteria – Mapping Document – Option 1

(Please note: This document was prepared as part of a broader comprehensive assessment process in relation to the possibility of . . . . being Autistic. It details areas in which . . . . met these criteria.)

Section 1

Area Number	Area Description	Information Gathered
1	Experience of social-emotional reciprocity, e.g., communication preferences, interaction preferences, 'small talk', conversation style, sharing of interests / emotions / affect, initiating and responding to social interactions.	→ Communication preferences: In this area – consider how the young person best communicates / interacts with others, how they prefer others to communicate / interact with them, or are they more comfortable not communicating / interacting with others? Do they experience masking (depending on age, they may not be consciously aware of this)? Do they engage in an Autistic communication style (clear, direct and honest communication) and find neurotypical communication styles confusing (e.g., sarcasm, not saying things directly so as not to appear rude, etc.)? Are they non-speaking or intermittently speaking?
2	Experience of non-spoken communication, e.g., eye contact / body language / gestures / facial expressions.	→ In this area, consider how a young person feels about engaging in non-spoken communication. Are they comfortable or uncomfortable with it? Do they appear confused by it? Is there a masking role here for them (i.e., are they masking discomfort in relation to eye contact because others have taught them to make it)?

cont.

Area Number	Area Description	Information Gathered
3	Experience of friendships and relationships.	→ Consider whether a young person has friendships or not. Are they comfortable with their friends – would they like more or fewer? Do they spend time alone? Would they prefer to spend time alone? Are their friendships more aligned with typical Autistic friendships (sporadic or irregular face-to-face contact, engaging in things side-by-side, etc.) or are they aligned with typical neurotypical friendships (spending regular face-to-face time together, engaging in activities directly)? Consider their connections with their pets.

Section 2

Area Number	Area Description	Information Gathered
1	Preference / need for particular or repeated motor movements, use of objects or vocalisations that might be balancing / regulating.	→ Consider whether a young person engages in any hand / body movements or vocalisations. Consider why they might do these things – is it for comfort and / or to express positive emotions?
2	Preference / need for routines, particular ways of doing things, managing change and transitions, thinking patterns, specific greetings, taking the same route or eating the same food every day.	→ Consider how a young person responds to changes in plans, routines or their surroundings. Are they very organised? Do they thrive within structure and routine? Do they have a strong sense of fairness and equality, or justice?
3	Interests / passions for particular topics or activities.	→ Consider a child's interests and passions. How do they engage with their interests? Are they able to hyperfocus on their interests? Do they have deep knowledge about their interests?
4	Sensory experiences.	→ Consider both sensory sensitivities and also sensory seeking. Autistic people can experience great joy with their sensory experiences, as well as have sensory experiences they find hard to tolerate.

Appendix 5: Neuro-Affirmative Autistic Criteria
– Mapping Document – Option 2

(Please note: This document was prepared as part of a broader comprehensive assessment process in relation to the possibility of . . . . being Autistic. It details areas in which . . . . met these criteria.)

Section 1

Experiences of communication and engagement with others. Consider how experiences might change across a person's lifespan, and whether they communicate via spoken and / or non-spoken methods. Consider the following areas:

Area Number	Area Description	Information Gathered
1	Experience of social communication with others, e.g., experience of spoken and non-spoken communication with others, and understanding of behaviour in different contexts.	→ Communication preferences:
2	Experience of non-spoken communication, e.g., eye contact, facial expression, body language, and gestures; and how the person experiences non-spoken communication in conjunction with spoken communication.	→
3	Experience of using spoken communication with others.	→

cont.

Area Number	Area Description	Information Gathered
4	Experience of masking.	→
5	Experience of developing, maintaining and understanding friendships and relationships.	→
6	Experience of emotion, empathy and compassion.	→
7	Experience of sharing experiences of the world with others.	→

Section 2

Calming and / or energising and balancing movements / activities, task engagement preferences, interests and sensory experiences. These may include:

Area Number	Area Description	Information Gathered
1	Preference and / or need for familiarity.	→
2	Preference and / or need for routines and specific routes.	→
3	Preference and / or need for specific ways of doing things.	→
4	Preference and / or need for rules to be followed.	→
5	Particular or repeated hand or body movements that a person may find balancing or self-regulating.	→
6	Interests and passions. Preferred objects.	→
7	Sensory experiences.	→

References

Acevedo, S., & Nusbaum, E. A. (2020). Autism, neurodiversity, and inclusive education. *Oxford Research Encyclopedia of Education*. https://doi.org/10.1093/acrefore/9780190264093.013.1260

Adams, M. (2023). *The myth of the untroubled therapist: Private life, professional practice*. Routledge.

Ahmed, S. (2021). *Complaint!* Duke University Press.

Aishworiya, R., Ma, V. K., Stewart, S., Hagerman, R., & Feldman, H. M. (2023). Meta-analysis of the Modified Checklist for Autism in Toddlers, Revised/Follow-up for screening. *Pediatrics, 151*(6), e2022059393. https://doi.org/10.1542/peds.2022059393

Alcorn, A. M., Fletcher-Watson, S., McGeown, S., Murray, F., Aitken, D., Peacock, L. J. J., & Mandy, W. (2022). *Learning about neurodiversity at school: A resource pack for primary school teachers and pupils*. University of Edinburgh.

Ali, D., O'Brien, S., Hull, L., Kenny, L., & Mandy, W. (2023). 'The key to this is not so much the technology. It's the individual who is using the technology': Perspectives on telehealth delivery for autistic adults during the COVID-19 pandemic. *Autism, 27*(2), 552–564. https://doi.org/10.1177/13623613221108010

Alvares, G. A., Bebbington, K., Cleary, D., Evans, K., Glasson, E. J., Maybery, M. T., Pillar, R., Uljarević, M., Varcin, K., Wray, J., & Whitehouse, A. J. (2020). The misnomer of 'high functioning autism': Intelligence is an imprecise predictor of functional abilities at diagnosis. *Autism, 24*(1), 221–232. https://doi.org/10.1177/1362361319852831

American Psychiatric Association. (2022). *Diagnostic and statistical manual of mental disorders: DSM-5-TR* (5th ed., text rev.). American Psychiatric Association Publishing.

American Speech-Language-Hearing Association. (n.d.). Augmentative and alternative communication. www.asha.org/Practice-Portal/Professional-Issues/Augmentative-and-Alternative-Communication/

Anderson, D. K., Lord, C., Risi, S., DiLavore, P. S., Shulman, C., Thurm, A., Welch, K., & Pickles, A. (2007). Patterns of growth in verbal abilities among children with autism spectrum disorder. *Journal of Consulting and Clinical Psychology, 75*(4), 594–604. https://doi.org/10.1037/0022-006X.75.4.594

Anderson, L. K. (2023). Autistic experiences of applied behavior analysis. *Autism: The International Journal of Research and Practice, 27*(3), 737–750. https://doi.org/10.1177/13623613221118216

Arias, V. D., Gomez, L. E., Moran, M. L., Alcedo, M. A., Monsalve, A., & Fontanil, Y. (2018). Does quality of life differ for children with autism spectrum disorder and intellectual disability compared to peers without autism? *Journal of Autism and Developmental Disorders, 48*(1), 123–136. https://doi.org/10.1007/s10803-017-3289-8

Arnold, S. R. C., Huang, Y., Hwang, Y. E., Richdale, A. L., Trollor, J. N., & Lawson, L. P. (2020). 'The single most important thing that happened to me in my life': Development of the Impact of Diagnosis Scale – Preliminary revision. *Autism in Adulthood, 2*(1), 34–41. https://doi.org/10.1089/aut.2019.0059

Association of Occupational Therapists of Ireland. (2024). *What is occupational therapy?* www.aoti.ie/what-is-ot/What-is-Occupational-Therapy

Assouline, S. G., Foley Nicpon, M., & Dockery, L. (2012). Predicting the academic achievement of gifted students with autism spectrum disorder. *Journal of Autism and Developmental Disorders, 42*(9), 1781–1789. https://doi.org/10.1007/s10803-011-1403-x

Autistic Science Person. (2022, 3 October). Adult misdiagnosis: The default path to an autistic identity. *Thinking Person's Guide to Autism*. https://thinkingautismguide.com/2022/10/adult-misdiagnosis-the-default-path-to-an-autistic-identity.html

Autistica. (2015). *Your questions: Shaping future autism research*. www.autistica.org.uk/downloads/files/Autism-Top-10-Your-Priorities-ForAutismResearch.pdf

Babalola, T., Sanguedolce, G., & Dipper, L. (2024). Barriers and facilitators of healthcare access for autistic children in the UK: A systematic review. *Review Journal of Autism and Developmental Disorders*. https://doi.org/10.1007/s40489-023-00420-3

Baggs, A. (2012). Untitled. In J. Bascom (Ed.), *Loud hands, autistic people speaking* (pp. 324–334). Autistic Self Advocacy Network, The Autistic Press.

Bal, V. H., Katz, T., Bishop, S. L., & Krasileva, K. (2016). Understanding definitions of minimally verbal across instruments: Evidence for subgroups within minimally verbal children and adolescents with autism spectrum disorder. *Journal of Child Psychology and Psychiatry, and Allied Disciplines, 57*(12), 1424–1433. https://doi.org/10.1111/jcpp.12609

Ball, S. J. (2003). The teacher's soul and the terrors of performativity. *Journal of Education Policy, 18*(2), 215–228. https://doi.org/10.1080/0268093022000043065

Bargiela, S., Steward, R., & Mandy, W. (2016). The experiences of late-diagnosed women with autism spectrum conditions: An investigation of the female autism phenotype. *Journal of Autism and Developmental Disorders, 46*, 3281–3294. https://doi.org/10.1007/s10803-016-2872-8

Baum, C. M., Christiansen, C. H., & Bass, J. D. (2015). The Person-Environment-Occupation-Performance (PEOP) model. In C. H. Christiansen, C. M. Baum, & J. D. Bass (Eds.), *Occupational therapy: Performance, participation, and well-being* (4th ed., pp. 49–56). SLACK Incorporated.

Beardon, L. (2017). *Autism and Asperger syndrome in adults.* Sheldon Press.

Beardon, L. (2020). *Avoiding anxiety in autistic children: A guide for autistic wellbeing.* Hachette UK.

Beardon, L. (2022). *What works for autistic children.* Sheldon Press.

Begeer, S., Bouk, S. E., Boussaid, W. et al. (2009). Underdiagnosis and Referral Bias of Autism in Ethnic Minorities. *J Autism Dev Disord, 39*, 142–148. https://doi.org/10.1007/s10803-008-0611-5

Benson, K. J. (2023). Perplexing presentations: Compulsory neuronormativity and cognitive marginalisation in social work practice with autistic mothers of autistic children. *The British Journal of Social Work, 53*(3), 1445–1464. https://doi.org/10.1093/bjsw/bcac229

Berg, K. L., Acharya, K., Shiu, C. S., & Msall, M. E. (2018). Delayed diagnosis and treatment among children with autism who experience adversity. *Journal of Autism and Developmental Disorders, 48*, 45–54. https://doi.org/10.1007/s10803-017-3294-y

Bernadi, F. (2023). Postponing humanity: Pathologizing autism, childhood and motherhood. In D. Milton & S. Ryan (Eds.), *The Routledge international handbook of critical autism studies.* Routledge.

Bertilsdotter Rosqvist, H., Hultman, L., Österborg Wiklund, S., Nygren, A., Storm, P., & Sandberg, G. (2023). Intensity and variable attention: Counter narrating ADHD, from ADHD deficits to ADHD difference. *The British Journal of Social Work, 53*(3), 1–18. https://doi.org/10.1093/bjsw/bcad138

Bertilsdotter Rosqvist, H., & Nygren, A. (2023). I am that name? Naming neurotypical imaginaries of the sole autist in autistic/autism fiction. *Canadian Journal of Disability Studies, 12*(1), 118–140. https://cjds.uwaterloo.ca/index.php/cjds/article/view/974

Bertilsdotter Rosqvist, H., Stenning, A., & Chown, N. (2020). Neurodiversity studies: Proposing a new field of inquiry. In H. Bertilsdotter Rosqvist, N. Chown & A. Stenning (Eds.), *Neurodiversity studies: A new critical paradigm* (pp. 1–12). Routledge.

Bhat, A. N. (2020). Is motor impairment in autism spectrum disorder distinct from developmental coordination disorder? A report from the SPARK study. *Physical Therapy, 100*(4), 633–644. https://doi.org/10.1093/ptj/pzz190

Binger, C., Renley, N., Babej, E., & Hahs-Vaughn, D. (2021). A survey of school-age children with highly unintelligible speech. *Augmentative and Alternative Communication, 37*(3), 194–205. https://doi.org/10.1080/07434618.2021.1947370

Bishop, S. L., & Lord, C. (2023). Commentary: Best practices and processes for assessment of autism spectrum disorder – The intended role of standardized diagnostic instruments. *Journal of Child Psychology and Psychiatry, 64*(8), 834–838. https://doi.org/10.1111/jcpp.13802

Black, M. H., Van Goidsenhoven, L., Hens, K., Bourgeron, T., & Bölte, S. (2023). Risk and resilience in developmental diversity: Protocol of developing ICF core sets. *Neurodiversity, 1*, 27546330231190235.

Blanc, M. (2012). *Natural language acquisition on the autism spectrum: The journey from echolalia to self-generated language.* Communication Development Center.

Blanc, M., Blackwell, A., & Elias, P. (2023). Using the Natural Language Acquisition Protocol to support gestalt language development. *Perspectives of the ASHA Special Interest Groups, 8*(6), 1279–1286. https://doi.org/10.1044/2023_PERSP-23-00098

Blank, R., Barnett, A. L., Cairney, J., Green, D., Kirby, A., Polatajko, H., Rosenblum, S., Smits-Engelsman, B., Sugden, D., Wilson, P., & Vinçon, S. (2019). International clinical practice recommendations on the definition, diagnosis, assessment, intervention, and psychosocial aspects of developmental coordination disorder. *Developmental Medicine and Child Neurology, 61*(3), 242–285. https://doi.org/10.1111/dmcn.14132

Bloom, P. (2017). *Against empathy: The case for rational compassion*. Vintage.

Bosman, R., & Thijs, J. (2023). Language preferences in the Dutch autism community: A social psychological approach. *Journal of Autism and Developmental Disorders*. https://doi.org/10.1007/s10803-023-05903-0

Botha, M., Chapman, R., Giwa Onaiwu, M., Kapp, S. K., Stannard, A., & Walker, N. (2024). The neurodiversity concept was developed collectively: An overdue correction on the origins of neurodiversity theory. *Autism: The International Journal of Research and Practice*. https://doi.org/10.1177/13623613241237871

Botha, M., Dibb, B., & Frost, D. M. (2020). 'Autism is me': An investigation of how autistic individuals make sense of autism and stigma. *PsyArXiv Preprints*. https://doi.org/10.31219/osf.io/gv2mw

Botha, M., Hanlon, J., & Williams, G. L. (2023). Does language matter? Identity-first versus person-first language use in autism research: A response to Vivanti. *Journal of Autism and Developmental Disorders, 53*, 870–878. https://doi.org/10.1007/s10803-020-04858-w

Braden, B. B., Smith, C. J., Thompson, A., Glaspy, T. K., Wood, E., Vatsa, D., Abbott, A. E., McGee, S. C., & Baxter, L. C. (2017). Executive function and functional and structural brain differences in middle-age adults with autism spectrum disorder. *Autism Research, 10*(12), 1945–1959. https://doi.org/10.1002/aur.1842

Brede, J., Cage, E., Trott, J., Palmer, L., Smith, A., Serpell, L., Mandy, W., & Russell, A. (2022). 'We have to try to find a way, a clinical bridge' – Autistic adults' experience of accessing and receiving support for mental health difficulties: A systematic review and thematic meta-synthesis. *Clinical Psychology Review, 93*, 102131. https://doi.org/10.1016/j.cpr.2022.102131

Brimo, K., Dinkler, L., Gillberg, C., Lichenstein, P., Lundström, S., & Asberg Johnels, J. (2021). The co-occurrence of neurodevelopmental problems in dyslexia. *Dyslexia: An International Journal of Research and Practice, 27*(3), 277–293. https://doi.org/10.1002/dys.1681

British Dyslexia Association (BDA). (2019). *Educational cost of dyslexia: Financial, standards and attainment cost to education of unidentified and poorly supported dyslexia, and a policy pathway to end the educational cost of dyslexia*. Report from the All-Party Parliamentary Group for Dyslexia and other SpLDs. https://cdn.bdadyslexia.org.uk/uploads/documents/About/APPG/Educational-cost-of-dyslexia-APPG-for-Dyslexia-and-other-SpLDs-October-2019.pdf?v=1632303330

British Psychological Society (2021). *Working with Autism: Best Practice for Psychologists*. https://doi.org/10.53841/bpsrep.2021.rep156

Brosnan, M., & Mills, E. (2016). The effect of diagnostic labels on the affective responses of college students towards peers with 'Asperger's syndrome' and 'autism spectrum disorder'. *Autism, 20*(4), 388–394. https://doi.org/10.1177/1362361315586721

Brownlow, C., O'Dell, L., & Abawi, R. (2023). Critically contextualising 'normal' development and the construction of the autistic individual. In D. Milton & S. Ryan (Eds.), *The Routledge international handbook of critical autism studies*. Routledge.

Bruni, T. P. (2014). Review of Social Responsiveness Scale–Second Edition (SRS-2) [Review of the software *Social Responsiveness Scale–Second Edition*, by J. N. Constantino & C. P. Gruber]. *Journal of Psychoeducational Assessment, 32*(4), 365–369. https://doi.org/10.1177/0734282913517525

Bryson, S. E., Bradley, E. A., Thompson, A., & Wainwright, A. (2008). Prevalence of autism among adolescents with intellectual disabilities. *Canadian Journal of Psychiatry, 53*(7), 449–459. https://doi.org/10.1177/070674370805300710

Buck, T. R., Viskochil, J., Farley, M., Coon, H., McMahon, W. M., Morgan, J., & Bilder, D. A. (2014). Psychiatric comorbidity and medication use in adults with autism spectrum disorder. *Journal of Autism and Developmental Disorders, 44*, 3063–3071. https://doi.org/10.1007/s10803-014-2170-2

Buckle, K. L., Leadbitter, K., Poliakoff, E., & Gowen, E. (2021). 'No way out except from external intervention': First-hand accounts of autistic inertia. *Frontiers in Psychology, 12*. https://doi.org/10.3389/fpsyg.2021.631596

Buijsman, R., Begeer, S., & Scheeren, A. M. (2023). 'Autistic person' or 'person with autism'? Person-first language preference in Dutch adults with autism and parents. *Autism, 27*(3), 788–795. https://doi.org/10.1177/13623613221117914

Burke, B. L., Hall, R. W., & The Section on Telehealth Care. (2015). Telemedicine: Pediatric applications. *Pediatrics, 136*(1), 293–308. https://doi.org/10.1542/peds.2015-1517

Cage, E., & Troxell-Whitman, Z. (2019). Understanding the reasons, contexts, and costs of camouflaging for autistic adults. *Journal of Autism and Developmental Disorders, 49*(5), 1899–1911. https://doi.org/10.1007/s10803-018-03878-x

Cage, E., De Andres, M., & Mahoney, P. (2020). Understanding the factors that affect university completion for autistic people. *Research in Autism Spectrum Disorders, 72*, 101519. https://doi.org/10.1016/j.rasd.2020.101519

Calder, S. D., Brennan-Jones, C. G., Robinson, M., Whitehouse, A. J. O., & Hill, E. (2022). The prevalence of and potential risk factors for developmental language disorder at 10 years in the Raine Study. *Journal of Paediatrics and Child Health, 58*(11), 2044–2050. https://doi.org/10.1111/jpc.16149

Canadian Paediatric Society. (2019). Standards of diagnostic assessment for autism spectrum disorder. *Paediatrics & Child Health, 24*(7), 444–451. https://doi.org/10.1093/pch/pxz117

Casanova, E. L., Sharp, J. L., Chakraborty, H., Sumi, N. S., & Casanova, M. F. (2016). Genes with high penetrance for syndromic and non-syndromic autism typically function within the nucleus and regulate gene expression. *Molecular Autism, 7*(1), 18. https://doi.org/10.1186/s13229-016-0082-z

Cederlöf, M., Larsson, H., Lichtenstein, P., Almqvist, C., Serlachius, E., & Ludvigsson, J. F. (2016). Nationwide population-based cohort study of psychiatric disorders in individuals with Ehlers-Danlos syndrome or hypermobility syndrome and their siblings. *BMC Psychiatry, 16*(1), 207. https://doi.org/10.1186/s12888-016-0922-6

Centers for Disease Control and Prevention. (2023). Spotlight on a new pattern in racial and ethnic differences emerges in autism spectrum disorder (ASD) identification among 8-year-old children. *Autism and Developmental Disabilities Monitoring (ADDM) Network.* www.cdc.gov/ncbddd/autism/addm-community-report/spotlight-on-racial-ethnic-differences.html

Chance, P., & Lovaas, I. (1974). 'After you hit a child, you just can't get up and leave him; you are hooked to that kid': Conversation with Ivar Lovaas. *Psychology Today,* January, 76–84.

Chapman, R. (2021). Neurodiversity and the social ecology of mental functions. *Perspectives on Psychological Science, 16*(6), 1360–1372.

Chapman, R. (2023). *Empire of normality: Neurodiversity and capitalism.* Pluto Press.

Chapman, R., & Botha, M. (2023). Neurodivergence-informed therapy. *Developmental Medicine and Child Neurology, 65*(3), 310–317. https://doi.org/10.1111/dmcn.15384

Chapman, R., & Carel, H. (2022). Neurodiversity, epistemic injustice, and the good human life. *Journal of Social Philosophy, 52,* 614–631. https://doi.org/10.1111/josp.12456

Chawarska, K., Klin, A., Paul, R., Macari, S., & Volkmar, F. (2009). A prospective study of toddlers with ASD: Short-term diagnostic and cognitive outcomes. *Journal of Child Psychology and Psychiatry, 50*(10), 1235–1245. https://doi.org/10.1111/j.1469-7610.2009.02077.x

Chen, K., Zhang, C., Gurley, A., Chen, L., & Srivastava, R. (2023). Appointment non-attendance for telehealth versus in-person primary care visits at a large public healthcare system. *Journal of General Internal Medicine, 38,* 922–928. https://doi.org/10.1007/s11606-022-07814-9

Chen, Y. L., Senande, L. L., Thorsen, M., & Patten, K. (2021). Peer preferences and characteristics of same-group and cross-group social interactions among autistic and non-autistic adolescents. *Autism, 25*(7), 1885–1900. https://doi.org/10.1177/13623613211005918

Chown, N. (2017). *Understanding and evaluating autism theory.* Jessica Kingsley Publishers.

Cidav, Z., Xie, M., & Mandell, D. S. (2018). Foster care involvement among Medicaid-enrolled children with autism. *Journal of Autism and Developmental Disorders, 48,* 176–183. https://doi.org/10.1007/s10803-017-3311-1

Clements, L., & Aiello, A. L. (2021). *Institutionalising parent carer blame: The experiences of families with disabled children in their interactions with English local authority children's services departments.* Cerebra, University of Leeds. https://cerebra.org.uk/download/institutionalising-parent-carer-blame/

CommunicationFIRST. (2023). The Words We Use. https://communicationfirst.org/the-words-we-use/

Constantino, J. N., & Frazier, T. W. (2013). Commentary: The observed association between autistic severity measured by the Social Responsiveness Scale (SRS) and general psychopathology – A response to Hus et al. *Journal of Child Psychology and Psychiatry, 54*(6), 695–697. https://doi.org/10.1111/jcpp.12064

Constantino, J. N., & Gruber, C. P. (2012). *Social Responsiveness Scale* (2nd ed.). Western Psychological Services.

Cooper, K., Smith, L. G. E., & Russell, A. J. (2018). Gender identity in autism: Sex differences in social affiliation with gender groups. *Journal of Autism and Developmental Disorders, 48*(12), 3995–4006. https://doi.org/10.1007/s10803-018-3590-1

Corsello, C., Hus, V., Pickles, A., Risi, S., Cook Jr., E. H., Leventhal, B. L., & Lord, C. (2007). Between a ROC and a hard place: Decision making and making decisions about using the SCQ. *Journal of Child Psychology and Psychiatry, 48*(9), 932–940. https://doi.org/10.1111/j.1469-7610.2007.01762.x

Crane, L., Jones, L., Prosser, R., Taghrizi, M., & Pellicano, E. (2019). Parents' views and experiences of talking about autism with their children. *Autism, 23*(8), 1969–1981. https://doi.org/10.1177/1362361319836257

Crane, L., Lui, L. M., Davies, J., & Pellicano, E. (2021). Autistic parents' views and experiences of talking about autism with their autistic children. *Autism, 25*(4), 1161–1167. https://doi.org/10.1177/1362361320981317

Cresswell, L., & Cage, E. (2019). 'Who am I?': An exploratory study of the relationships between identity, acculturation, and mental health in autistic adolescents. *Journal of Autism and Developmental Disorders, 49,* 2901–2912. https://doi.org/10.1007/s10803-019-04016-x

Crompton, C. J., DeBrabander, K., Heasman, B., Milton, D., & Sasson, N. J. (2021). Double empathy: Why autistic people are often misunderstood. *Frontiers for Young Minds, 9,* 554875. https://doi.org/10.3389/frym.2021.554875

Crompton, C. J., Ropar, D., Evans-Williams, C. V., Flynn, E. G., & Fletcher-Watson, S. (2020). Autistic peer-to-peer information transfer is highly effective. *Autism, 24*(7), 1704–1712. https://doi.org/10.1177/1362361320919286

Cruz, S., Zubizarreta, S. C. P., Costa, A. D. et al. (2024). Is There a Bias Towards Males in the Diagnosis of Autism? A Systematic Review and Meta-Analysis. *Neuropsychol Rev.* https://doi.org/10.1007/s11065-023-09630-2

Curnow, E., Utley, I., Rutherford, M., Johnston, L., & Maciver, D. (2023). Diagnostic assessment of autism in adults – Current considerations in neurodevelopmentally informed professional learning with reference to ADOS-2. *Frontiers in Psychiatry, 14,* 1258204. https://doi.org/10.3389/fpsyt.2023.1258204

Dahiya, A. V., McDonnell, C., DeLucia, E., & Scarpa, A. (2020). A systematic review of remote telehealth assessments for early signs of autism spectrum disorder: Video and mobile applications. *Practice Innovations, 5*(2), 150–164. https://doi.org/10.1037/pri0000117

David, A. S., & Heeley, Q. (2024). Dangers of self-diagnosis in neuropsychiatry. *Psychological Medicine.* https://doi.org/10.1017/S0033291724000308

Davidovitch, M., Levit-Binnun, N., Golan, D., & Manning-Courtney, P. (2015). Late diagnosis of autism spectrum disorder after initial negative assessment by a multidisciplinary team. *Journal of Developmental and Behavioral Pediatrics, 36*(4), 227–234. https://doi.org/10.1097/DBP.0000000000000133

Davis, J., Watson, N., & Cunningham-Burley, S. (2000). Learning the lives of disabled children: Developing a reflexive approach. *University of Edinburgh Research Explorer.* www.research.ed.ac.uk/en/publications/learning-the-lives-of-disabled-children-developing-a-reflexive-ap

Dawkins, T., Meyer, A. T., & Van Bourgondien, M. E. (2016). The relationship between the Childhood Autism Rating Scale: Second edition and clinical diagnosis utilizing the DSM-IV-TR and the DSM-5. *Journal of Autism and Developmental Disorders, 46*(10), 3361–3368. https://doi.org/10.1007/s10803-016-2860-z/tables/5

De Laet, H., Nijhof, A. D., & Wiersema, J. R. (2023). Adults with autism prefer person-first language in Dutch: A cross-country study. *Journal of Autism and Developmental Disorders.* https://doi.org/10.1007/s10803-023-06192-3

de Vaan, G., Vervloed, M. P. J., Hoevenaars-van den Boom, M., Anotnissen, A., Knoors, H., & Verhoeven, L. (2016). A critical review of screening and diagnostic instruments for autism spectrum disorders in people with sensory impairments in addition to intellectual disabilities. *Journal of Mental Health Research in Intellectual Disabilities, 9*(1–2), 36–59. https://doi.org/10.1080/19315864.2015.1119917

de Vignemont, F., & Singer, T. (2006). The empathic brain: How, when and why? *Trends in Cognitive Sciences, 10*(10), 435–441. https://doi.org/10.1016/j.tics.2006.08.008

Dewinter, J., De Graaf, H., & Begeer, S. (2017). Sexual orientation, gender identity, and romantic relationships in adolescents and adults with autism spectrum disorder. *Journal of Autism and Developmental Disorders, 47*(9), 2927–2934. https://doi.org/10.1007/s10803-017-3199-9

Dijkhuis, R., de Sonneville, L., Ziermans, T., Staal, W., & Swaab, H. (2020). Autism symptoms, executive functioning and academic progress in higher education students. *Journal of Autism and Developmental Disorders, 50*(4), 1353–1363. https://doi.org/10.1007/s10803-019-04267-8

Dodson, W. (2022). Secrets of your ADHD brain. *ADDitude.* www.additudemag.com/secrets-of-the-adhd-brain/

Doherty, M., McCowen, S., & Shaw, S. (2023). Autistic SPACE: A novel framework for meeting the needs of autistic people in healthcare settings. *British Journal of Hospital Medicine, 84*(4). https://doi.org/10.12968/hmed.2023.0006

Doherty, M., Neilson, S., O'Sullivan, J., Carravallah, L., Johnson, M., Cullen, W., & Shaw, S. C. K. (2022). Barriers to healthcare and self-reported adverse outcomes for autistic adults: A cross-sectional study. *BMJ Open, 12*(2), e056904. https://doi.org/10.1136/bmjopen-2021-056904

Donaldson, A. L., Zisk, A. H., Eddy, B., Corbin, E., Ugianskis, M., Ford, E., & Strickland, O. (2023). Autistic communication: A survey of school-based professionals. *Perspectives of the ASHA Special Interest Groups, 8*(6), 1248–1264. https://doi.org/10.1044/2023_PERSP-23-00107

Du, K., & McDaniel, E. (2016). When an autism diagnosis comes in adulthood. *NPR.* www.npr.org/sections/health-shots/2016/03/27/471600733/when-an-autism-diagnosis-comes-in-adulthood

Edgar, H. (2024). Autistic burnout – Supporting young people at home & school. *Autistic Realms*. www.autisticrealms.com/post/autistic-burnout-at-home-school

Elder, J. H., Kreider, C. M., Brasher, S. N., & Ansell, M. (2017). Clinical impact of early diagnosis of autism on the prognosis and parent–child relationships. *Psychology Research and Behavior Management, 10*, 283–292. https://doi.org/10.2147/PRBM.S117499

Elias, R., & Lord, C. (2022). Diagnostic stability in individuals with autism spectrum disorder: Insights from a longitudinal follow-up study. *Journal of Child Psychology and Psychiatry, 63*(9), 973–983. https://doi.org/10.1111/jcpp.13551

Emma. (2020). Autism and diagnosis – A personal opinion. *Undercover Autism*. https://undercoverautism.org/2020/07/12/autism-and-diagnosis-a-personal-opinion/

Evans, J. A., Krumrei-Mancuso, E. J., & Rouse, S. (2023). What you are hiding could be hurting you: Autistic masking in relation to mental health, interpersonal trauma, authenticity, and self-esteem. *Autism in Adulthood*. https://doi.org/10.1089/aut.2022.0115

Farahar, C. (2023). Autistic identity, culture, community and space for well-being. In D. Milton & S. Ryan (Eds.), *The Routledge international handbook of critical Autism studies*. Routledge.

Fein, D., Barton, M., Eigsti, I. M., Kelley, E., Naigles, L., Schultz, R. T., Stevens, M., Helt, M., Orinstein, A., Rosenthal, M., Troyb, E., & Tyson, K. (2013). Optimal outcome in individuals with a history of autism. *Journal of Child Psychology and Psychiatry, 54*(2), 195–205. https://doi.org/10.1111/jcpp.12037

Fisher, N. (2023). *A different way to learn: Neurodiversity and self-directed education*. Jessica Kingsley Publishers.

Fletcher, R., Barnhill, J., & Cooper, A. (2017). *DM-ID-2: Diagnostic manual, intellectual disability: A textbook of diagnosis of mental disorders in persons with intellectual disability*. NADD.

Fletcher-Watson, S., & Bird, G. (2020). Autism and empathy: What are the real links? *Autism, 24*(1), 3–6. https://doi.org/10.1177/1362361319883506

Foley Nicpon, M., Allmon, A., Sieck, B., & Stinson, R. D. (2011). Empirical investigation of twice-exceptionality: Where have we been and where are we going? *Gifted Child Quarterly, 55*(1), 3–17. https://doi.org/10.1177/0016986210382575

Fountain, C., Winter, A. S., & Bearman, P. S. (2012). Six developmental trajectories characterize children with autism. *Pediatrics, 129*(5), e1112–e1120. https://doi.org/10.1542/peds.2011-1601

Frazier, T. W., Thompson, L., Youngstrom, E. A., Law, P., Hardan, A. Y., Eng, C., & Morris, N. (2014). A twin study of heritable and shared environmental contributions to autism. *Journal of Autism and Developmental Disorders, 44*(8), 2013–2025. https://doi.org/10.1007/s10803-014-2081-2

Freudenstein, O., Shimoni, H. N., Gindi, S., & Leitner, Y. (2020). Disagreement between assessment of ASD utilizing the ADOS-2 and DSM-5 – A preliminary study. *Annales Universitatis Paedagogicae Cracoviensis. Studia Psychologica, 13*, 17–26. https://doi.org/10.24917/20845596.13.1

Fricker, M. (2007). *Epistemic injustice: Power and the ethics of knowing*. Oxford University Press.

Frizelle, P., Tolonen, A. K., Tulip, J., Murphy, C. A., Saldana, D., & McKean, C. (2021). The influence of quantitative intervention dosage on oral language outcomes for children with developmental language disorder: A systematic review and narrative synthesis. *Language, Speech, and Hearing Services in Schools, 52*(2), 738–754. https://doi.org/10.1044/2020_LSHSS-20-00058

Ganz, J. B., Earles-Vollrath, T. L., Heath, A. K., Parker, R. I., Rispoli, M. J., Duran, J. B. (2012). A meta-analysis of single case research studies on aided augmentative and alternative communication systems with individuals with autism spectrum disorders. *Journal of Autism and Developmental Disorders, 42*(1), 60–74. doi:10.1007/s10803-011-1212-2.

Garau, V. (2023). The Monotropism questionnaire. *Open Science Framework*. https://doi.org/10.17605/OSF.IO/WPX5G

Garau, V., Murray, A. L., Woods, R., Chown, N., Hallett, S., Murray, F., Wood, R., & Fletcher-Watson, S. (2023). Development and validation of a novel self-report measure of monotropism in autistic and non-autistic people: The Monotropism questionnaire. *Open Science Framework*. https://doi.org/10.31219/osf.io/ft73y

Garau, V., Woods, R., Chown, N., Hallett, S., Murray, F., Wood, R., Murray, A., & Fletcher-Watson, S. (2023). The Monotropism questionnaire. *Open Science Framework*. https://doi.org/10.17605/OSF.IO/WPX5G

Gelbar, N. W., Cascio, A. A., Madaus, J. W., & Reis, S. M. (2022). A systematic review of the research on gifted individuals with autism spectrum disorder. *Gifted Child Quarterly, 66*(4), 266–276.

Georgiou, N., & Spanoudis, G. (2021). Developmental language disorder and autism: Commonalities and differences on language. *Brain Sciences, 11*(5), 589. https://doi.org/10.3390/brainsci11050589

Gernsbacher, M. A. (2017). Editorial perspective: The use of person-first language in scholarly writing may accentuate stigma. *Journal of Child Psychology and Psychiatry, 58*(7), 859–861. https://doi.org/10.1111/jcpp.12706

Gjevik, E., Eldevik, S., Fjæran-Granum, T., & Sponheim, E. (2011). Kiddie-SADS reveals high rates of DSM-IV disorders in children and adolescents with autism spectrum disorders. *Journal of Autism and Developmental Disorders, 41*(6), 761–769. https://doi.org/10.1007/s10803-010-1095-7

Gobrial, E. (2019). Comorbid mental health disorders in children and young people with intellectual disabilities and autism spectrum disorders. *Advances in Mental Health and Intellectual Disabilities, 13*(5), 173–181. https://doi.org/10.1108/AMHID-05-2018-0026

George, R., & Stokes, M. A. (2018). Gender identity and sexual orientation in autism spectrum disorder. *Autism: The International Journal of Research and Practice, 22*(8), 970–982. https://doi.org/10.1177/1362361317714587

Goodall, E., Dargue, N., Hinze, E., Sulek, R., Varcin, K., et al. (2023). *A national guideline for the assessment and diagnosis of autism in Australia: 2023 update* [Draft updated guideline for public consultation]. Autism CRC.

Gotham, K., Brunwasser, S. M., & Lord, C. (2015). Depressive and anxiety symptom trajectories from school age through young adulthood in samples with autism spectrum disorder and developmental delay. *Journal of the American Academy of Child and Adolescent Psychiatry, 54*(5), 369–376.e3. https://doi.org/10.1016/j.jaac.2015.02.005

Gray-Hammond, D. (2022). *The new normal: Autistic musings on the threat of a broken society.* Independently published.

Gray-Hammond, D. (2024). *CAMHS in crisis: Writing on the failure of CAMHS to support autistic people.* Independently published.

Gray-Hammond, D., & Adkin, T. (2022). Creating autistic suffering: Fabricated or induced illness, state-sanctioned bullying. *Emergent Divergence.* https://emergentdivergence.com/2022/01/25/creatingautistic-sufferingfabricatedorinduced-illness-state-sanctioned-bullying/

Greene, R. W. (1998). *The explosive child: A new approach for understanding and parenting easily frustrated, 'chronically inflexible' children.* HarperCollins.

Griffiths, S., Allison, C., Kenny, R., Holt, R., Smith, P., & Baron-Cohen, S. (2019). The Vulnerability Experiences Quotient (VEQ): A study of vulnerability, mental health, and life satisfaction in autistic adults. *Autism Research, 12*(10), 1516–1528. https://doi.org/10.1002/aur.2162

Guerra-Farfan, E., Garcia-Sanchez, Y., Jornet-Gibert, M., Huñez, J. H., Balaguer-Castro, M., & Madden, K. (2022). Clinical practice guidelines: The good, the bad, and the ugly. *Injury, 54*(3), 1–7. https://doi.org/10.1016/j.injury.2022.01.047

Guthrie, W., Swineford, L. B., Nottke, C., & Wetherby, A. M. (2013). Early diagnosis of autism spectrum disorder: Stability and change in clinical diagnosis and symptom presentation. *Journal of Child Psychology and Psychiatry, 54*(5), 582–590. https://doi.org/10.1111/jcpp.12008

Haberstroh, S., & Shulte-Körne, G. (2019). The diagnosis and treatment of dyscalculia. *Deutsches Ärzteblatt International, 116*(7), 107–114. https://doi.org/10.3238/arztebl.2019.0107

Hall-Lande, J., Hewitt, A., Mishra, S., Piescher, K., & LaLiberte, T. (2015). Involvement of children with autism spectrum disorder (ASD) in the child protection system. *Focus on Autism and Other Developmental Disabilities, 30*(4), 237–248. https://doi.org/10.1177/1088357614539834

Harrison, K. (2013). Counselling psychology and power: Considering therapy and beyond. *Counselling Psychology Review, 28*(2), 107–177. https://doi.org/10.53841/bpscpr.2013.28.2.107

Hartman, D., Day, A., O'Donnell-Killen, T., Doyle, J. K., Kavanagh, M., & Azevedo, J. (2024). What does it mean to be neurodiversity affirmative (with a focus on the autistic experience) and how can professionals and services adapt? Special issue on neurodiversity. *British Psychological Society.* www.bps.org.uk/psychologist/what-does-it-mean-be-neurodiversity-affirmative

Hartman, D., O'Donnell-Killen, T., Doyle, J. K., Kavanagh, M., Day, A., & Azevedo, J. (2023). *The adult autism assessment handbook: A neurodiversity affirmative approach.* Jessica Kingsley Publishers.

Havdahl, K. A., Bishop, S. L., Surén, P., Øyen, A. S., Lord, C., et al. (2017). The influence of parental concern on the utility of autism diagnostic instruments. *Autism Research, 10*(10), 1672–1686. https://doi.org/10.1002/aur.1817

Heasman, B., & Gillespie, A. (2019). Neurodivergent intersubjectivity: Distinctive features of how autistic people create shared understanding. *Autism: The International Journal of Research and Practice, 23*(4), 910–921. https://doi.org/10.1177/1362361318785172

Hens, K. (2021). *Towards an ethics of autism: A philosophical exploration.* Open Book Publishers. https://doi.org/10.11647/OBP.0261

Hens, K., & Van Goidsenhoven, L. (2023). Developmental diversity: Putting the development back into research about developmental conditions. *Frontiers in Psychiatry, 13*, 986732. https://doi.org/10.3389/fpsyt.2022.986732

Herrán Salcedo, B. (2021, 10 April). Autista Construyendo: Neurotypical people are not trash. *Neuroclastic.* https://neuroclastic.com/neurotypical-people-are-not-trash/

Higgins, J. M., Arnold, S. R., Weise, J., Pellicano, E., & Trollor, J. N. (2021). Defining autistic burnout through experts by lived experience: Grounded Delphi method investigating #AutisticBurnout. *Autism, 25*(8), 2356–2369. https://doi.org/10.1177/13623613211019858

Hill, A. (2024, 4 March). What's behind the UK's increase in autism diagnoses. *The Guardian*. www.theguardian.com/society/2024/mar/04/uk-increase-autism-diagnoses-neurodiversity

Hill, C. V., Pérez-Stable, E. J., Anderson, N. A., & Bernard, M. A. (2015). The National Institute on Aging health disparities research framework. *Ethnicity & Disease, 25*(3), 245–254. https://doi.org/10.18865/ed.25.3.245

Hillier, A., Gallop, N., Mendes, E., Tellez, D., Buckingham, A., Nizami, A., & O'Toole, D. (2020). LGBTQ+ and autism spectrum disorder: Experiences and challenges. *International Journal of Transgender Health, 21*(1), 98–110. https://doi.org/10.1080/15532739.2019.1594484

Hobson, H. M., Toseeb, U., & Gibson, J. L. (2024). Developmental language disorder and neurodiversity: Surfacing contradictions, tensions and unanswered questions. *International Journal of Language and Communication Disorders*. https://doi.org/10.1111/1460-6984.13009

Hobson, P. (2011). *The cradle of thought: Exploring the origins of thinking*. Pan Macmillan.

Holingue, C., Pfeiffer, D., Ludwig, N. N., Reetzke, R., Hong, J. S., Kalb, L. G., & Landa, R. (2023). Prevalence of gastrointestinal symptoms among autistic individuals, with and without co-occurring intellectual disability. *Autism Research, 16*(8), 1609–1618. https://doi.org/10.1002/aur.2972

Hollocks, M. J., Casson, R., White, C., Dobson, J., Beazley, P., & Humphrey, A. (2019). Brief report: An evaluation of the social communication questionnaire as a screening tool for autism spectrum disorder in young people referred to child & adolescent mental health services. *Journal of Autism and Developmental Disorders, 49*(6), 2618–2623. https://doi.org/10.1007/s10803-019-03982-6

Holyfield, C., Drager, K. D. R., Kremkow, J. M. D., & Light, J. (2017). Systematic review of AAC intervention research for adolescents and adults with autism spectrum disorder. *Augmentative and Alternative Communication, 33*(4), 201–212. doi:10.1080/07434618.2017.1370495.

Honeybourne, V. (2018). *The neurodiverse classroom: A teachers' guide to individual learning needs and how to meet them*. Jessica Kingsley Publishers.

Howlin, P., Savage, S., Moss, P., Tempier, A., & Rutter, M. (2014). Cognitive and language skills in adults with autism: A 40-year follow-up. *Journal of Child Psychology and Psychiatry, and Allied Disciplines, 55*(1), 49–58. https://doi.org/10.1111/jcpp.12115

Huang, Y., Arnold, S. R., Foley, K.-R., & Trollor, J. N. (2020). Diagnosis of autism in adulthood: A scoping review. *Autism, 24*(6), 1311–1327. https://doi.org/10.1177/1362361320903128

Huke, V., Turk, J., Saeidi, S., Kent, A., & Morgan, J. F. (2013). Autism spectrum disorders in eating disorder populations: A systematic review. *European Eating Disorders Review: The Journal of the Eating Disorders Association, 21*(5), 345–351. https://doi.org/10.1002/erv.2244

Hull, L., Mandy, W., Lai, M. C., Baron-Cohen, S., Allison, C., Smith, P., & Petrides, K. V. (2019). Development and validation of the camouflaging autistic traits questionnaire (CAT-Q). *Journal of Autism and Developmental Disorders, 49*(3), 819–833. https://doi.org/10.1007/s10803-018-3792-6

Hull, L., Petrides, K. V., & Mandy, W. (2020). The female autism phenotype and camouflaging: A narrative review. *Review Journal of Autism and Developmental Disorders, 7*, 306–317.

Hupfeld, K. E., Abagis, T. R., & Shah, P. (2019). Living 'in the zone': Hyperfocus in adult ADHD. *Attention Deficit and Hyperactivity Disorders, 11*(2), 191–208. https://doi.org/10.1007/s12402-018-0272-y

Hus, V., Bishop, S., Gotham, K., Huerta, M., & Lord, C. (2013). Factors influencing scores on the social responsiveness scale. *Journal of Child Psychology and Psychiatry, 54*(2), 216–224. https://doi.org/10.1111/j.1469-7610.2012.02589.x

Hyman, S. L., Levy, S. E., Myers, S. M., Kuo, D. Z., Apkon, C. S., et al. (2020). Identification, evaluation, and management of children with autism spectrum disorder. *Pediatrics, 145*(1), Article e20193447. https://doi.org/10.1542/PEDS.2019-3447

Iannone, P., Montano, N., Minardi, M., Doyle, J., Cavagnaro, P., & Cartabellotta, A. (2017). Wrong guidelines: Why and how often they occur. *BMJ Evidence-Based Medicine, 22*(1), 1–3. https://doi.org/10.1136/ebmed-2016-110606

Intriago, K. E. C., Rodríguez, L. M. A., & Cevallos, L. A. T. (2021). Specific learning difficulty: Autism, dyscalculia, and dysgraphia. *International Journal of Engineering, IT & Scientific Research, 7*(3), 97–106. https://doi.org/10.21744/irjeis.v7n3.1539

Isaksson, J., Pettersson, E., Kostrzewa, E., Diaz Heijtz, R., & Bölte, S. (2017). Brief report: Association between autism spectrum disorder, gastrointestinal problems, and perinatal risk factors within sibling pairs. *Journal of Autism and Developmental Disorders*. https://doi.org/10.1007/s10803-017-3169-2

Jaarsma, P., & Welin, S. (2012). Autism as a natural human variation: Reflections on the claims of the Neurodiversity Movement. *Health Care Analysis, 20*, 20–30. https://doi.org/10.1007/s10728-011-0169-9

Jack, J. (2012). Gender copia: Feminist rhetorical perspectives on an autistic concept of sex/gender. *Women's Studies in Communication, 35*(1), 1–17. https://doi.org/10.1080/07491409.2012.667519

Jackson-Perry, D., Bertilsdotter Rosqvist, H., Annable, J. L., & Kourti, M. (2020). Sensory strangers: Travels in normate sensory worlds. In H. Bertilsdotter Rosqvist, N. Chown & A. Stenning (Eds.), *Neurodiversity studies: A new critical paradigm*. Routledge.

Jagoe, C., & Wharton, T. (2021). Meaning non-verbally: The neglected corners of the bidimensional continuum communication in people with aphasia. *Journal of Pragmatics, 178*, 21–30. https://doi.org/10.1016/j.pragma.2021.02.027

Jones, J. L., Gallus, K. L., Viering, K. L., & Oseland, L. M. (2015). 'Are you by chance on the spectrum?' Adolescents with autism spectrum disorder making sense of their diagnoses. *Disability & Society, 30*(10), 1490–1504. https://doi.org/10.1080/09687599.2015.1108902

Joshi, G., Wozniak, J., Petty, C., et al. (2013). Psychiatric comorbidity and functioning in a clinically referred population of adults with autism spectrum disorders: A comparative study. *Journal of Autism and Developmental Disorders, 43*, 1314–1325. https://doi.org/10.1007/s10803-012-1679-5

Kaihlanen, A.-M., Hietapakka, L., & Heponiemi, T. (2019). Increasing cultural awareness: Qualitative study of nurses' perceptions about cultural competence training. *BMC Nursing, 18*(1), 38. https://doi.org/10.1186/s12912-019-0363-x

Kamp-Becker, I., Tauscher, J., Wolff, N., Küpper, C., Poustka, L., Roepke, S., Roessner, V., Heider, D., & Stroth, S. (2021). Is the combination of ADOS and ADI-R necessary to classify ASD? Rethinking the 'gold standard' in diagnosing ASD. *Frontiers in Psychiatry, 12*, Article 727308. https://doi.org/10.3389/fpsyt.2021.727308

Kanner, L. (1943). Autistic disturbances of affective contact. *Nervous Child, 2*, 217–250.

Kapp, S. K., Steward, R., Crane, L., Elliott, D., Elphick, C., Pellicano, E., & Russell, G. (2019). 'People should be allowed to do what they like': Autistic adults' views and experiences of stimming. *Autism: The International Journal of Research and Practice, 23*(7), 1782–1792. https://doi.org/10.1177/1362361319829628

Kedar, I. (2012). *Ido in Autismland: Climbing out of autism's silent prison*. Sharon Kedar.

Kenny, L., Hattersley, C., Molins, B., Buckley, C., Povey, C., & Pellicano, L. (2015). Which terms should be used to describe autism? Perspectives from the UK autism community. *Autism, 20*(4), 442–462. https://doi.org/10.1177/1362361315588200

Kindgren, E., Quiñones Perez, A., & Knez, R. (2021). Prevalence of ADHD and autism spectrum disorder in children with hypermobility spectrum disorders or hypermobile Ehlers-Danlos syndrome: A retrospective study. *Neuropsychiatric Disease and Treatment, 17*, 379–388. https://doi.org/10.2147/NDT.S290494

King, M., & Bearman, P. (2009). Diagnostic change and the increased prevalence of autism. *International Journal of Epidemiology, 38*(5), 1224–1234. https://doi.org/10.1093/ije/dyp261

Klaiman, C., White, S., Richardson, S., McQueen, E., Walum, H., et al. (2024). Expert clinician certainty in diagnosing autism spectrum disorder in 16–30-month-olds: A multi-site trial secondary analysis. *Journal of Autism and Developmental Disorders, 54*, 393–408. https://doi.org/10.1007/s10803-022-05812-8

Klusek, J., Martin, G. E., & Losh, M. (2014). Consistency between research and clinical diagnoses of autism among boys and girls with fragile X syndrome. *Journal of Intellectual Disability Research, 58*(10), 940–952. https://doi.org/10.1111/jir.12121

Koenen, K. C., Ratanatharathorn, A., Ng, L., McLaughlin, K. A., Bromet, E. J., et al. (2017). Posttraumatic stress disorder in the World Mental Health Surveys. *Psychological Medicine, 47*(13), 2260–2274. https://doi.org/10.1017/S0033291717000708

Kourti, M., & MacLeod, A. (2019). 'I don't feel like a gender, I feel like myself': Autistic individuals raised as girls exploring gender identity. *Autism in Adulthood: Challenges and Management, 1*(1), 52–59. https://doi.org/10.1089/aut.2018.0001

Kuo, S. S., van der Merwe, C., Fu, J. M., Carey, C. E., Talkowski, M. E., Bishop, S. L., & Robinson, E. B. (2022). Developmental variability in autism across 17,000 autistic individuals and 4,000 siblings without an autism diagnosis: Comparisons by cohort, intellectual disability, genetic etiology, and age at diagnosis. *JAMA Pediatrics, 176*(9), 915–923. https://doi.org/10.1001/jamapediatrics.2022.2423

Kuyken, W., Padesky, C. A., & Dudley, R. (2009). *Collaborative case conceptualisation*. Guilford Press.

Lachambre, C., Proteau-Lemieux, M., Lepage, J.-F., Bussières, E.-L., & Lippé, S. (2021). Attentional and executive functions in children and adolescents with developmental coordination disorder and the influence of comorbid disorders: A systematic review of the literature. *PLoS ONE, 16*(6), e0252043. https://doi.org/10.1371/journal.pone.0252043

Lai, M. C., Kassee, C., Besney, R., Bonato, S., Hull, L., Mandy, W., Szatmari, P., & Ameis, S. H. (2019). Prevalence of co-occurring mental health diagnoses in the autism population: A systematic review and meta-analysis. *The Lancet Psychiatry, 6*(10), 819–829. https://doi.org/10.1016/S2215-0366(19)30289-5

Lai, M. C., Lombardo, M. V., Chakrabarti, B., Ruigrok, A. N., Bullmore, E. T., et al. (2019). Neural self-representation in autistic women and association with 'compensatory camouflaging'. *Autism, 23*(5), 1210–1223.

Lai, M. C., Lombardo, M. V., Ruigrok, A. N., Chakrabarti, B., Auyeung, B., Szatmari, P., Happé, F., Baron-Cohen, S., & MRC AIMS Consortium. (2017). Quantifying and exploring camouflaging in men and women with autism. *Autism, 21*(6), 690–702. https://doi.org/10.1177/1362361316671012

Landa, R. J., Gross, A. L., Stuart, E. A., & Faherty, A. (2013). Developmental trajectories in children with and without autism spectrum disorders: The first 3 years. *Child Development, 84*(2), 429–442. https://doi.org/10.1111/j.1467-8624.2012.01870.x

Lawson, W. (2011). *The passionate mind: How individuals with autism learn.* Jessica Kingsley Publishers.

Leadbitter, K., Buckle, K. L., Ellis, C., & Dekker, M. (2021). Autistic self-advocacy and the Neurodiversity Movement: Implications for autism early intervention research and practice. *Frontiers in Psychology, 12*, 635690. https://doi.org/10.3389/fpsyg.2021.635690

Leader, G., Abberton, C., Cunningham, S., Gilmartin, K., Grudzien, M., Higgins, E., Joshi, L., Whelan, S., & Mannion, A. (2022). Gastrointestinal symptoms in autism spectrum disorder: A systematic review. *Nutrients, 14*(7), 1471. https://doi.org/10.3390/nu14071471

Lebenhagen, C. (2020). Including speaking and nonspeaking autistic voice in research. *Autism in Adulthood, 2*(2), 128–131. https://doi.org/10.1089/aut.2019.0002

Lebersfeld, J. B., Swanson, M., Clesi, C. D., & O'Kelley, S. E. (2021). Systematic review and meta-analysis of the clinical utility of the ADOS-2 and the ADI-R in diagnosing autism spectrum disorders in children. *Journal of Autism and Developmental Disorders, 51*(11), 4101–4114. https://doi.org/10.1007/s10803-020-04839-z

Le Couteur, A., Haden, G., Hammal, D., & McConachie, H. (2008). Diagnosing autism spectrum disorders in pre-school children using two standardised assessment instruments: The ADI-R and the ADOS. *Journal of Autism and Developmental Disorders, 38*, 362–372. https://doi.org/10.1007/s10803-007-0403-3

Lee, C. M., Altschuler, M. R., Esler, A. N., Burrows, C. L., & Hudock, R. L. (2023). Why are only some children with autism spectrum disorder misclassified by the social communication questionnaire? An empirical investigation of individual differences in sensitivity and specificity in a clinic-referred sample. *Journal of Neurodevelopmental Disorders, 15*, 28. https://doi.org/10.1186/s11689-023-09497-7

Levesque, J. F., Harris, M. F., & Russell, G. (2013). Patient-centred access to health care: Conceptualising access at the interface of health systems and populations. *International Journal for Equity in Health, 12*(18). https://doi.org/10.1186/1475-9276-12-18

Lewis, A. (2009). Silence in the context of 'Child Voice'. *Children & Society, 24*(1), 14–23. https://doi.org/10.1111/j.1099-0860.2008.00200.x

Leyfer, O. T., Folstein, S. E., Bacalman, S., Davis, N. O., Dinh, E., Morgan, J., Tager-Flusberg, H., & Lainhart, J. E. (2006). Comorbid psychiatric disorders in children with autism: Interview development and rates of disorders. *Journal of Autism and Developmental Disorders, 36*(7), 849–861. https://doi.org/10.1007/s10803-006-0123-0

Liu, X., Sun, X., Sun, C., Zou, M., Chen, Y., Huang, J., Wu, L., & Chen, W.-X. (2021). Prevalence of epilepsy in autism spectrum disorders: A systematic review and meta-analysis. *Autism,* 136236132110450. https://doi.org/10.1177/13623613211045029

Lockwood, A. (2023). This common diagnostic assessment tool is failing adults with suspected autism: Here's how. *The Mighty.* https://themighty.com/topic/autism-spectrum-disorder/adult-autism-humiliated-assessment-ados-2/

Logan, K., Iacono, T., & Trembath, D. (2017). A systematic review of research into aided AAC to increase social-communication functions in children with autism spectrum disorder. *Augmentative and Alternative Communication, 33*(1), 51–64. doi:10.1080/07434618.2016.1267795.

Long, R. M. (2024). Access points: Understanding special interests through autistic narratives. *Autism in Adulthood.* https://doi.org/10.1089/aut.2023.0157

López, B., & Keenan, L. (2014). Barriers to employment in autism: Future challenges to implementing the Adult Autism Strategy. *Autism Research Network.* www.autismrpphub.org/sites/default/files/articles/employment_report.pdf

Lord, C., Luyster, R. J., Gotham, K., & Guthrie, W. (2012). *Autism Diagnostic Observation Schedule, Second Edition: Part II: Toddler Module.* Western Psychological Services.

Lord, C., Rutter, M., DiLavore, P.C., & Risi, S. (1999). *Autism diagnostic observation schedule-WPS (ADOS-WPS).* Western Psychological Services.

Lord, C., Rutter, M., DiLavore, P. C., Risi, S., Gotham, K., & Bishop, S. L. (2012). *Autism Diagnostic Observation Schedule, Second Edition (ADOS-2) Modules 1–4.* Western Psychological Services.

Lord, C., Rutter, M., & Le Couteur, A. (1994). Autism Diagnostic Interview-Revised: A revised version of a diagnostic interview for caregivers of individuals with possible pervasive developmental disorders. *Journal of Autism and Developmental Disorders, 24*(5), 659–685. https://doi.org/10.1007/BF02172145

Lugo-Marín, J., Magán-Maganto, M., Rivero-Santana, A., Cuellar-Pompa, L., Alviani, M., Jenaro-Rio, C., Díez, E., & Canal-Bedia, R. (2019). Prevalence of psychiatric disorders in adults with autism spectrum disorder: A systematic review and meta-analysis. *Research in Autism Spectrum Disorders, 59*, 22–33. https://doi.org/10.1016/j.rasd.2018.12.004

Lundin Remnélius, K., & Bölte, S. (2023). Camouflaging in autism: Age effects and cross-cultural validation of the Camouflaging Autistic Traits Questionnaire (CAT-Q). *Journal of Autism and Developmental Disorders*. https://doi.org/10.1007/s10803-023-05909-8

Lyall, K., Van de Water, J., Ashwood, P., & Hertz-Picciotto, I. (2015). Asthma and allergies in children with autism spectrum disorders: Results from the CHARGE study. *Autism Research, 8*(3), 167–174. https://doi.org/10.1002/aur.1471

Maddox, B. B., Dickson, K. S., Stadnick, N. A., Mandell, D. S., & Brookman-Frazee, L. (2021). Mental health services for autistic individuals across the lifespan: Recent advances and current gaps. *Current Psychiatry Reports, 23*(10), 66. https://doi.org/10.1007/s11920-021-01278-0

Maenner, M. J., Shaw, K. A., & Baio, J. (2020). Prevalence of autism spectrum disorder among children aged 8 years – Autism and developmental disabilities monitoring network, 11 sites, United States, 2016. *MMWR Surveillance Summaries, 69*(4), 1–12. https://doi.org/10.15585/mmwr.ss6904a1

Mahler, K. (2016). *Interoception: The eighth sensory system*. AAPC Publishing.

Malik-Soni, N., Shaker, A., Luck, H., Mullin, A. E., Wiley, R. E., Lewis, M. E. S., Fuentes, J., & Frazier, T. W. (2022). Tackling healthcare access barriers for individuals with autism from diagnosis to adulthood. *Pediatric Research, 91*(5), 1028–1035. https://doi.org/10.1038/s41390-021-01465-y

Mandy, W., Midouhas, E., Hosozawa, M., Cable, N., Sacker, A., & Flouri, E. (2022). Mental health and social difficulties of late-diagnosed autistic children, across childhood and adolescence. *Journal of Child Psychology and Psychiatry, and Allied Disciplines, 63*(11), 1405–1414. https://doi.org/10.1111/jcpp.13587

Matthews, N. L., Ly, A. R., & Goldberg, W. A. (2015). College students' perceptions of peers with autism spectrum disorder. *Journal of Autism and Developmental Disorders, 45*, 90–99. https://doi.org/10.1007/s10803-014-2195-6

May, T., Brignell, A., & Williams, K. (2021). Parent-reported autism diagnostic stability and trajectories in the longitudinal study of Australian children. *Autism Research, 14*(4), 773–786. https://doi.org/10.1002/aur.2470

Mazefsky, C. A., Oswald, D. P., Day, T. N., Eack, S. M., Minshew, N. J., & Lainhart, J. E. (2012). ASD, a psychiatric disorder, or both? Psychiatric diagnoses in adolescents with high-functioning ASD. *Journal of Clinical Child and Adolescent Psychology: The Official Journal for the Society of Clinical Child and Adolescent Psychology, 41*(4), 516–523. https://doi.org/10.1080/15374416.2012.686102

McAlonan, G. M. (2004). Mapping the brain in autism: A voxel-based MRI study of volumetric differences and intercorrelations in autism. *Brain, 128*(2), 268–276. https://doi.org/10.1093/brain/awh332

McCabe, P., Murray, E., & Thomas, D. (2024). *Evidence summary – Childhood apraxia of speech January 2024*. https://rest.sydney.edu.au/wp-content/uploads/2024/01/CAS_evidence_brief_2024.pdf

McCauley, J. B., Elias, R., & Lord, C. (2020). Trajectories of co-occurring psychopathology symptoms in autism from late childhood to adulthood. *Development and Psychopathology, 32*(4), 1287–1302. https://doi.org/10.1017/S0954579420000826

McCormack, L., Wong, S. W., & Campbell, L. E. (2023). 'If I don't do it, I'm out of rhythm and I can't focus as well': Positive and negative adult interpretations of therapies aimed at 'fixing' their restricted and repetitive behaviours in childhood. *Journal of Autism and Developmental Disorders, 53*(9), 3435–3448. https://doi.org/10.1007/s10803-022-05644-6

McDermott, C. (2022). Theorising the neurotypical gaze: Autistic love and relationships in *The Bridge*. *Medical Humanities, 48*(1), 51–62. https://doi.org/10.1136/medhum-2020-011906

McDonnell, A., & Milton, D. (2014). Going with the flow: Reconsidering 'repetitive behaviour' through the concept of 'flow states'. In G. Jones & E. Hurley (Eds.), *Good autism practice: Autism, happiness and wellbeing* (pp. 38–47). BILD.

McGreevy, E., Quinn, A., Law, R., Botha, M., Evans, M., Rose, K., Moyse, R., Boyens, T., Matejko, M., & Pavlopoulou, G. (2024). An experience sensitive approach to care with and for autistic children and young people in clinical services. *Journal of Humanistic Psychology*. https://doi.org/10.1177/00221678241232442

McNicholl, E. (2020). *A kind of spark*. Knights Of.

Menezes, M., Soland, J., & Mazurek, M. (2023). Screen time and diagnoses of anxiety and depression in autistic versus neurotypical youth. *Research in Autism Spectrum Disorders, 107*(102222). https://doi.org/10.1016/j.rasd.2023.102222

Mesa, S., & Hamilton, L. G. (2022). 'We are different, that's a fact, but they treat us like we're different-er': Understanding of autism and adolescent identity development. *Advances in Autism, 8*(3), 217–231.

Miller, H. L., Sherrod, G. M., Mauk, J. E., Fears, N. E., Hynan, L. S., & Tamplain, P. M. (2021). Shared features or co-occurrence? Evaluating symptoms of developmental coordination disorder in children and adolescents with autism spectrum disorder. *Journal of Autism and Developmental Disorders, 51*(10), 3443–3455. https://doi.org/10.1007/s10803-020-04766-z

Milton, D. (2012). On the ontological status of autism: The 'double empathy problem'. *Disability & Society, 27*(6), 883–887. https://doi.org/10.1080/09687599.2012.710008

Miserandino, C. (2017). The spoon theory. In L. J. Davis (Ed.), *Beginning with disability* (pp. 174–178). Routledge.

Mogensen, L., & Mason, J. (2015). The meaning of a label for teenagers negotiating identity: Experiences with autism spectrum disorder. *Sociology of Health & Illness, 37*(2), 255–269. https://doi.org/10.1111/1467-9566.12208

Mohd Nordin, A., Ismail, J., & Kamal Nor, N. (2021). Motor development in children with autism spectrum disorder. *Frontiers in Paediatrics, 9*, Article 598276. https://doi.org/10.3389/fped.2021.598276

Monteiro, M. J., & Stegall, S. (2018). *Monteiro interview guidelines for diagnosing the autism spectrum, Second Edition (MIGDAS-2)*. Western Psychological Services.

Moody, E. J., Reyes, N., Ledbetter, C., Wiggins, L., Di Guiseppi, C., Alexander, A., Jackson, S., Lee, L. C., Levy, S. E., & Rosenberg, S. A. (2017). Screening for autism with the SRS and SCQ: Variations across demographic, developmental, and behavioral factors in preschool children. *Journal of Autism and Developmental Disorders, 47*(11), 3550–3561. https://doi.org/10.1007/s10803-017-3255-5

Moon, S. J., Hwang, J. S., Shin, A. L., Kim, J. Y., Bae, S. M., Sheehy-Knight, J., & Kim, J. W. (2019). Accuracy of the Childhood Autism Rating Scale: A systematic review and meta-analysis. *Developmental Medicine and Child Neurology, 61*(9), 1030–1038. https://doi.org/10.1111/dmcn.14246

Morgan, F., & Costello, E. (2022). *Square pegs: Inclusivity, compassion and fitting in – A guide for schools*. Independent Thinking Press.

Morgan, S., & Dipper, L. (2018). Is the communication pyramid a useful model of language development? *Royal College of Speech & Language Therapists Bulletin*, May, 26–28. www.rcslt.org/docs/bulletin/2018/may_2018

Morsanyi, K., van Bers, B. M. C. W., McCormack, T., & McGourty, J. (2018). The prevalence of specific learning disorder in mathematics and comorbidity with other developmental disorders in primary school-age children. *British Journal of Psychology, 109*(4), 917–940. https://doi.org/10.1111/bjop.12322

Mueller, V. T. (2021). Total communication (TC) approach. In F. R. Volkmar (Ed.), *Encyclopedia of autism spectrum disorders* (pp. 4869–4874). Springer. https://doi.org/10.1007/978-3-319-91280-6_1708

Mukherjee, S., & Beresford, B. (2023). Factors influencing the mental health of autistic children and teenagers: Parents' observations and experiences. *Autism, 27*(8), 2324–2336. https://doi.org/10.1177/13623613231158959

Murphy, K. (2022). *Neurodiversity in the early years: Neurodiversity and ableism reflection tool*. https://assets-global.websitefiles.com/5f903cbab2ae71f26cf02400/638a04bcc5a15c6fda2c02b1_AUDIT_Kerry%20Murphy.pdf

Murphy, K. (2023). *A beginner's guide to self-directed neurodivergent play*. Tapestry UK. https://tapestry.info/a-beginners-guide-to-self-directed-neurodivergent-play-2.html

Murphy, S. (2021). The pros and cons of being an autistic parent. *Good Autism Practice, 22*(1), 87–96.

Murray, D., Lesser, M., & Lawson, W. (2005). Attention, monotropism, and the diagnostic criteria for autism. *Autism, 9*(2), 139–156. https://doi.org/10.1171/1362361305051398

Murray, F. (2017). Autism as a disability. *Medium*. https://oolong.medium.com/autism-as-a-disability-14790520ef81

Murray, F. (2019). Me and monotropism: A unified theory of autism. *The Psychologist, 32*, 44–49.

Murray, F. (2023). Monotropism and wellbeing. Scottish Autism Research Group Meeting October 2023. https://monotropism.org/wellbeing/

Nadesan, M. H. (2005). *Constructing autism: Unravelling the 'truth' and understanding the social*. Routledge.

Neihart, M. (2008). Identifying and providing services to twice exceptional children. In S. I. Pfeiffer (Ed.), *Handbook of giftedness in children: Psychoeducational theory, research, and best practices* (pp. 115–137). Springer Science + Business Media. https://doi.org/10.1007/978-0-387-74401-8_7

Neumeier, S. M. (2018, 9 February). 'To Siri with Love' and the problem with neurodiversity lite. *Rewire News*. https://rewirenewsgroup.com/2018/02/09/siri-love-problem-neurodiversity-lite/

NeuroClastic. (2021, 11 February). Nonspeaker perspectives on representation. *NeuroClastic*.

NICE. (2017). Autism spectrum disorder in under 19's: Recognition, referral and diagnosis. *NICE Clinical Guideline [CG128]*. National Institute for Health and Care Excellence. www.nice.org.uk/guidance/cg128

NICE. (2021). Autism spectrum disorder in under 19's: Support and management. *NICE Clinical Guidelines [CG170]*. National Institute for Health and Care Excellence. www.nice.org.uk/guidance/cg170

NICE. (2023). Clinical knowledge summary attention deficit hyperactivity disorder. National Institute for Health and Care Excellence. https://cks.nice.org.uk/topics/attention-deficit-hyperactivity-disorder/

Nicolaidis, C., Milton, D., Sasson, N. J., Sheppard, E., & Yergeau, M. (2019). An expert discussion on autism and empathy. *Autism in Adulthood, 1*(1), 4–11. https://doi.org/10.1089/aut.2018.29000.cjn

Nimbley, E., Gillespie-Smith, K., Duffy, F., Maloney, E., Ballantyne, C., & Sharpe, H. (2023). 'It's not about wanting to be thin or look small, it's about the way it feels': An IPA analysis of social and sensory differences in autistic and non-autistic individuals with anorexia and their parents. *Journal of Eating Disorders, 11*(1), 89. https://doi.org/10.1186/s40337-023-00813-z

Norbury, C. F., Gooch, D., Wray, C., Baird, G., Charman, T., Simonoff, E., Vamvakas, G., & Pickles, A. (2016). The impact of nonverbal ability on prevalence and clinical presentation of language disorder: Evidence from a population study. *Journal of Child Psychology and Psychiatry, 57*(11), 1247–1257. https://doi.org/10.1111/jcpp.12573

Nordahl-Hansen, A., Kaale, A., & Ulvund, S. E. (2014). Language assessment in children with autism spectrum disorder: Concurrent validity between report-based assessments and direct tests. *Research in Autism Spectrum Disorders, 8*(9), 1100–1106.

NSAI (National Standards Authority of Ireland). (2024). Universal design and inclusion. www.nsai.ie/standards/sectors/universal-design-and-inclusion/#:~:text=Universal%20Design%20is%20the%20process,%2C%20size2C%20ability%20or%20disability

O'Donnell-Killen, T., & Zadurian, N. (2023). *Exploring wellbeing in neurodiversity affirming families*. International Society for Autism Research Annual Meeting (INSAR).

Oredipe, T., Kofner, B., Riccio, A., Cage, E., Vincent, J., Kapp, S. K., Dwyer, P., & Gillespie-Lynch, K. (2023). Does learning you are autistic at a younger age lead to better adult outcomes? A participatory exploration of the perspectives of autistic university students. *Autism, 27*(1), 200–212. https://doi.org/10.1177/13623613221086700

Orsini, M., & Smith, M. (2010). Social movements, knowledge and public policy: The case of autism activism in Canada and the US. *Critical Policy Studies, 4*(1), 38–57. https://doi.org/10.1080/19460171003714989

Ostrolenk, A., Forgeot d'Arc, B., Jelenic, P., Samson, F., & Mottron, L. (2017). Hyperlexia: Systematic review, neurocognitive modelling, and outcome. *Neuroscience and Biobehavioral Reviews, 79*, 134–149. https://doi.org/10.1016/j.neubiorev.2017.04.029

Ozonoff, S., Young, G. S., Brian, J., Charman, T., Shephard, E., Solish, A., & Zwaigenbaum, L. (2018). Diagnosis of autism spectrum disorder after age 5 in children evaluated longitudinally since infancy. *Journal of the American Academy of Child & Adolescent Psychiatry, 57*(11), 849–857. https://doi.org/10.1016/j.jaac.2018.06.022

Ozonoff, S., Young, G. S., Landa, R. J., Brian, J., Bryson, S., Charman, T., Chawarska, K., Macari, S. L., Messinger, D., Stone, W. L., Zwaigenbaum, L., & Iosif, A. M. (2015). Diagnostic stability in young children at risk for autism spectrum disorder: A baby siblings research consortium study. *Journal of Child Psychology and Psychiatry, 56*(9), 988–998. https://doi.org/10.1111/jcpp.12421

Parks, K. M. A., Hannah, K. E., Moreau, C. N., Brainin, L., & Joanisse, M. F. (2023). Language abilities in children and adolescents with DLD and ADHD: A scoping review. *Journal of Communication Disorders, 106*, 106381. https://doi.org/10.1016/j.jcomdis.2023.106381

Pavlopoulou, G. (2021). A good night's sleep: Learning about sleep from autistic adolescents' personal accounts. *Frontiers in Psychology, 22*(11), 583868. https://doi.org/10.3389/fpsyg.2020.583868

Payne, K. (2022). *Supporting the wellbeing of children with SEND: Essential ideas for early years educators*. Little Minds Matter.

Pearson, A., & Rose, K. (2021). A conceptual analysis of autistic masking: Understanding the narrative of stigma and the illusion of choice. *Autism in Adulthood, 3*(1), 52–60. https://doi.org/10.1089/aut.2020.0043

Pearson, A., & Rose, K. (2023). *Autistic masking: Understanding identity management and the role of stigma*. Pavilion.

Pecora, L. A., Hancock, G. I., Mesibov, G. B., & Stokes, M. A. (2019). Characterising the sexuality and sexual experiences of autistic females. *Journal of Autism and Developmental Disorders, 49*(12), 4834–4846. https://doi.org/10.1007/s10803-019-04204-9

Peters, A. M. (1977). Language learning strategies: does the whole equal the sum of the parts? *Language, 53*, 5673.

Peters, A. M. (1983). *The Units of Language Acquisition*. Cambridge University Press.

Pham, H. H., Sandberg, N., Trinkl, J., & Thayer, J. (2022). Racial and ethnic differences in rates and age of diagnosis of autism spectrum disorder. *JAMA Network Open, 5*(10), e2239604. https://doi.org/10.1001/jamanetworkopen.2022.39604

Phung, J., Penner, M., Pirlot, C., & Welch, C. (2021). What I wish you knew: Insights on burnout, inertia, meltdown, and shutdown from autistic youth. *Frontiers in Psychology, 12*, 741421. https://doi.org/10.3389/fpsyg.2021.741421

Pierce, K., Gazestani, V. H., Bacon, E., Barnes, C. C., Cha, D., Nalabolu, S., Lopez, L., Moore, A., Pence-Stophaeros, S., & Courchesne, E. (2019). Evaluation of the diagnostic stability of the early autism spectrum disorder phenotype in the general population starting at 12 months. *JAMA Pediatrics, 173*(6), 578–587. https://doi.org/10.1001/jamapediatrics.2019.0624

Pohl, A., Blakemore, M., & Allison, C. (2016). Positive and negative experiences of mothers with autism. Poster presentation, IMFAR, Baltimore.

Polyak, A., Kubina, R. M., & Girirajan, S. (2015). Comorbidity of intellectual disability confounds ascertainment of autism: Implications for genetic diagnosis. *American Journal of Medical Genetics Part B: Neuropsychiatric Genetics, 168*(7), 600–608. https://doi.org/10.1002/ajmg.b.32338

Posner, J., Polanczyk, G. V., & Sonuga-Barke, E. (2020). Attention-deficit hyperactivity disorder. *The Lancet, 395*(10222), 450–462. https://doi.org/10.1016/S0140-6736(19)33004-1

Prizant, B. M. (1983). Language acquisition and communicative behavior in autism: Toward an understanding of the 'whole' of it. *Journal of Speech and Hearing Disorders, 48*(3), 296–307. https://doi.org/10.1044/jshd.4803.296

Prizant, B. M., Wetherby, A. M., Rubin, E., Laurent, A. C., & Rydell, P. J. (2006). *The SCERTS model: A comprehensive educational approach for children with autism spectrum disorders* (Vol. 1). Paul H. Brookes Publishing.

Proctor, G. (2002). *The dynamics of power in counselling and psychotherapy.* PCCS Books.

Psychological Society of Ireland (PSI). (2022). *Professional practice guidelines for the assessment, formulation, and diagnosis of autism in children and adolescents* (2nd ed.). PSI.

Purkis, Y. (2022, 24 March). Why empathy is not as simple as it seems. *Yenn Purkis Autism Page.* https://yennpurkis.home.blog/

Ram, J. (2020). I am a disillusioned BCBA: Autistics are right about ABA. *Neuroclastic.* https://neuroclastic.com/i-am-a-disillusioned-bcba-autistics-are-right-about-aba/

Randall, M., Egberts, K. J., Samtani, A., Scholten, R., Hooft, L., Livingstone, N., et al. (2018). Diagnostic tests for autism spectrum disorder (ASD) in preschool children. *Cochrane Database of Systematic Reviews, 7.* https://doi.org/10.1002/14651858.CD009044

Rapaport, H., Clapham, H., Adams, J., Lawson, W., Porayska-Pomsta, K., & Pellicano, E. (2023). 'In a state of flow': A qualitative examination of autistic adults' phenomenological experiences of task immersion. *Autism in Adulthood.* https://doi.org/10.1089/aut.2023.0032

Raymaker, D. M., Teo, A. R., Steckler, N. A., Lentz, B., Scharer, M., Delos Santos, A., Kapp, S. K., Hunter, M., Joyce, A., & Nicolaidis, C. (2020). 'Having all of your internal resources exhausted beyond measure and being left with no clean-up crew': Defining autistic burnout. *Autism in Adulthood, 2*(2). https://doi.org/10.1089/aut.2019.0079

Raznahan, A., Toro, R., Daly, E., Robertson, D., Murphy, C., Deeley, Q., Bolton, P. F., Paus, T., & Murphy, D. G. M. (2010). Cortical anatomy in autism spectrum disorder: An in vivo MRI study on the effect of age. *Cerebral Cortex, 20*(6), 1332–1340. https://doi.org/10.1093/cercor/bhp198

Reilly, S., Wake, M., Ukoumunne, O. C., Bavin, E., Prior, M., Cini, E., Bretherton, L. (2010). Predicting language outcomes at 4 years of age: Findings from Early Language in Victoria study. *Pediatrics, 126*(6), e1530-e1537.

Reis, S. M., Gelbar, N. W., & Madaus, J. W. (2022). Understanding the academic success of academically talented college students with autism spectrum disorders. *Journal of Autism and Developmental Disorders, 52*(10), 4426–4439. https://doi.org/10.1007/s10803-021-05290-4

Reuben, K. E., Stanzione, C. M., & Singleton, J. L. (2021). Interpersonal trauma and posttraumatic stress in autistic adults. *Autism in Adulthood, 3*(3), 247–256. https://doi.org/10.1089/aut.2020.0073

Riccio, A., Kapp, S. K., Jordan, A., Dorelien, A. M., & Gillespie-Lynch, K. (2021). How is autistic identity in adolescence influenced by parental disclosure decisions and perceptions of autism? *Autism, 25*(2), 374–388. https://doi.org/10.1177/1362361320958214

Rice-Adams, E. (2023). Autistic young people's sense of self and the social world: A challenge to deficit-based characteristics. In D. Milton & S. Ryan (Eds.), *The Routledge international handbook of critical autism studies.* Routledge.

Richards, C., Jones, C., Groves, L., Moss, J., & Oliver, C. (2015). Prevalence of autism spectrum disorder phenomenology in genetic disorders: A systematic review and meta-analysis. *The Lancet Psychiatry, 2*(10), 909–916. https://doi.org/10.1016/S2215-0366(15)00376-4

Richman, K. (2020). Neurodiversity and autism advocacy: Who fits under the autism tent? *American Journal of Bioethics, 20*(4), 33–34. https://doi.org/10.1080/15265161.2020.1730493

Reiersen, A. M., Constantino, J. N., Volk, H. E., & Todd, R. D. (2007). Autistic traits in a population-based ADHD twin sample. *Journal of Child Psychology and Psychiatry, and Allied Disciplines, 48*(5), 464–472. https://doi.org/10.1111/j.1469-7610.2006.01720.x

Rimland, B. (1964). *Infantile autism: The syndrome and its implications for a neural theory of behavior.* Appleton-Century-Crofts.

Risi, S., Lord, C., Gotham, K., Corsello, C., Chrysler, C., Szatmari, P., et al. (2006). Combining information from multiple sources in the diagnosis of autism spectrum disorders. *Journal of the American Academy of Child and Adolescent Psychiatry, 45*(9), 1094–1103. https://doi.org/10.1097/01.chi.0000227880.42780.0e

Robins, D. L., Casagrande, K., Barton, M., Chen, C. M. A., Dumont-Mathieu, T., & Fein, D. (2014). Validation of the modified checklist for autism in toddlers, revised with follow-up (M-CHAT-R/F). *Pediatrics, 133*(1), 37–45. https://doi.org/10.1542/peds.2013-1813

Robins, D. L., Fein, D., & Barton, M. (1999). *The modified checklist for autism in toddlers (M-CHAT).* Self-published.

Roche, L., Adams, D., & Clark, M. (2020). Research priorities of the autism community: A systematic review of key stakeholder perspectives. *Autism, 25*(2), 336–348. https://doi.org/10.1177/1362361320967790

Rose, J. (2009). *Identifying and teaching children and young people with dyslexia and literacy difficulties.* Department for Children, Schools, and Families.

Rose, K. (2018, May 21). An autistic burnout – The autistic advocate. *The Autistic Advocate.* https://theautisticadvocate.com/an-autistic-burnout/

Rosen, T. E., Mazefsky, C. A., Vasa, R. A., & Lerner, M. D. (2018). Co-occurring psychiatric conditions in autism spectrum disorder. *International Review of Psychiatry, 30*(1), 40–61. https://doi.org/10.1080/09540261.2018.1450229

Russell, G., Mandy, W., Elliott, D., White, R., Pittwood, T., & Ford, T. (2019). Selection bias on intellectual ability in autism research: A cross-sectional review and meta-analysis. *Molecular Autism, 10*(1), 1–13. https://doi.org/10.1186/s13229-019-0260-x

Rutherford, M., & Johnston, L. (2023). Rethinking autism assessment, diagnosis, and intervention within a neurodevelopmental pathway framework. In M. Carotenuto (Ed.), *Autism spectrum disorders – Recent advances and new perspectives.* IntechOpen. https://doi.org/10.5772/intechopen.108784

Rutter, M., Bailey, A., & Lord, C. (2003). *Social communication questionnaire.* Western Psychological Services.

Rutter, M., LeCouteur, A., & Lord, C. (2003). *Autism diagnostic interview-revised (ADI-R).* Western Psychological Services.

Sala, G., Pecora, L., Hooley, M., & Stokes, M. A. (2020). As diverse as the spectrum itself: Trends in sexuality, gender, and autism. *Current Developmental Disorders Reports, 7*(2), 59–68. https://doi.org/10.1007/s40474-020-00190-1

Sandin, S., Lichtenstein, P., Kuja-Halkola, R., Hultman, C., Larsson, H., & Reichenberg, A. (2017). The heritability of autism spectrum disorder. *JAMA, 318*(12), 1182–1184. https://doi.org/10.1001/jama.2017.12141

Santinele Martino, A. (2017). Cripping sexualities: An analytic review of theoretical and empirical writing on the intersection of disabilities and sexualities. *Sociology Compass, 11*(5), e12471. https://doi.org/10.1111/soc4.12471

Sasson, N. J., & Morrison, K. E. (2019). First impressions of adults with autism improve with diagnostic disclosure and increased autism knowledge of peers. *Autism, 23*(1), 50–59. https://doi.org/10.1177/1362361317729526

Sasson, N. J., Faso, D. J., Nugent, J., Lovell, S., Kennedy, D. P., & Grossman, R. B. (2017). Neurotypical peers are less willing to interact with those with autism based on thin slice judgments. *Scientific Reports, 7*, 40700. https://doi.org/10.1038/srep40700

Sayal, K., Prasad, V., Daley, D., Ford, T., & Coghill, D. (2018). ADHD in children and young people: Prevalence, care pathways, and service provision. *The Lancet Psychiatry, 5*(2), 175–186. https://doi.org/10.1016/S2215-0366(17)30167-0

Schopler, E., Van Bourgondien, M. E., Wellman, G. J., & Love, S. R. (2010). *CARS-2: Childhood Autism Rating Scale–Second edition.* Western Psychological Services.

Scottish Intercollegiate Guidelines Network. (2016). *SIGN 145: Assessment, diagnosis and interventions for autism spectrum disorders: A national clinical guideline.* www.sign.ac.uk/assets/sign145.pdf

Seli, P., Wammes, J. D., Risko, E. F., & Smilek, D. (2015). On the relation between motivation and retention in educational contexts: The role of intentional and unintentional mind wandering. *Psychonomic Bulletin & Review, 23*(4), 1280–1287. https://doi.org/10.3758/s13423-015-0979-0

Sheppard, E., Pillai, D., Wong, G. T. L., Ropar, D., & Mitchell, P. (2016). How easy is it to read the minds of people with autism spectrum disorder? *Journal of Autism and Developmental Disorders, 46*(4), 1247–1254. https://doi.org/10.1007/s10803-015-2662-8

Shriberg, L. D., Paul, R., Black, L. M., & van Santen, J. P. (2011). The hypothesis of apraxia of speech in children with autism spectrum disorder. *J Autism Dev Disord, 41*(4), 405–426. doi: 10.1007/s10803-010-1117-5

Silberman, S. (2016). *Neurotribes: The legacy of autism and the future of neurodiversity*. Avery.

Simmonds, M. (2023). Through the lens of (Black) Critical Race Theory. In D. Milton & S. Ryan (Eds.), *The Routledge international handbook of critical autism studies*. Routledge.

Simonoff, E., Pickles, A., Charman, T., Chandler, S., Loucas, T., & Baird, G. (2008). Psychiatric disorders in children with autism spectrum disorders: Prevalence, comorbidity, and associated factors in a population-derived sample. *Journal of the American Academy of Child and Adolescent Psychiatry, 47*(8), 921–929. https://doi.org/10.1097/CHI.0b013e318179964f

Sinclair, J. (1993). Don't mourn for us. *Our Voice, 1*(3). www.autreat.com/dont_mourn.html

Slade, G. (2014). *Diverse perspectives: The challenges for families affected by autism from Black, Asian, and minority ethnic communities*. The National Autistic Society. https://positiveaboutautism.co.uk/uploads/9/7/4/5/97454370/nas-diverseperspectivesreport-1.pdf

Soares, N., & Patel, D. R. (2015). Dyscalculia. *International Journal of Child and Adolescent Health, 8*(1), 15–26.

Spence, S., & Schneider, M. (2009). The role of epilepsy and epileptiform EEGs in autism spectrum disorders. *Pediatric Research*. https://doi.org/10.1203/PDR.0b013e31819e7168

Stagnitti, K., & Cooper, R. (2009). *Play as therapy: Assessment and therapeutic interventions*. Jessica Kingsley Publishers.

Stearns, P. N. (2004). *Anxious parents: A history of modern childrearing in America*. NYU Press.

Steffenburg, H., Steffenburg, S., Gillberg, C., & Billstedt, E. (2018). Children with autism spectrum disorders and selective mutism. *Neuropsychiatric Disorders Treatment, 7*(14), 1163–1169. https://doi.org/10.2147/NDT.S154966

Stoll, M. M., Bergamo, N., & Rossetti, K. G. (2021). Analyzing modes of assessment for children with autism spectrum disorder (ASD) using a culturally sensitive lens. *Advances in Neurodevelopmental Disorders, 5*(3), 233–244. https://doi.org/10.1007/s41252-021-00210-0

Straiton, D., & Sridhar, A. (2022). Short report: Call to action for autism clinicians in response to anti-Black racism. *Autism, 26*(4), 988–994. https://doi.org/10.1177/13623613211043643

Sturm, A., Kuhfeld, M., Kasari, C., & McCracken, J. T. (2017). Development and validation of an item response theory-based Social Responsiveness Scale short form. *Journal of Child Psychology and Psychiatry, 58*(9), 1053–1061. https://doi.org/10.1111/jcpp.12731

Sturner, R., Howard, B., Bergmann, P., Attar, S., Stewart-Artz, L., Bet, K., Allison, C., & Baron-Cohen, S. (2022). Autism screening at 18 months of age: A comparison of the Q-CHAT-10 and M-CHAT screeners. *Molecular Autism, 13*(2). https://doi.org/10.1186/s13229-021-00480-4

Sturner, R., Howard, B., Bergmann, P., Morrel, T., Landa, R., Walton, K., & Marks, D. (2017). Accurate autism screening at the 18-month well-child visit requires different strategies than at 24 months. *Journal of Autism and Developmental Disorders, 31*(1), 1–5. https://doi.org/10.1007/s10803-017-3231-0

Sutherland, R., Trembath, D., & Roberts, J. (2018). Telehealth and autism: A systematic search and review of the literature. *International Journal of Speech-Language Pathology, 20*(3), 324–336. https://doi.org/10.1080/17549507.2018.1465123

Therapist Neurodiversity Collective. (2018–2024). *Non-ABA evidence-based practice*. https://therapistndc.org/therapy/non-aba-evidence-based-practice/

Thomas, N., Blake, S., Morris, C., & Moles, D. (2018). Autism and primary care dentistry: Parents' experiences of taking children with autism or working diagnosis of autism for dental examinations. *International Journal of Paediatric Dentistry, 28*(2), 226–238. https://doi.org/10.1111/ipd.12345

Thompson-Hodgetts, S., Ryan, J., Coombs, E., Brown, H. M., Xavier, A., Devlin, C., Lee, A., Kedmy, A., & Borden, A. (2023). Toward understanding and enhancing self-determination: A qualitative exploration with autistic adults without co-occurring intellectual disability. *Frontiers in Psychiatry, 14*, 1250391. https://doi.org/10.3389/fpsyt.2023.1250391

Thresher, K. (2019). Young people's experience of an autism assessment. Service evaluation project prepared as part of the Leeds D.Clin. Psychology Programme. https://dclinpsych.leeds.ac.uk/wp-content/uploads/sites/26/2020/06/kate_thresher_sep_online.pdf

Thurm, A., Farmer, C., Salzman, E., Lord, C., & Bishop, S. (2019). State of the field: Differentiating intellectual disability from autism spectrum disorder. *Frontiers in Psychiatry, 10*. https://doi.org/10.3389/fpsyt.2019.00526

Timimi, S., Milton, D., Bovell, V., Kapp, S., & Russell, G. (2019). Deconstructing diagnosis: Four commentaries on a diagnostic tool to assess individuals for autism spectrum disorders. *Autonomy, 1*(6), AR26.

Todres, L., Galvin, K. T., & Holloway, I. (2009). The humanization of healthcare: A value framework for qualitative research. *International Journal of Qualitative Studies on Health and Wellbeing, 4*(2), 68–77. https://doi.org/10.1080/17482620802646204

Toft, A. (2023). 'These made-up things mean nothing to me': Exploring the intersection of autism and bisexuality in the lives of young people. *Journal of Bisexuality, 23*(3), 229–249. https://doi.org/10.1080/15299716.2023.2214134

Toft, A., Franklin, A., & Langley, E. (2020). 'You're not sure that you are gay yet': The perpetuation of the 'phase' in the lives of young disabled LGBT+ people. *Sexualities, 23*(4), 516–529. https://doi.org/10.1177/1363460719842135

Toh, T. H., Tan, V. W., Lau, P. S., & Kiyu, A. (2017). Accuracy of Modified Checklist for Autism in Toddlers (M-CHAT) in detecting autism and other developmental disorders in community clinics. *Journal of Autism and Developmental Disorders, 2*, 1–8.

Tomblin, J. B., Records, N. L., Buckwalter, P., Zhang, X., Smith, E., & O'Brien, M. (1997). Prevalence of specific language impairment in kindergarten children. *Journal of Speech, Language and Hearing Research, 40*(6), 1245–1260. https://doi.org/10.1044/jslhr.4006.1245

Totton, N. (2015). *Embodied relating: The ground of psychotherapy.* Routledge.

Totton, N. (2023). *Different bodies: Deconstructing normality.* PCCS Books.

Treffert, D. A., & Rebedew, D. L. (2015). The Savant Syndrome Registry: A preliminary report. *WMJ: Official Publication of the State Medical Society of Wisconsin, 114*(4), 158–162.

Triana, A. J., Gusforf, R. E., Kaustav, P. S., & Horst, S. N. (2020). Technology literacy as a barrier to telehealth during COVID-19. *Telemedicine and e-Health, 26*(9), 1118–1119. https://doi.org/10.1089/tmj.2020.0155

Tromans, S., Chester, V., Gemegah, E., Roberts, K., Morgan, Z., Yao, G. L., & Brugha, T. (2021). Autism identification across ethnic groups: A narrative review. *Advances in Autism, 7*(3), 241–255. https://doi.org/10.1108/AIA-03-2020-0017

Uddin, L. Q. (2022). Exceptional abilities in autism: Theories and open questions. *Current Directions in Psychological Science, 31*(6), 509–517. https://doi.org/10.1177/09637214221113760

Underhill, J. C., Ledford, V., & Adams, H. (2019). Autism stigma in communication classrooms: Exploring peer attitudes and motivations toward interacting with atypical students. *Communication Education, 68*(2), 175–192. https://doi.org/10.1080/03634523.2019.1569247

Valvano, L., & Shelton, J. (2021). Existing outside of gender: Autism and gender identity: A conversation with Liliana Valvano. In J. Shelton & G. P. Mallon (Eds.), *Social work practice with transgender and gender expansive youth* (pp. 153–159). Routledge.

Vogindroukas, I., Stankova, M., Chelas, E. N., & Proedrou, A. (2022). Language and speech characteristics in autism. *Neuropsychiatric Disorders Treatment, 14*(18), 2367–2377. https://doi.org/10.2147/NDT.S331987

Wakefield, D. A., & McCarthy, A. M. (2020). Ethical concerns with Applied Behaviour Analysis for autism spectrum disorder. *Kennedy Institute of Ethics Journal, 30*(1), 36–69. https://doi.org/10.1353/ken.2020.0000

Walker, N. (2019). Somatics and autistic embodiment. In D. H. Johnson (Ed.), *Diverse bodies, diverse practices: Towards an inclusive somatics.* North Atlantic Books.

Walker, N. (2021). *Neuroqueer heresies.* Autonomous Press.

Waltz, M. (2020). The production of the normal child. In H. Bertilsdotter Rosqvuist, N. Chown, & A. Stenning (Eds.), *Neurodiversity studies: A new critical paradigm.* Routledge.

Warrier, V., Greenberg, D. M., Weir, E., Buckingham, C., Smith, P., Lai, M. C., Allison, C., & Baron-Cohen, S. (2020). Elevated rates of autism, other neurodevelopmental and psychiatric diagnoses, and autistic traits in transgender and gender-diverse individuals. *Nature Communications, 11*(1), 1–12. https://doi.org/10.1038/s41467-020-17794-1

Wassell, C., & Burke, E. (2022). *Autism, girls, & keeping it all inside.* Autistic Girls Network. https://autisticgirlsnetwork.org/keeping-it-all-inside.pdf

Weir, E., Allison, C., & Baron-Cohen, S. (2020). Increased prevalence of non-communicable physical health conditions among autistic adults. *Autism, 25*(3), 681–694. https://doi.org/10.1177/1362361320953652

Weir, E., Allison, C., & Baron-Cohen, S. (2021). The sexual health, orientation, and activity of autistic adolescents and adults. *Autism Research: Official Journal of the International Society for Autism Research, 14*(11), 2342–2354. https://doi.org/10.1002/aur.2604

Wenger, T. L., Miller, J. S., De Polo, L. M., de Marchena, A. B., Clements, C. C., et al. (2016). 22q11.2 duplication syndrome: Elevated rate of autism spectrum disorder and need for medical screening. *Molecular Autism, 7*(27). https://doi.org/10.1186/s13229-016-0097-5

Westwood, H., & Tchanturia, K. (2017). Autism spectrum disorder in anorexia nervosa: An updated literature review. *Current Psychiatry Reports, 19*(41). https://doi.org/10.1007/s11920-017-0791-9

Wieckowski, A. T., Williams, L. N., Rando, J., Lyall, K., & Robins, D. L. (2023). Sensitivity and specificity of the Modified Checklist for Autism in Toddlers (Original and Revised): A systematic review and meta-analysis. *JAMA Pediatrics, 177*(4), 373–383. https://doi.org/10.1001/jamapediatrics.2022.5975

Wiggins, L. D., Nadler, C., Hepburn, S., Rosenberg, S., Reynolds, A., & Zubler, J. (2022). Toileting resistance among preschool-age children with and without autism spectrum disorder. *Journal of Developmental and Behavioural Paediatrics, 43*(4), 216–223. https://doi.org/10.1097/DBP.0000000000001036

Wilcock, A. A., & Townsend, E. A. (2009). Occupational justice. In E. B. Crepeau, E. S. Cohn, & B. A. Boyt Schell (Eds.), *Willard & Spackman's occupational therapy* (11th ed., pp. 192–199). Lippincott Williams & Wilkins.

Williams, D. (1996). *Autism: An inside-out approach.* Jessica Kingsley Publishers.

Wing, L. (1981). Asperger's syndrome: A clinical account. *Psychological Medicine, 11*(1), 115–129. https://doi.org/10.1017/S0033291700053332

Wise, S. J. (2024). *We're all neurodiverse.* Jessica Kingsley Publishers.

Wodka, E. L., Mathy, P., & Kalb, L. (2013). Predictors of phrase and fluent speech in children with autism and severe language delay. *Pediatrics, 131*(4), e1128–e1134. https://doi.org/10.1542/peds.2012-2221

Wood, R. (2019a). Autism, intense interests and support in school: From wasted efforts to shared understandings. *Educational Review, 73*(1), 34–54. https://doi.org/10.1080/00131911.2019.1566213

Wood, R. (2019b). *Inclusive education for autistic children.* Jessica Kingsley Publishers.

Woods, S. E. O., & Estes, A. (2023). Toward a more comprehensive autism assessment: The survey of autistic strengths, skills, and interests. *Frontiers in Psychiatry, 14*, 1264516. https://doi.org/10.3389/fpsyt.2023.1264516

Woolf, S. H., Grol, R., Hutchinson, A., Eccles, M., & Grimshaw, J. (1999). Potential benefits, limitations, and harms of clinical guidelines. *British Medical Journal, 318*(7182), 527–530. https://doi.org/10.1136/bmj.318.7182.527

World Federation of Occupational Therapists. (2019). *Occupational therapy and human rights.* https://wfot.org/resources/occupational-therapy-and-human-rights

Wu, I. C., Lo, C. O., & Tsai, K. F. (2019). Learning experiences of highly able learners with ASD: Using a success case method. *Journal for the Education of the Gifted, 42*(3), 216–242. https://doi.org/10.1177/0162353219855681

Wu, S., Zhao, J., de Villiers, J., Liu, X. L., Rolfhus, E., Sun, X., Li, X., Pan, H., Wang, H., Zhu, Q., Dong, Y., Zhang, Y., & Jiang, F. (2023). Prevalence, co-occurring difficulties, and risk factors of developmental language disorder: First evidence for Mandarin speaking children in a population-based study. *The Lancet Regional Health, West Pacific, 17*, 100713. https://doi.org/10.1016/j.lanwpc.2023.100713

Yergeau, M. (2018). *Authoring autism: On rhetoric and neurological queerness.* Duke University Press.

Yilmaz-Yenioglu, B., & Melekoglu, M. A. (2021). Review of Studies for Twice Exceptional Individuals with Learning Disabilities and Giftedness. *Ankara University Faculty of Educational Sciences Journal of Special Education, 22*(4), 999–1024.

Yu, B., & Sterponi, L. (2023). Toward neurodiversity: How conversation analysis can contribute to a new approach to social communication assessment. *Language, Speech, and Hearing Services in Schools, 54*(1), 27–41. https://doi.org/10.1044/2022_LSHSS-22-00041

Yu, Y., Ozonoff, S., & Miller, M. (2024). Assessment of autism spectrum disorder. *Assessment, 31*(1), 24–41. https://doi.org/10.1177/10731911231173089

Yuen, T., Penner, M., Carter, M. T., Szatmari, P., & Ungar, W. J. (2018). Assessing the accuracy of the Modified Checklist for Autism in Toddlers: A systematic review and meta-analysis. *Developmental Medicine and Child Neurology, 60*(11), 1093–1100. https://doi.org/10.1111/dmcn.13964

Zhu, X., Need, A. C., Petrovski, S., & Goldstein, D. B. (2014). One gene, many neuropsychiatric disorders: Lessons from Mendelian diseases. *Nature Neuroscience, 7*(6), 773–781. https://doi.org/10.1038/nn.3713

Zisk, A. H., & Dalton, E. (2019). Augmentative and alternative communication for speaking autistic adults: Overview and recommendations. *Autism in Adulthood, 1*(2), 93–100. https://doi.org/10.1089/aut.2018.0007

Zisk, A. H., Konyn, L., & Neimeijer, D. (2023). What AAC terminology should I use? Insights from a community survey. *AssistiveWare.* www.assistiveware.com/blog/aactermiology-survey

Subject Index

AAC (augmentative and alternative
    communication) 32–4, 204–6,
    258–60 264, 294, 295
ableism 25, 29, 44, 76, 171, 205, 251, 271, 315
abuse 35, 38, 164
acceptance 84, 197, 200, 222, 223
ADHD 69, 144–9
    assessment 149
    and autism 144–5
    cognitive deficit approach 146–7
    cognitive difference 147–9
    co-occurrence with
        dyspraxia 152–3
        dyscalculia 152
        Ehlers-Danlos Syndrome 266
    DSM-5-TR criteria for 145–6
    and monotropism 235, 297
adverse childhood experiences
    (ACEs) 166, 176, 177
agency 73, 75, 76, 261, 288, 293, 305, 319
alexithymia 114, 306, 310, 314, 326
animals, deep connection with 101–2, 104, 236
anxiety 107, 109, 161, 184, 236, 325, 243,
    247, 265, 266, 294, 306, 307, 314
    misdiagnosed Autistic burnout 162
    reducing 303–4, 311, 313
anxiety-based
    demand avoidance 292
    school avoidance 289
Applied Behaviour Analysis (ABA) 38,
    39–41, 49–51, 55 72, 77, 314
Asperger, Hans 36–7, 39
Asperger's disorder 217
Asperger's syndrome 36, 43, 45, 217
assessment
    collaborative 15, 249
    cognitive 154, 277, 278
        necessity for 140
    deficit-based 17, 57, 81, 222, 241, 322

education, multi-modal 293
language of 20
perspectives a parent and
    professional of 59–63, 63–7
measures
    see assessment tools
medical model 16, 20, 72, 73, 167, 178, 211
neuro-affirmative 67, 246, 253
see also identification/exploration process
Assessment of Functioning and
    Medial Evaluation 277
assessment process
    see identification/exploration process
assessment tools
    adapting 240
    Autism Diagnostic Interview–
        Revised (ADI–R) 231, 233
    Autism Diagnostic Observation
        Schedule, 2nd Edition (ADOS–2)
        224, 225, 247, 231–3
    Childhood Autism Rating Scale–2
        (CARS–2) 233–4
    Child Occupational Self
        Assessment (COSA) 240
    current, issues with 222, 230
        constraints in age/cognitive
            level adaptability 225
        limited scope 225
        overlooked personal experiences 226
        pathologising Autistic neurology 223,
            240
        results, discrepancies in interpretation
            224
        rigid use of 223–4
        'test scores' as barriers to
            accessing services 226–7
    and intersectionality 174–5
    Model of Human Occupation
        (MOHO) 239–40

Monteiro Interview Guidelines for
  Diagnosing the Autism Spectrum
  2nd Edition (MIGDAS-2)
neurodiversity principles, aligning with
Occupational Self Assessment (OSA) 240
questionnaires
  Camouflaging Autistic Traits
    Questionnaire (CAT-Q) 235
  Monotropism Questionnaire (MQ) 235
  Survey of Autistic Strengths, Skills
    and Interests (SASSI) 235-6
standardised
  and best practice guidelines 215-16
  OT perspectives on 239-40
attention 115, 116, 117, 118, 269, 297, 310
  ADHD 147-8
  focused/focusing 98, 117, 128, 129, 133
  interest-led 138, 139
  inattentiveness 146
  monotropic 129, 138, 235
    see also ADHD, hyperfocus,
      monotropism
auditory 181
  assessment 183, 326, 328
  processing 42, 107, 150
  see also misophonia
augmentative and alternative
  communication 204-6
autism diagnosis 57, 88, 174, 178
  history of 35-43
  self-diagnosis 179
Autism + Environment = Outcome 69, 286,
  296
autism identification process
  see identification/exploration process
autism theory 88
Autistic
  activists and scholars 46-8
  advocates 44, 52, 55, 69
  communication 31, 96, 127, 219, 263, 324,
    337
  culture 66, 74, 75, 90, 158, 220, 221, 285
  inertia 119, 142, 297
    see also inertia
  -led organisations 46-8
  play 99-100, 141, 263, 268
  pathology 37
  perception 106, 181, 182, 194, 198
  savant 41, 156
  well-being 54, 55
    see also well-being
Autistic burnout 162, 163, 293, 298, 299, 301
  see also burnout

Autistic development 134
  vs. neurotypical development/
    developmental trajectory 31,
    50, 54-5, 131-43, 139-40
Autistic experience 28, 40, 41, 51, 52-3,
    56-9, 59-63, 63-7, 120-1
  alexithymia 114
  animals, deep connection
    with 101-2, 104, 236
  being Autistic, 91-6
  child's voice (narratives) 5, 103-4, 236-8,
    243-4, 245-6, 251-2, 280-1, 322-3
  clinician/practitioner knowledge base 84-5
  deficit-based framing of 73-5
  defining 'normal' 87-9
  double empathy 121-5
  executive functioning 114-19
  gender identity/variance 171-3, 271-2
  intersectionality 173-4
  labelling 82-3
  masking 125-8
  meltdowns and shutdowns 104-6
  mental health 161-3
  monotropism 128-30
  and other neurodivergencies
    ADHD 144-5
    childhood apraxia of speech
      (CAS) 135, 155-6
    dyscalculia 151-2
    dyslexia 150-1
    dyspraxia 15-3
    intellectual disabilities 153-4
    giftedness 156-7
  passions and interests 102
  play 99-100
  researchers/academics/
    advocates, work on 98-9
  routine 100
  sensory needs
    body 112-13
    body in relation to environment 110-12
    environment 107-9
  speaking 96-8
  stimming as non-spoken
    communication 98-9
  trauma 163-5
Autistic identity, exploring
  see identification/exploration process
Autistic neurology
  age for identification 176
  assessment tools
    see assessment tools
  and best practice guidelines 214-16

Autistic neurology *cont.*
 children in care 176–8
 exploring
  see identification/exploration process
 vs. giftedness 157–8
 and intellectual disability 153–5
 and trauma 163–6
Autistic occupation(s) 141–2, 318
Autistic people, history of 35–42, 49–50
Autistic SPACE framework 198–202
Autistic ways of being 58, 122, 260, 275
 cognitive ability, assessing 278
 gender and sexuality, entwined with 172
 monotropism 297
 neuro-affirmative practice 73
 pathologising 74, 87, 99, 283
 autonomy 78, 89, 100, 281, 309, 315, 321
 vs. independence 319
 pervasive drive/desire for 313
 post-identification support 287, 288
  education/school 291, 293, 298,
   299, 302, 304, 306
atypical autism 217
aversives/aversive techniques 38, 39, 287
avoidant/restrictive food intake
  disorder (AFRID) 312
 see also eating disorders

balance
 sensory 109, 181, 184, 190, 194, 330, 332
 vestibular 111, 191, 183, 326, 330, 333, 334
Beardon's golden equation 69
 see also Autism + Environment = Outcome
behaviour
 compliance-based 49, 50, 51, 73,
  75, 77, 89, 281–2, 314
 inhibitory control 117–18
 modifying/modification 70, 72
 social 232, 265, 326
behavioural therapy, intensive 39–41
being Autistic, experience of 91–6
best practice guidelines
 Autistic identity, identification/assessment
  96, 130, 140, 178, 210, 214, 220, 242
 Autistic neurology 154, 225
 cognitive and other assessments 277–9
 mapping identification information
  272–3, 324 –7
 multidisciplinary professional teams 276–7
 neurodiversity affirmative practice
  and 215, 216, 230
 standardised tools and 227, 230, 240–1
 see also assessment tools

Black Autistic children 126, 174, 175
bodily/body signals 112, 113, 310, 334
 see also alexithymia, emotional
  states, interoception
body movements 125, 217, 248, 253
 hand or 155, 268, 325, 338, 341
body position
 see proprioception
burnout 29, 105, 106, 126, 142, 164,
  197, 293, 297, 307, 316
 see also Autistic burnout

camouflaging 235, 307
 see also masking
Camouflaging Autistic Traits
  Questionnaire (CAT–Q) 235
capitalism and concepts of normality 70, 87,
  88
Child Guidance Movements 88–9
childhood autism 217
childhood development 88, 131
 early and monotropism 138
 measuring 139
 schizophrenia 35–6
 see also Autistic developmental trajectory
childhood apraxia of speech
  (CAS) 135, 155–6, 225
childhood disintegrative disorder 217
childversity 13
classifications systems for autism 216–18
 issues with 218–20
 mapping identification information
  to 272–3, 324–7
 medical model 74
 neuro-affirmative process, use within 220–1
clinical practice guidelines
 see assessment tools, best
  practice guidelines
clutter
 lighting 187
 visual 109, 184, 187
cluttering 136
cognition 236
 monotropic 235
 and sensory experience 182
cognitive
 ability/ies 87, 139, 140, 154, 156,
  157, 225, 278, 304
 assessments 139, 140, 143, 154, 277–9
 deficit vs. difference 146–7
 development 131, 141, 307
 difference 146, 147–9
 disability 72

empathy 123
flexibility 115, 118
inhibition 117
processing 97, 115
style 139, 225 306
   gestalt 136
   monotropic 235
systems, functions and executive
   functions 114, 115
Comfort Zone 78–9
communication 124, 201
adjustments 203–6
cross-neurotype 77, 128
disability/ies 32, 34, 73, 264
home/school 290
milestones 134
mismatch 122, 130, 201
non-spoken 98, 246, 257, 262,
   264, 335, 337, 339
preferences 31, 32, 33, 65, 242, 287, 292, 337
spoken 140, 205–6, 207, 246, 252, 262, 339
supports 32, 97, 203, 205, 263
   see also AAC
communication methods 204, 252, 258–60
various, using 127, 192, 203, 207, 221, 241
see also AAC
communication, social 15, 93, 94,
   154, 159, 265, 287, 324, 339
communication space 183, 193–4, 264, 328
communication, non-spoken 98,
   221, 257, 262, 264, 325, 327
methods 211, 253, 339
stimming 98
communication, spoken 29, 140,
   205, 209, 211, 257, 262, 339
communication style(s) 69, 74, 78, 125,
   170, 202, 203, 269, 285, 287, 324, 337
   see also Autistic communication styles
compassion 83, 123–4, 254, 260, 326, 340
compliance-based behaviour therapy
   49–51, 73, 75, 77, 89, 281, 282, 314
concentrate/concentration 106,
   147, 150, 268, 269, 298
   see also focus (and others)
consent 169, 172, 254, 259, 262, 287
co-occurring
conditions 24, 121, 133, 147, 189, 224,
   229, 230, 232, 234, 277, 312, 315
disability 156
dyscalculia 152
dyspraxia (DCD) 152, 153
Ehlers-Danlos syndrome,
   hypermobility syndrome 266

learning disability 86, 315
medical conditions 264, 265
mental health challenges,
   diagnoses 161, 162, 314
neurodivergences 115
physical conditions 314
culturally competent (clinicians) 173, 175
Curious Zone 78 –9

deficit-based
approach/assessment 17, 31, 57,
   58, 81, 303, 321, 322
assessment tools 222, 231
diagnostic criteria 102
interventions 314
knowledge about autism 84–5
language about autism 96
narratives
   ADHD 144, 147
   autistic experience 73, 74, 122, 302
depression 69, 161, 162, 314
developmental
coordination disorder (DCD)
   see dyspraxia
delay vs. developmental difference 133
language disorder (DLD) 159
milestones/norms 31, 88, 132, 138
developmental trajectory
Autistic 74, 138, 225
neurodivergent 134
neurotypical 138, 315
diagnostic criteria 85
development of 19, 43, 86, 217–8
evaluating 216–17
re-framed in neuro-affirmative
   framework 324–7
reworking (thought experiment) 92–5
'widening' of 178
using in a best practice framework 220–1
see also assessment tools, best
   practice guidelines
diagnostic overshadowing 153, 161,
   163, 164, 176, 177, 312
disability, social model of 53, 68, 78
disabled person/people 26 –7
double empathy/double empathy problem
   72, 77, 82, 98, 121–5, 201, 248, 287, 303,
   315
embedding in practice 127–8
key ideas 124–5
dyscalculia 151–2
dyslexia 69, 150–1, 152
dyspraxia 69, 152–3

eating 110, 113, 188, 189, 310,
    312, 318, 331, 332, 338
  see also misophonia
eating disorders 161, 266, 312
echolalia 36, 65, 137
  delayed 137
education
  see school
educational placement 299–301
Ehlers-Danlos Syndrome (EDS)
    190, 265, 266, 314
electroshock therapy (EST) 37, 49
embodiment 97, 98
emotion(s) 93, 137, 195, 243
  alexithymia 114
  connection to smell and taste 109
  and empathy/hyperempathy 123
  experience of 64, 65, 123, 230, 324, 326,
    340
  express 124, 310, 325, 338
  inhibitory control 117
  intense 98, 123, 325
emotional regulation 89, 115, 306, 317
  see also regulation
emotional space 202, 250, 251
emotional states 98, 112, 113, 326
emotional support 101, 157, 278
empathy 122 –3, 201, 326, 340
  affective 122, 123
  cognitive 122, 123
  hyper-empathy 102, 123, 201
  see also double empathy
employment 117, 142, 152, 286
  see also occupation
environment 90–1
energy accounting 316–17
  Spoon Theory/management 316
epilepsy 135, 196, 265
epistemic
  injustice 96, 120, 314
  privilege, authority 51, 85, 87, 114, 120
  violence 19, 58
ethical listening 98, 262
ethics, professional codes of 224
ethnic minorities 173–5
  see also intersectionality
eugenics 48
exams (school) 293
executive function 119, 141, 299, 309
executive functioning 114–21
  Autistic burnout and 167, 297
  and sensory experiences 157
executive functions 115, 116, 117, 118–9

exhaustion 162, 184
  see also Autistic burnout, burnout
eye contact 93, 94, 126, 168, 201,
    258, 323, 325, 335, 337, 339

families
  mealtimes and food considerations 312
  needs, competing 311–12
  routines, schedules 304–5, 303–9
  screentime 309–11
  stimming 311
  support for 303–12
  working with 169–71
fidgeting 105, 112
fidget toys/objects 105, 112, 252, 280, 306
fine motor skills 110, 112, 190, 332
florescent lights
  see lighting
flow state 297, 298, 306
focus
  attentional 117, 133, 310
  intense 128, 147
  see also hyperfocus, monotropism
food
  avoidant/restrictive food intake
    disorder (AFRID) 312
  choice 100, 111, 189, 332
  preferences 10, 325
  same 100, 101, 338
  sensory considerations 106, 109,
    110, 111, 188, 312, 331
functioning, high/low 28–30, 53, 79

gender
  gender-affirming 171, 172, 211, 271–2
  binaries 92
  identity 89, 211, 271–2, 279, 315, 337
  variance and GSRD 171–3, 174 223, 272
gestalt language acquisition 136–7
gestalt language processing 137, 314
gestures 33, 94, 125, 201, 205, 325, 337, 339
giftedness 156–8
Growth Zone 79, 80
GSRD (gender, sexuality, and
    relationship diversity) 171–3
gustatory 110
  assessment 189, 332
  see also taste

habituation 89, 180, 320
hand/body movements 97, 112,
    155, 268, 325, 328, 341

head movement 97, 111
healthcare access, barriers to 163, 196–8,
     198–202, 204–5, 206, 226–7,
     264, 266–7, 283–4
hearing 107, 154, 295, 226, 334
heterosexual 92, 172
home, support recommendations for 303–12
homework, post-identification
     support for 290–1
hyperactivity 146, 148
hyperactivity-impulsivity 145
hyperacusis 107, 114
hyper-empathy 102, 123, 201
     see also empathy
hyperfocus 127, 129, 147, 148, 219, 236,
     254, 260, 269, 270, 326, 338
     see also monotropic state, monotropism
hyperlexia 136, 158

identification/exploration process
     (assessment) 249
  AAC mediated 258–61
  accessibility
     advance information 108–9
     approach transparency: neuro-
          affirming vs. medical model 211
     communication adjustments 203–6
     clinical spaces 198
     environmental design 197
     information gathering 210–11
     information options 207–8
     introducing clinical team 206–7
     lack of neurodivergent professionals 197
     referral pathways 197
     remote sessions 209–10
     service adaptation/SPACE
          framework 199–202
     service availability 197
  autism
     collaborative information gathering
        experience of the world 260–2
        gender identity/variance 171–3, 271–2
        on inner experience 247–9, 253–8
        lifeworld framework 262–4
        mapping to best practice
             criteria 272–3, 324–7
        medical history 264–6
        mental health history 266–7
        selecting tools/instruments 246–7
        significant life events/trauma 267–71
     collaborative preparation,
          professionals' role in 242–6
     children in care 176–8

     children/young people reluctant
          to engage 275–6
     cognitive, other assessments 277–9
     creating a safe space 250–2
     emotions experienced by
          families prior to 243
     experience sensitive 261–4
     families with difficult service experiences
          history, working with 169–71
     intersectionality and ethnic minorities 173–5
     multi-disciplinary teams, involving 276–7
     other neurodivergencies
        ADHD 149
        childhood apraxia of speech (CAS) 156
        dyscalculia 152
        dyslexia 151
        dyspraxia 153
        intellectual disabilities 154–5
        giftedness 157–8
     outcome session 273–5
     power dynamics/differences/
          imbalances 73, 75, 165, 167–9, 195,
          196, 207, 219, 230, 247, 262, 270
     practice points 175
     professionals, role in 245
     reports, documentation 279–84
        letter for older children/adolescents 283
        letter for state benefits, education
             support 283–4
        main report 281–2
        report for younger children 282–3
        short letter 282
     trauma-informed process 270–1
     young person/family participation/
          collaboration 244–5
     young person who cannot rely
          on speech alone 258–60
identification piece
     see identification/exploration process
identity-first language 23–8,
     289, 315
inclusion 181, 263, 321
     strategies 295–6
inertia 105, 106, 297
     see also Autistic inertia
infantile autism 36, 39, 217
information processing 115, 151, 169
inhibition (task, response) 115
     see also cognitive inhibition
inhibitory control 117–8
initiation/initiating 115, 324, 337
info/information dumping 74, 94, 96
institutions/institutionalisation 37, 38, 41, 88

intellectual disability/ies 134, 140,
    153–5, 225, 227, 265, 277, 278
    and childhood apraxia of speech
        (CAS) 135, 155–6
intelligence 29, 30
interest groups 296
interest-led/based
    attention 139
    development 138–9
    groups/activities 298
    learning 118, 139, 301
    motivation 147
interoception 112–13, 142, 181,
    306, 310, 314, 318, 326
interoceptive
    accessibility 192
    assessment 192, 334
    awareness 113, 116
    differences 113, 114, 142
    input 113
intersectionality 173–5, 271
invalidation 166, 171, 172

knowledge about autism/Autistic experience
    61, 82, 85, 86, 130, 168, 248

labels vs. identity 82–4
labelled/labelling 29, 84, 92, 312
language
    ableist to avoid 31
    acquisition, gestalt 136–7
    of assessments 20
    body 248, 264, 325, 335, 337, 339
    gender-affirming 171, 271
    identity-first 23–8, 289, 315
    neurodiversity affirmative 32–4
    person-first 23–9, 79
    spoken 86, 134, 135, 140, 248
learning
    difficulties, specific 150–3
    disability/ies 86, 288, 293, 295, 315
    interest-based 118, 139
    opportunities, adapted (multimodal) 294–5
    perspectives of an educator 301–2
    self-directed 298
learning about neurodiversity in schools 289
learning style
    interest-led 139
    monotropic 298
    polytropic 139, 140
Learning Zone 79–80
LEANS (Learning About Neurodiversity
    at School) 83, 128, 289

LED lights
    see lighting
LGBTQIA+ 43, 52, 71, 171, 172, 211, 272
    see also gender, sexuality
lifeworld framework 261
    application in a SLT/autism
        assessment 262–4
light(s)
    bright 106, 109, 187, 198, 199, 208
    concealing 188
    florescent 185, 186, 329
        alternatives to 330
    intensity 184
    LED
        addressing issues with 186–7
        impact of 187–8
    RGB 320
    sensitivity 105
    soft/softening 184, 187
lighting 109, 185
    balance 183
listening, ethical 98, 262

marginalisation 79, 175
masking 50, 77, 84, 125, 162, 164, 186, 232, 235,
    248, 249, 254, 260, 269, 282, 290, 293,
    299, 307, 315, 324, 325, 326, 337, 340
mealtimes 93, 312
medical conditions co-occurring
    with autism 196, 264, 265
medical history 250, 253, 261, 264–6
medical model 17, 73
    deficit-based) 32, 68, 72, 74, 211, 233, 321
    power dynamics 167, 178–9
meltdown(s) 104–6, 107, 108, 118, 126
memory 115, 117, 119, 130, 150, 269
    working 115, 118, 119, 140
mental health 50, 51, 161–3, 336
    history 266–7
    trauma 163–5, 267–70
    see also Autistic burnout, burnout,
        diagnostic overshadowing
minimally speaking 33, 77, 205
misophonia 107, 312
mitigations (gestalt language) 137
Model of Human Occupation
    (MOHO) 239–40, 320
monitoring 115, 116, 117
monologuing 96, 269
monotropic 138, 297
    attention 74, 129
    cognition 235
    learning 297, 298, 302

processing 192, 297
state117, 129, 147, 148
monotropism 98, 128–30, 138–9,
225, 264, 306, 310, 315
and early childhood development 138
teaching educators about 297–8
theory of 47, 128, 302, 304
mothers 171
as 'cold' parents 37
see also Autistic mothers
motor challenges/difficulties 153
motor coordination 150, 317
fine and/or gross 152
motor disorders 152, 278
motor skill(s) 89, 110, 134, 152, 154, 278
mouth words 33, 259

narratives
of deficiency 87
first-hand (child's voice) 5, 103–4, 236–8,
243–4, 245–6, 251–2, 280–1, 322–3
how stories shape us 56–9
parent/professional perspective 30,
59–63
OT perspectives 63–7
sexuality and gender identity 173
see also Autistic experience
Natural Language Acquisition protocol
136–7
neuro-affirmative/neurodiversity
affirmative identification process
see identification/exploration process
neuro-affirming/neurodiversity affirmative
language 30, 32–4, 74, 79, 81, 303
neuro-affirmative/neurodiversity affirmative
approach 17, 73–4, 210, 234, 321
and diagnostic criteria 96, 215–16, 233
see also neuro-affirmative/neurodiversity
affirmative practice
neuro-affirmative/neurodiversity
affirmative assessments
see identification/exploration process
neuro-affirmative/neurodiversity affirmative
practice 73–80, 133, 183, 276, 320, 322
and best practice guidelines 215–16
key principles 74–80
shifts to 19, 58
see also neuro-affirmative/neurodiversity
affirmative approach
neuro-affirmative services 70–2
neurodevelopmental disability/
disorder 72, 135, 155
see also childhood apraxia of speech (CAS)

neurodivergent 23, 47, 69–70
language and communication profiles 158–9
professionals, lack of 197
neurodiversity 23, 42, 43, 68–9, 70, 75–6
Neurodiversity and Ableism
Reflection Tool, The 78–80
neurodiversity affirmative 74–8, 78–9
neurodiversity affirmative assessments,
conducting 72–3
see also identification/exploration process
neurodiversity affirmative framework
15, 68, 149, 221, 253, 272, 276, 321
see also Neurodiversity Paradigm
neurodiversity affirmative model
see Neurodiversity Paradigm
neurodiversity affirmative practitioner,
becoming a 78–80
neurodiversity-lite 52, 73, 79, 303
see also Neurodiversity Paradigm
Neurodiversity Movement
history 35–9, 70
criticisms of 52–5
and rights, human/disability/social 69, 76
Neurodiversity Paradigm 68–70
cognitive deficit model vs.
cognitive difference 147
criticisms of 52–5
mainstream assessment tools,
critique of 222–7
philosophy 69
self-identification 178–9
neurodiversity practice 73–80
key principles 74–8
neurotypical 23
development/developmental trajectory
57, 131, 132, 133, 134, 138, 141, 315
vs. Autistic development 139–40
gaze 59, 68, 78
milestones/developmental milestones 31
perception 181, 182
social behaviours/expectations 158
social skills training 55, 73, 77, 125, 128, 282
spectrum disorder (thought exercise) 92–5
NICE guidance 145, 146, 214, 276, 277
noise(s)
ambient 183, 328
excessive 183, 329
loud 107, 108
recurrent beeping 199
sensitive to 105
unexpected 329
see also sensory audit
non-binary 171, 337

non-speaking Autistic children 53,
76, 77, 86, 92, 101, 135, 140, 205,
225, 248, 257, 259, 293, 337
non-speaking vs non-verbal 32–3
normal 88
child, construction of 88–9
notion of 87

obsessive compulsive disorder (OCD)
23, 24, 69, 161, 266, 314
occupational justice 90, 308–9, 318
occupational therapist (OT)
72, 276, 277, 310, 311
perspectives of an OT
Autistic Occupations across
the Lifespan 141–2
Autistic Play 99–100
Autistic Space (Healthcare) 198–202
Meaningful Occupation 308–9
My Personal Experience 63–7
Neuro-Affirmative Services 70–2
The PEOP Model 89–91
Post-Identification Support 317–20
Standardised Assessment Tools 238–40
occupational therapy 89, 100, 114,
182, 239, 278, 308, 314, 317–20
occupation(s) 89–91, 99
meaningful 72, 91, 308–9, 317, 318
odours 188, 331
see also smell(s)
olfactory 109, 110, 326
assessment 188–9, 331
see also odours, smell(s)
online
community/ies 77, 310
session/meeting 191, 192
spaces/environments/platforms 77,
180, 186, 191, 193, 203, 328, 333
organisation/organising (skill) 115,
116, 118, 146, 150, 151, 152, 336
overwhelm 113, 163, 195, 256, 289, 304, 306, 307
managing 306
masking 126
meltdowns/shutdowns 104,
105, 106, 118, 266
monotropism 128
sensory 107, 108, 109, 184, 312
stimming 311
triggers 269–70, 248

parent/carer blame 170–1
parent blaming 38

parenting, low-demand 313
passions vs. special interests 31, 102
pathological demand avoidance (PDA) 313
pathologising
assessment/screening tools
227–8, 233, 234, 236–9
Autistic identity (gender/sexuality)171, 271
Autistic neurology 132, 223, 233
Autistic ways of being 74, 99–100
classification systems 217, 218, 220, 221
early development 133, 138
report language 281–2, 283
pathology paradigm 48, 72, 73, 88
personal journey 263, 288
person-centered
approach 89–91, 318
best practices 71–2
care 196, 202
Person-Environment-Occupation-Performance
Model (PEOP Model) 89–91
person-first language 23–9, 79
pervasive developmental disorder 37, 44, 217
physical health/conditions 198, 202, 299, 314
see also medical conditions
physical space/environment 90, 184, 188,
190, 191, 192, 202, 250, 251, 328
planning 115, 116, 118, 141, 152
plants 188, 190–1, 329, 330, 331
play 99, 141, 253, 255, 256, 257, 268, 299, 325, 327
Positive Behavior Support (PBS)
49, 51, 72, 77, 306, 314
post-identification support 74,
148, 160, 262, 317–20
neuro-affirming framework, within 286–8
principles 287–8
mental health 163
recommendations
clinical 314–320
home 303–13
education/school 289–3, 301–2
power dynamic(s)/differences/
imbalances 73, 75, 167–9
in Autistic identity exploration
165, 195, 196, 207
in formal Autistic identification 167–9,
219, 230, 247, 262, 264, 270
predictable 100, 325, 330
predictability 184, 186, 200, 204,
203, 304, 309, 334–7
presentation 247, 278
gender 192
home vs. school 290
see also masking

problem-solving 114, 115, 118, 150
processing
    differences 314
    space/time 202, 294
pronouns 173, 211, 272, 279
proprioception/proprioceptive 110,
        112, 181, 190, 266, 326, 332
    assessment 189–91, 332
    input 112, 189, 190, 332
PSI guidelines 214, 278
psychiatric disorders, misidentified 161
PTSD (post-traumatic stress
        disorder) 23, 69, 163–4, 267

quality of life 48, 55, 77–8, 83, 265, 286, 308

race consciousness 173
    see also intersectionality
reciprocity, social-emotional 93, 94, 324, 337
refrigerator mother theory 37, 38
reflective practice 251
regulate 88, 191, 220, 259, 268, 269,
        291, 294, 299, 304, 310, 311, 312
    co-regulate 113, 292
    self-regulate 113, 186, 306
regulation 29, 115, 163, 164, 253
    co-regulation 98, 291, 306
    self-regulation 145, 182, 298, 309, 311
relationships 70, 73, 90, 93, 124, 167,
        172, 216–17, 232, 260–1, 298, 310,
        313, 315, 325, 335–6, 338, 340
repetitive movements 95, 311
    see also stimming
Rett's disorder 217
routine(s) 101, 304–5, 307, 325, 338
    changes in 104, 298
    preference for 95, 100
    and schedules 303–5

safe space, create/creating 245, 248, 250–2,
        255, 257, 271–2, 275–6, 292, 321
savant 156
    see also Autistic savant
scents 109, 188
schedules
    see routine(s)
school 142
    assessments, multi-modal 293
    anxiety-based avoidance 289
    and Autistic burnout 162
    -home communication 290
    detentions, exclusions 298–9

executive functioning 115–16, 119
events 293–4
exam time 293
inclusion strategies 295–6
multi-modal, adapted learning 294–5
perspectives of an educator 301–2
post-identification support 289–302
sensory environment 296–7
support plans 292
total communication approach 295
screening tools 227–8
    Modified Checklist for Autism in
        Toddlers, Revised (M-CHAT-R) 228
    Social Communication
        Questionnaire (SCQ) 229
    Social Responsiveness Scale, 2nd
        Edition (SRS-2) 229
screentime 309–11
selective mutism 5, 97
self-advocacy 51, 74, 75, 77, 78,
        259, 281, 282, 285, 319
self-advocating 41–2
self-awareness 55, 113, 148, 168, 317
self-care 113, 141–2, 307, 316, 317, 318, 326
self-control/monitoring 117
self-determination 74, 77, 121, 313, 319
self-identification 120, 178–9
self-understanding 59, 83, 144, 179, 263
sense-making 137, 263
sense of place 263
sensory audit
        assessment
        appointments and space settings 192–4
        auditory assessment 183
        gustatory assessment 189
        interoceptive assessment 192
        olfactory assessment 188–9
        proprioceptive and tactile
            assessment 189–91
        vestibular assessment 191–2
        visual assessment 183–6
    checklist 328–34
    consultant criteria 182
    preparation and key people 181–3
sensory balance(s) 161, 182, 184, 194, 329
sensory differences 74, 106, 227
sensory domains 181, 183
sensory distress, what can help
    auditory/hearing 108
    gustatory/taste 110
    interoception/body signals 113
    olfactory/smell 109
    proprioception/sense of body position 112

sensory distress, what can help *cont.*
  tactile/touch 111
  vestibular/head movement 112
  visual/seeing 109
sensory environment(s) 107, 184, 191
  school 296–7
sensory experience 106, 110, 157, 182,
    188, 195, 217, 239, 253, 260–1,
    269, 315, 325, 334–5, 338, 341
sensory habituation 180
sensory information 117, 181, 199, 326, 334–5
sensory input 106, 184, 185, 311, 326
sensory needs
  body 112–14
  body in relation to the environment 110–12
  environment 107–9
sensory overload/overwhelm 104,
    107, 109, 113, 202, 292, 329
  reducing 181, 328
sensory processing 89, 106, 199, 297, 309, 317
  assessment 239
  differences 141, 199, 304, 312
sensory regulation 276, 314
sensory systems 30, 110,1 182, 299
sensory toolbox 306
sequencing 115, 116, 118, 141
sexuality 89, 171–3, 315
  see also gender, LGBTQIA+
shame 35, 41, 77, 83, 148, 247
shutdowns 29, 104–6, 108, 118, 266, 292
SIGN guidelines 267, 277–8
smell(s) 106,109, 136, 188, 189, 199,
    203, 269, 312, 326, 331, 334
social-emotional reciprocity 93, 94, 324, 337
social interaction(s) 72, 83, 94, 225, 324, 337
social justice 68, 124, 236, 308, 325
social skills training 31, 55, 70, 94, 125
  rejecting 72, 73, 77, 128, 282
solitude 307
sound(s) 97, 98, 107, 108, 183, 311, 325, 329
  vocal 33, 336
  see also misophonia, noise
SPACE framework 198–202
special interests vs. passions 102
spectrum concept 30
speech
  apraxia 155–6, 225
    see also childhood apraxia of speech
      (CAS)
  disability vs. speech/
      communication deficit 34
  insufficient 97
  intermittent 96

unable to rely on 97, 258–60
unreliable 96
speech, language and communication
    needs (SLCN) 158–9
speech, language and communication
    profiles 135–6
speech and language development
  see communication milestones,
      developmental milestones
speech and language therapist (SLT)
    132, 276, 277, 278, 295
  perspectives of
    augmentative and alternative
        communication 204–6
    Autistic experiences of speaking 96–7
    conducting neurodiversity
        affirmative assessments 72–3
    considerations for conducting an
        assessment of a child/young person
        who cannot rely on speech alone
        to be heard or understood 258–60
    experience sensitive approach
        to assessment 261–2
    gestalt language acquisition 136–7
    neurodiversity affirmative language
        and terminology 32–4
    role of speech and language therapy in
        identifying neurodivergent language
        and communication profiles 158–9
    speech, language and communication
        profiles of Autistic children 135–6
    stimming as non-spoken
        communication 98
speech and language therapy 314
speech sound disorders 135–6
SPINs (special interests) 305
spoon management 316–17
Spoon Theory 316
stereotype(s) 44, 82, 92, 223
stigma 24, 27, 45, 82, 83, 182 196, 197, 205
stim(s) 97, 112, 125, 142, 307
stimming 50, 98, 1:05, 164, 182, 190,
    191, 225, 263, 298, 311, 328, 333,
stress/overwhelming stress
  see Autistic burnout, burnout,
      masking, stimming
Subject Access Request 170
surfaces, materials for 190
support needs, high and low 28–30

tactile 110–11, 326
  assessment, proprioceptive and 189–91, 332
  see also touch

taste 100, 109, 110, 189, 312, 326, 332, 334
Tendril Theory 129
terminology
    see language
theory of Heilpädagogik (therapeutic
    education) 36
Theory of Mind 60 75, 94, 121
time blindness 304
timetable 303
    visual 292
    see also schedules
togetherness 264, 288
touch 110, 111, 190, 269, 326, 334
Tourette's 69
toys 255, 256, 327
trauma 51, 89, 160, 163–5, 176
    adverse childhood experiences 176–7
    and children in care 176–8
    history, gathering information about 267–70
    see also Autistic burnout, burnout

trauma-informed process/approach
    165–6, 252, 270–1
triad of impairments 38

uniqueness 263, 283

vaccines 44
ventilation 188, 331
vestibular 111–12, 326
    assessment 191–2, 333
    see also head movement, balance
visual 109, 326
    assessment 183–6, 320–30
    clutter 109, 184, 187
    schedules/timetables 292, 304, 305, 310

well-being 57, 76, 106, 107, 181, 182, 188,
    192, 201, 202, 261, 286, 288, 290, 306,
    307, 308, 311, 313, 315, 316, 320, 321

Author Index

Abagis, T. R. 349
Abawi, R. 344
Abberton, C. 351
Abbott, A. E. 344
Acevedo, S. 222, 342
Acharya, K. 343
Adams, D. 356
Adams, H. 358
Adams, J. 355
Adams, M. 342
Adkin, T. 348
Aiello, A. L. 170, 345
Aishworiya, R. 228, 342
Aitken, D. 342
Alcedo, M. A. 342
Alcorn, A. M. 83, 128, 342
Alexander, A. 353
Ali, D. 209, 342
Allison, C. 348, 349, 355, 357, 358
Allmon, A. 347
Almqvist, C. 345
Altschuler, M. R. 351
Alvares, G. A. 29, 342
Alviani, M. 352
Ameis, S. H. 350
American Psychiatric Association
        151, 152, 158, 225, 342
American Speech-Language-Hearing
        Association 204, 342
Anderson, D. K. 134, 135, 342
Anderson, L. K. 51, 342
Anderson, N. A. 349
Annable, J. L. 350
Anotnissen, A. 346
Ansell, M. 347
Apkon, C. S. 349
Arias, V. D. 153, 342
Arnold, S. R. 349
Arnold, S. R. C. 83, 342

Asberg Johnels, J. 344
Ashwood, P. 352
Association of Occupational
        Therapists of Ireland 308, 342
Assouline, S. G. 156, 342
Attar, S. 357
Autistic Science Person 266, 342
Autistica, 161, 342
Azevedo, J. 348

Babalola, T. 196, 343
Babej, E. 343
Bacalman, S. 351
Bacon, E. 355
Bae, S. M. 353
Baggs, A. 98, 343
Bailey, A. 229, 356
Baio, J. 352
Baird, G. 354, 357
Bal, V. H. 225, 343
Balaguer-Castro, M. 348
Ball, S. J. 299, 343
Ballantyne, C. 354
Bargiela, S. 161, 343
Barnes, C. C. 355
Barnett, A. L. 343
Barnhill, J. 347
Baron-Cohen, S. 348, 349, 351, 357, 358
Barton, M. 347, 356
Bass, J. D. 343
Baum, C. M. 89, 343
Bavin, E. 355
Baxter, L. C. 346
Beardon, L. 69, 297, 343
Bearman, P. 153, 350
Bearman, P. S. 347
Beazley, P. 349
Bebbington, K. 342
Begeer, S. 223, 343, 344, 346, 346

Benson, K. J. 170, 171, 343
Beresford, B. 162, 163, 353
Berg, K. L. 177, 343
Bergamo, N. 357
Bergmann, P. 357
Bernadi, F. 57, 58, 343
Bernard, M. A. 349
Bertilsdotter Rosqvist, H. 58, 68, 146,
    147, 148, 343, 350, 357, 358
Besney, R. 350
Bet, K. 357
Bhat, A. N. 153, 343
Bilder, D. A. 344
Billstedt, E. 357
Binger, C. 205, 343
Bird, G. 123, 347
Bishop, S. 349, 357
Bishop, S. L. 224, 225, 226, 227, 230,
    232, 233, 343, 348, 350, 351
Black, L. M. 357
Black, M. H. 134, 343
Blackwell, A. 343
Blake, S. 357
Blakemore, M. 355
Blanc, M. 136, 343
Blank, R. 153, 343
Bloom, P. 122, 123, 124, 344
Bölte, S. 235, 243, 249, 252
Bolton, P. F. 355
Bonato, S. 350
Borden, A. 357
Bosman, R. 24, 344
Botha, M. 24, 43, 69, 72, 223, 344, 345, 352
Bouk, S. E. 343
Bourgeron, T. 343
Boussaid, W. 343
Bovell, V. 358
Boyens, T. 352
Braden, B. B. 265, 344
Bradley, E. A. 344
Brainin, L. 354
Brasher, S. N. 347
Brede, J. 267, 344
Brennan-Jones, C. G. 345
Bretherton, L. 355
Brian, J. 354
Brignell, A. 352
Brimo, K. 150, 344
British Dyslexia Association, 150, 344
British Psychological Society, 214, 344, 348
Bromet, E. J. 350
Brookman-Frazee, L. 352
Brosnan, M. 83, 344

Brown, H. M. 357
Brownlow, C. 88, 344
Brugha, T. 358
Bruni, T. P. 299, 344
Brunwasser, S. M. 348
Bryson, S. 354
Bryson, S. E. 153, 348
Buck, T. R. 161, 344
Buckingham, A. 349
Buckingham, C. 358
Buckle, K. L. 297, 344, 351
Buckley, C. 350
Buckwalter, P. 358
Buijsman, R. 24, 344
Bullmore, E. T. 351
Burke, B. L. 209, 344
Burke, E. 92, 358
Burrows, C. L. 351
Bussières, E.-L. 350

Cable, N. 352
Cage, E. 125, 163, 197, 344, 346, 354
Cairney, J. 343
Calder, S. D. 159, 345
Campbell, L. E. 352
Canadian Paediatric Society 215, 345
Canal-Bedia, R. 352
Carel, H. 86, 345
Carey, C. E. 350
Carravallah, L. 346
Cartabellotta, A. 349
Carter, M. T. 359
Casagrande, K. 356
Casanova, E. L. 153, 345
Casanova, M. F. 153, 345
Cascio, A. A. 347
Casson, R. 349
Cavagnaro, P. 349
Cederlöf, M. 266, 345
Centers for Disease Control and
    Prevention, 45, 175, 345
Cevallos, L. A. T. 349
Cha, D. 355
Chakrabarti, B. 351
Chakraborty, H. 345
Chance, P. 39, 345
Chandler, S. 357
Chapman, R. 15, 73, 72, 86, 87, 88, 223, 286, 344
Charman, T. 354, 357
Chawarska, K. 176, 345, 354
Chelas, E. N. 359
Chen, C. M. A. 209, 356
Chen, K. 209, 357

Chen, L. 345
Chen, W.-X. 351
Chen, Y. 347, 351
Chen, Y. L. 121, 345
Chester, V. 358
Chown, N. 115, 343, 345, 347, 350, 358
Christiansen, C. H. 343
Chrysler, C. 356
Cidav, Z. 176, 345
Cini, E. 355
Clapham, H. 355
Clark, M. 356
Cleary, D. 342
Clements, C. C. 358
Clements, L. 70, 345
Clesi, C. D. 351
Coghill, D. 356
CommunicationFIRST, 32, 33, 345
Constantino, J. N. 229, 344, 345, 356
Cook Jr. E. H. 345
Coombs, E. 357
Coon, H. 344
Cooper, A. 347
Cooper, K. 171, 345
Cooper, R. 141, 357
Corbin, E. 346
Corsello, C. 229, 345, 356
Costa, A. D. 346
Costello, E. 291, 299, 353
Courchesne, E. 355
Crane, L. 83, 345, 350
Cresswell, L. 163, 346
Crompton, C. J. 121, 346
Cruz, S. 223, 346
Cuellar-Pompa, L. 352
Cullen, W. 346
Cunningham, S. 351
Cunningham-Burley, S. 346
Curnow, E. 233, 346

Dahiya, A. V. 209, 346
Daley, D. 356
Dalton, E. 96, 359
Daly, E. 355
Dargue, N. 348
David, A. S. 179, 346
Davidovitch, M. 176, 346
Davies, J. 345
Davis, J. 346, 353
Davis, N. O. 295, 351
Dawkins, T. 233, 346
Day, A. 59, 348
Day, T. N. 352

De Andres, M. 344
De Graaf, H. 346
De Laet, H. 24, 346
de Marchena, A. B. 358
De Polo, L. M. 358
de Sonneville, L. 346
de Vaan, G. 227, 346
de Vignemont, F. 122, 346
de Villiers, J. 359
DeBrabander, K. 346
Deeley, Q. 355
Dekker, M. 42, 351
Delos Santos, A. 355
DeLucia, E. 346
Devlin, C. 357
Dewinter, J. 171, 346
Diaz Heijtz, R. 349
Dibb, B. 344
Dickson, K. S. 352
Díez, E. 352
Dijkhuis, R. 116, 346
DiLavore, P. S. 351
DiLavore, P.C. 342
Dinkler, L. 344
Dipper, L. 205 343, 353
Dobson, J. 349
Dockery, L. 342
Dodson, W. 147, 346
Doherty, M. 46, 196, 198, 199, 264, 346
Donaldson, A. L. 205, 346
Dong, Y. 359
Dorelien, A. M. 355
Doyle, J. 349
Doyle, J. K. 348
Drager, K. D. R. 349
Du, K. 196, 346
Dudley, R. 350
Duffy, F. 354
Dumont-Mathieu, T. 356
Duran, J. B. 347
Dwyer, P. 354

Eack, S. M. 352
Earles-Vollrath, T. L. 347
Eccles, M. 359
Eddy, B. 346
Edgar, H. 297, 301, 346
Egberts, K. J. 355
Eigsti, I. M. 347
Elder, J. H. 176, 347
Eldevik, S. 348
Elias, P. 343
Elias, R. 233, 347, 352

Elliott, D. 350, 356
Ellis, C. 351
Elphick, C. 350
Emma, 196, 236
Eng, C. 347
Esler, A. N. 351
Estes, A. 359
Evans, J. A. 164, 347
Evans, K. 342
Evans, M. 352
Evans-Williams, C. V. 346

Faherty, A. 351
Farahar, C. 57, 347
Farley, M. 344
Farmer, C. 357
Faso, D. J. 356
Fears, N. E. 353
Fein, D. 351, 356
Feldman, H. M. 342
Fisher, N. 298, 299, 347
Fjæran-Granum, T. 348
Fletcher, R. 154, 347
Fletcher-Watson, S. 123, 342, 346, 347
Flouri, E. 352
Flynn, E. G. 346
Foley Nicpon, M. 157, 342, 347
Foley, K.-R. 349
Folstein, S. E. 359
Fontanil, Y. 342
Ford, E. 346
Ford, T. 356
Forgeot d'Arc, B. 354
Fountain, C. 133, 347
Franklin, A. 358
Frazier, T. W. 229, 245, 247, 352
Freudenstein, O. 230, 233, 247
Fricker, M. 19, 86, 347
Frizelle, P. 72, 347
Frost, D. M. 344
Fu, J. M. 350
Fuentes, J. 352

Gallop, N. 349
Gallus, K. L. 350
Galvin, K. T. 358
Ganz, J. B. 205, 347
Garau, V. 139, 235, 297, 347
Garcia-Sanchez, Y. 353
Gazestani, V. H. 355
Gelbar, N. W. 355, 156, 347
Gemegah, E. 358

George, R. 171, 348
Georgiou, N. 159, 347
Gernsbacher, M. A. 24, 347
Gibson, J. L. 349
Gillberg, C. 344, 357
Gillespie, A. 121, 348
Gillespie-Lynch, K. 354, 355
Gillespie-Smith, K. 354
Gilmartin, K. 351
Gindi, S. 347
Girirajan, S. 355
Giwa Onaiwu, M. 48, 344
Gjevik, E. 161, 348
Glaspy, T. K. 344
Glasson, E. J. 342
Gobrial, E. 196 348
Golan, D. 346
Goldberg, W. A. 352
Goldstein, D. B. 359
Gomez, L. E. 342
Gooch, D. 354
Goodall, E. 215, 348
Gotham, K. 161, 224, 348, 349, 351, 356
Gowen, E. 344
Gray-Hammond, D. 19, 160, 197, 348
Green, D. 343
Greenberg, D. M. 358
Greene, R. W. 313, 348
Griffiths, S. 161, 348
Grimshaw, J. 359
Grol, R. 359
Gross, A. L. 351
Grossman, R. B. 356
Groves, L. 355
Gruber, C. P. 229, 344, 345
Grudzien, M. 351
Guerra-Farfan, E. 213, 348
Gurley, A. 345
Gusforf, R. E. 358
Guthrie, W. 176, 348, 351

Haberstroh, S. 151, 152, 348
Haden, G. 351
Hagerman, R. 342
Hahs-Vaughn, D. 343
Hall, R. W. 344
Hallett, S. 347
Hall-Lande, J. 176, 348
Hamilton, L. G. 353
Hammal, D. 351
Hancock, G. I. 354
Hanlon, J. 344
Hannah, K. E. 354

Happé, F. 351
Hardan, A. Y. 347
Harris, M. F. 351
Harrison, K. 168, 348
Hartman, D. 17, 21, 35, 58, 92, 114, 120,
    144, 145, 167, 171, 173, 198, 324, 348
Hattersley, C. 350
Havdahl, K. A. 231, 348
Heasman, B. 121, 346, 348
Heath, A. K. 347
Heeley, Q. 179, 346
Heider, D. 350
Helt, M. 347
Hens, K. 19, 86, 88, 134, 343, 348
Hepburn, S. 359
Heponiemi, T. 350
Herrán Salcedo, B. 57, 348
Hertz-Picciotto, I. 352
Hewitt, A. 348
Hietapakka, L. 350
Higgins, E. 351
Higgins, J. M. 162, 349
Hill, A. 178, 349
Hill, C. V. 196, 349
Hill, E. 345
Hillier, A. 171, 349
Hinze, E. 348
Hobson, H. M. 159, 349
Hobson, P. 57, 349
Hoevenaars-van den Boom, M. 346
Holingue, C. 265, 349
Hollocks, M. J. 161, 229, 349
Holloway, I. 358
Holt, R. 348
Holyfield, C. 205, 349
Honeybourne, V. 290, 349
Hong, J. S. 349
Hooft, L. 355
Hooley, M. 356
Horst, S. N. 358
Hosozawa, M. 352
Howard, B. 357
Howlin, P. 28, 349
Huang, J. 84, 342, 351
Huang, Y. E. 84, 342, 349
Hudock, R. L. 351
Huke, V. 161, 349
Hull, L. 223, 235, 342, 349, 350
Hultman, C. 356
Hultman, L. 343
Humphrey, A. 349
Huñez, J. H. 348
Hunter, M. 355

Hupfeld, K. E. 129, 349
Hus, V. 229, 345, 349
Hutchinson, A. 348, 359
Hwang, J. S. 353
Hwang, Y. E. 342
Hyman, S. L. 176, 349
Hynan, L. S. 353

Iacono, T. 351
Iannone, P. 213, 349
Intriago, K. E. C. 150, 349
Iosif, A. M. 354
Isaksson, J. 196, 349
Ismail, J. 353

Jaarsma, P. 131, 349
Jack, J. 350
Jackson, S. 353
Jackson-Perry, D. 58, 172, 350
Jagoe, C. 73, 350
Jelenic, P. 354
Jenaro-Rio, C. 352
Jiang, F. 359
Joanisse, M. F. 354
Johnson, M. 346
Johnston, L. 222, 346, 356
Jones, C. 82, 355
Jones, J. L. 350
Jones, L. 345
Jordan, A. 355
Jornet-Gibert, M. 348
Joshi, G. 161, 350
Joshi, L. 351
Joyce, A. 355

Kaale, A. 354
Kaihlanen, A.-M. 173, 350
Kalb, L. 359
Kalb, L. G. 349
Kamal Nor, N. 353
Kamp-Becker, I. 231, 350
Kanner, L. 36, 37, 88, 350
Kapp, S. 358
Kapp, S. K. 98, 131, 223, 211, 344, 350, 354, 355
Kasari, C. 357
Kassee, C. 196, 350
Katz, T. 343
Kaustav, P. S. 358
Kavanagh, M. 348
Kedar, I. 135, 350
Kedmy, A. 353
Keenan, L. 197, 351

Kelley, E. 347
Kennedy, D. P. 356
Kenny, L. 315, 350
Kenny, R. 348
Kent, A. 349
Kim, J. W. 353
Kim, J. Y. 353
Kindgren, E. 266, 350
King, M. 153, 350
Kirby, A. 343
Kiyu, A. 358
Klaiman, C. 233, 358
Klin, A. 345
Klusek, J. 154, 350
Knez, R. 350
Knoors, H. 346
Koenen, K. C. 164, 267, 350
Kofner, B. 354
Konyn, L. 359
Kostrzewa, E. 349
Kourti, M. 173, 350
Krasileva, K. 343
Kreider, C. M. 347
Kremkow, J. M. D. 349
Krumrei-Mancuso, E. J. 347
Kubina, R. M. 355
Kuhfeld, M. 357
Kuja-Halkola, R. 356
Kuo, D. Z. 349
Kuo, S. S. 134, 350
Küpper, C. 350
Kuyken, W. 350

Lachambre, C. 152, 350
Lai, M. C. 196, 232, 349, 350, 351, 358
Lainhart, J. E. 351, 352
LaLiberte, T. 348
Landa, R. 349, 357
Landa, R. J. 176, 351, 354
Langley, E. 358
Larsson, H. 345, 356
Lau, P. S. 348
Laurent, A. C. 355
Law, P. 347
Law, R. 352
Lawson, L. P. 342
Lawson, W. 47, 128, 297, 351, 353, 355
Le Couteur, A. 231, 351, 352
Leadbitter, K. 31, 222, 344, 351
Leader, G. 265, 351
Lebenhagen, C. 98, 351
Lebersfeld, J. B. 231, 233, 351
LeCouteur, A. 154, 356

Ledbetter, C. 353
Ledford, V. 358
Lee, A. 357
Lee, C. M. 227, 229, 351
Lee, L. C. 353
Leitner, Y. 347
Lentz, B. 355
Lepage, J.-F. 350
Lerner, M. D. 356
Lesser, M. 47, 128, 353
Leventhal, B. L. 345
Levesque, J. F. 196, 351
Levit-Binnun, N. 346
Levy, S. E. 349, 353
Lewis, A. 295, 351
Lewis, M. E. S. 352
Leyfer, O. T. 161, 351
Li, X. 359
Lichenstein, P. 344
Lichtenstein, P. 345, 356
Light, J. 349
Lippé, S. 350
Liu, X. 265, 351
Livingstone, N. 355
Lo, C. O. 359
Lockwood, A. 196, 247, 351
Logan, K. 201, 351
Lombardo, M. V. 232, 351
Long, R. M. 305, 351
López, B. 197, 351
Lopez, L. 355
Lord, C. 154, 224, 225, 226, 227, 230, 231, 232, 233, 343, 345, 347, 348, 349, 351, 352, 356, 357
Losh, M. 350
Loucas, T. 357
Lovaas, I. 39, 40, 345
Love, S. R. 356
Lovell, S. 356
Luck, H. 352
Ludvigsson, J. F. 345
Ludwig, N. N. 349
Lugo-Marín, J. 161, 352
Lui, L. M. 345
Lundin Remnélius, K. 235, 352
Lundström, S. 344
Luyster, R. J. 154, 231, 232, 351
Ly, A. R. 352
Lyall, K. 196, 352, 359

Ma, V. K. 342
Macari, S. 345
Macari, S. L. 354
Maciver, D. 346

MacLeod, A. 173, 350
Madaus, J. W. 347, 355
Madden, K. 348
Maddox, B. B. 163, 352
Maenner, M. J. 153, 352
Magán-Maganto, M. 352
Mahler, K. 116, 352
Mahoney, P. 344
Malik-Soni, N. 196, 197, 352
Maloney, E. 354
Mandell, D. S. 345, 352
Mandy, W. 163, 342, 343, 344, 349, 356
Manning-Courtney, P. 346
Mannion, A. 351
Marks, D. 352
Martin, G. E. 350
Mason, J. 83, 353
Matejko, M. 352
Mathy, P. 359
Matthews, N. L. 83, 352
Mauk, J. E. 353
May, T. 161, 352,
Maybery, M. T. 342
Mazefsky, C. A. 161, 352, 356
Mazurek, M. 352
McAlonan, G. M. 352, 265
McCabe, P. 135, 352
McCarthy, A. M. 51, 358
McCauley, J. B. 161, 352
McConachie, H. 351
McCormack, L. 311, 352
McCormack, T. 353
McCowen, S. 334
McCracken, J. T. 357
McDaniel, E. 196, 346
McDermott, C. 78, 352
McDonnell, A, 298, 313, 352
McDonnell, C. 346
McGee, S. C. 344
McGeown, S. 342
McGourty, J. 353
McGreevy, E. 32, 72, 96, 98, 135, 136, 158, 204, 258, 259, 261, 262, 288, 307, 352
McKean, C. 347
McLaughlin, K. A. 350
McMahon, W. M. 344
McNicholl, E. 56, 352
McQueen, E. 350
Melekoglu, M. A. 157, 359
Mendes, E. 349
Menezes, M. 309, 352
Mesa, S. 163, 353
Mesibov, G. B. 354

Messinger, D. 354
Meyer, A. T. 346
Midouhas, E. 352
Miller, H. L. 153, 353
Miller, J. S. 358
Miller, M. 359
Mills, E. 83, 344
Milton, D. 47, 72, 98, 122, 226, 287, 298, 313, 343, 344, 346, 347, 352, 353, 354, 355, 357, 358
Minardi, M. 349
Minshew, N. J. 352
Miserandino, C. 316, 353
Mishra, S. 348
Mitchell, P. 357
Mogensen, L. 83, 353
Mohd Nordin, A. 134, 353
Moles, D. 357
Molins, B. 350
Monsalve, A. 342
Montano, N. 349
Monteiro, M. J. 234, 353
Moody, E. J. 229, 353
Moon, S. J. 233, 353
Moore, A. 355
Moran, M. L. 342
Moreau, C. N. 354
Morgan, F. 291, 299, 353
Morgan, J. 344, 349, 351
Morgan, S. 205, 353
Morgan, Z. 358
Morrel, T. 357
Morris, C. 357
Morris, N. 347
Morrison, K. E. 82, 356
Morsanyi, K. 152, 353
Moss, J. 355
Moss, P. 349
Mottron, L. 354
Moyse, R. 352
MRC AIMS Consortium 351
Msall, M. E. 343
Mueller, V. T. 353
Mukherjee, S. 162, 163, 353
Mullin, A. E. 352
Murphy, C. 355
Murphy, C. A. 347
Murphy, D. G. M. 355
Murphy, K. 78, 79, 80, 296, 353
Murphy, S. 290, 353
Murray, A. L. 296, 347
Murray, D. 47, 128, 138, 139, 302, 304, 353
Murray, E. 352
Murray, F. 98, 235, 296, 297, 298, 342, 353

Myers, S. M. 349

Nadesan, M. H. 88, 353
Nadler, C. 359
Naigles, L. 347
Nalabolu, S. 355
Need, A. C. 359
Neilson, S. 346
Neimeijer, D. 359
Neumeier, S. M. 303, 353
NeuroClastic 348, 353, 355
Ng, L. 350
NICE, 145, 146, 147, 159, 214, 276, 277, 353, 354
Nicolaidis, C. 122, 354, 355
Nijhof, A. D. 346
Nimbley, E. 312, 354
Nizami, A. 349
Norbury, C. F. 3158, 159, 354
Nordahl-Hansen, A. 248, 354
Nottke, C. 348
NSAI (National Standards Authority of Ireland) 197, 354
Nugent, J. 356
Nusbaum, E. A. 222, 342
Nygren, A. 58, 343

O'Brien, M. 358
O'Brien, S. 342
O'Dell, L. 344
O'Donnell-Killen, T. 348, 354
O'Kelley, S. E. 351
O'Sullivan, J. 346
O'Toole, D. 349
Oliver, C. 355
Oredipe, T. 83, 354
Orinstein, A. 347
Orsini, M. 311, 354
Oseland, L. M. 350
Österborg Wiklund, S. 343
Ostrolenk, A. 136, 158, 354
Oswald, D. P. 352
Øyen, A. S. 348
Ozonoff, S. 176, 354, 359

Padesky, C. A. 350
Palmer, L. 344
Pan, H. 359
Parker, R. I. 347
Parks, K. M. A. 159, 354
Patel, D. R. 152, 357
Patten, K. 345
Paul, R. 345, 357

Paus, T. 355
Pavlopoulou, G. 261, 352, 354
Payne, K. 296, 354
Peacock, L. J. J. 342
Pearson, A. 232, 293, 307, 354
Pecora, L. 356
Pecora, L. A. 171, 354
Pellicano, E. 345, 349, 350, 355
Pellicano, L. 350
Pence- Stophaeros, S. 355
Penner, M. 355, 359
Pérez-Stable, E. J. 349
Peters, A. M. 136, 354
Petrides, K. V. 349
Petrovski, S. 359
Pettersson, E. 349
Petty, C. 350
Pfeiffer, D. 349
Pham, H. H. 355
Phung, J. 355
Pickles, A. 345, 354, 357
Pierce, K. 176, 355
Piescher, K. 348
Pillai, D. 357
Pillar, R. 342
Pirlot, C. 355
Pittwood, T. 356
Pohl, A. 171, 355
Polanczyk, G. V. 355
Polatajko, H. 343
Poliakoff, E. 344
Polyak, A. 355
Porayska-Pomsta, K. 355
Posner, J. 146, 355
Poustka, L. 350
Povey, C. 350
Prasad, V. 356
Prior, M. 355
Prizant, B. M. 134, 136, 355
Proctor, G. 355
Proedrou, A. 358
Prosser, R. 345
Proteau-Lemieux, M. 350
Purkis, Y. 123, 355

Quinn, A. 352
Quiñones Perez, A. 350

Ram, J. 51, 355
Randall, M. 154, 355
Rando, J. 359
Rapaport, H. 298, 306, 355

Ratanatharathorn, A. 350
Raymaker, D. M. 162, 355
Raznahan, A. 265, 355
Rebedew, D. L. 156, 358
Records, N. L. 358
Reetzke, R. 349
Reichenberg, A. 356
Reiersen, A. M. 229, 356
Reilly, S. 159, 355
Reis, S. M. 152, 347, 355
Renley, N. 343
Reuben, K. E. 163, 267, 255
Reyes, N. 353
Reynolds, A. 359
Riccio, A. 83, 354, 355
Rice-Adams, E. 126, 355
Richards, C. 154, 355
Richardson, S. 350
Richdale, A. L. 342
Richman, K. 222, 356
Rimland, B. 38, 356
Risi, S. 154, 342, 345, 351, 356
Risko, E. F. 356
Rispoli, M. J. 347
Rivero-Santana, A. 352
Roberts, J. 357
Roberts, K. 358
Robertson, D. 355
Robins, D. L. 228, 356, 359
Robinson, E. B. 350
Robinson, M. 345
Roche, L. 161, 356
Rodríguez, L. M. A. 349
Roepke, S. 350
Roessner, V. 350
Rolfhus, E. 359
Ropar, D. 346, 357
Rose, J. 150, 356
Rose, K. 162, 232, 293, 307, 352, 354, 356
Rosen, T. E. 356
Rosenberg, S. 359
Rosenberg, S. A. 353
Rosenblum, S. 343
Rosenthal, M. 347
Rossetti, K. G. 357
Rouse, S. 347
Rubin, E. 355
Ruigrok, A. N. 351
Russell, A. J. 344, 345
Russell, G. 155, 350, 351, 356, 358
Rutherford, M. 222, 346, 356
Rutter, M. 154, 229, 231, 232, 349, 351, 352, 356
Ryan, J. 357

Rydell, P. J. 355

Sacker, A. 352
Saeidi, S. 349
Sala, G. 265, 356
Saldana, D. 347
Salzman, E. 357
Samson, F. 354
Samtani, A. 355
Sandberg, G. 343
Sandberg, N. 355
Sandin, S. 311, 356
Sanguedolce, G. 343
Santinele Martino, A. 172, 356
Sasson, N. J. 82, 121, 346, 364, 356
Savage, S. 349
Sayal, K. 145, 256
Scarpa, A. 346
Scharer, M. 355
Scheeren, A. M. 344
Schneider, M. 357
Scholten, R. 355
Schopler, E. 233, 256
Schultz, R. T. 347
Scottish Intercollegiate Guidelines
        Network 215, 356
Seli, P. 3298, 356
Senande, L. L. 345
Serlachius, E. 345
Serpell, L. 344
Shah, P. 349
Shaker, A. 352
Sharp, J. L. 345
Sharpe, H. 354
Shaw, K. A. 352
Shaw, S. 346
Shaw, S. C. K. 346
Sheehy-Knight, J. 353
Shelton, J. 172, 358
Shephard, E. 354
Sheppard, E. 121, 354, 357
Sherrod, G. M. 353
Shimoni, H. N. 347
Shin, A. L. 353
Shiu, C. S. 343
Shriberg, L. D. 135, 357
Shulman, C. 342
Shulte-Körne, G. 151, 152, 348
Sieck, B. 347
Silberman, S. 36, 55, 357
Simmonds, M. 125–6, 357
Simonoff, E. 161, 196, 354, 357
Sinclair, J. 24, 42, 357

Singer, T. 122, 346
Singleton, J. L. 355
Slade, G. 197, 357
Smilek, D. 356
Smith, A. 344
Smith, C. J. 344
Smith, E. 358
Smith, L. G. E. 345
Smith, M. 311, 354
Smith, P. 348, 349, 358
Smits-Engelsman, B. 343
Soares, N. 357
Soland, J. 352
Solish, A. 354
Sonuga-Barke, E. 255
Spanoudis, G. 159, 347
Spence, S. 196, 357
Sponheim, E. 348
Sridhar, A. 174, 175, 357
Srivastava, R. 345
Staal, W. 346
Stadnick, N. A. 352
Stagnitti, K. 141, 357
Stankova, M. 358
Stannard, A. 344
Stanzione, C. M. 355
Stearns, P. N. 88, 357
Steckler, N. A. 355
Steffenburg, H. 97, 357
Steffenburg, S. 357
Stegall, S. 234, 353
Stenning, A. 343, 350, 358
Sterponi, L. 222, 359
Stevens, M. 347
Steward, R. 343, 350
Stewart, S. 342
Stewart-Artz, L. 357
Stinson, R. D. 347
Stokes, M. A. 171, 348, 354, 356
Stoll, M. M. 174, 357
Stone, W. L. 354
Storm, P. 343
Straiton, D. 174, 175, 357
Strickland, O. 346
Stroth, S. 350
Stuart, E. A. 351
Sturm, A. 229, 357
Sturner, R. 227, 357
Sugden, D. 343
Sulek, R. 351
Sumi, N. S. 345
Sun, C. 351
Sun, X. 351, 359

Surén, P. 348
Sutherland, R. 357, 209
Swaab, H. 346
Swanson, M. 351
Swineford, L. B. 348
Szatmari, P. 350, 351, 356, 359

Tager-Flusberg, H. 351
Taghrizi, M. 345
Talkowski, M. E. 350
Tamplain, P. M. 353
Tan, V. W. 358
Tauscher, J. 350
Tchanturia, K. 161, 359
Tellez, D. 349
Tempier, A. 349
Teo, A. R. 355
Thayer, J. 355
The Section on Telehealth Care 344
Therapist Neurodiversity Collective 46, 51, 357
Thijs, J. 24, 344
Thomás, D. 352
Thomas, N. 192, 357
Thompson, A. 344
Thompson, L. 347
Thompson-Hodgetts, S. 306, 357
Thorsen, M. 345
Thresher, K. 247, 257
Thurm, A. 154, 342, 357
Timimi, S. 230, 233, 358
Todd, R. D. 356
Todres, L. 358, 261
Toft, A. 171, 172, 358
Toh, T. H. 227, 358
Tolonen, A. K. 347
Tomblin, J. B. 159, 358
Toro, R. 355
Toseeb, U. 349
Totton, N. 76, 87, 169, 358
Townsend, E. A. 308, 359
Treffert, D. A. 156, 358
Trembath, D. 351, 357
Triana, A. J. 209, 358
Trinkl, J. 355
Trollor, J. N. 342, 349
Tromans, S. 174, 223, 358
Trott, J. 344
Troxell-Whitman, Z. 125, 344
Troyb, E. 347
Tsai, K. F. 359
Tulip, J. 347
Turk, J. 348
Tyson, K. 347

Uddin, L. Q. 156, 156, 358
Ugianskis, M. 346
Ukoumunne, O. C. 355
Uljarević, M. 342
Ulvund, S. E. 354
Underhill, J. C. 82, 358
Ungar, W. J. 359
Utley, I. 346

Valvano, L. 172, 358
Vamvakas, G. 354
van Bers, B. M. C. W. 353
Van Bourgondien, M. E. 346, 356
Van de Water, J. 352
van der Merwe, C. 350
Van Goidsenhoven, L. 134, 343, 348
van Santen, J. P. 357
Varcin, K. 342, 348
Vasa, R. A. 356
Vatsa, D. 344
Verhoeven, L. 346
Vervloed, M. P. J. 346
Viering, K. L. 350
Vincent, J. 354
Vinçon, S. 343
Viskochil, J. 344
Vogindroukas, I. 358
Volk, H. E. 356
Volkmar, F. 345

Wainwright, A. 344
Wake, M. 355
Wakefield, D. A. 358
Walker, N. 23, 47, 72, 80, 97, 106, 344
Walton, K. 357
Waltz, M. 88, 358
Walum, H. 350
Wammes, J. D. 356
Wang, H. 359
Warrier, V. 171, 358
Wassell, C. 92, 358
Watson, N. 346
Weir, E. 171, 198, 358
Weise, J. 349
Welch, C. 367
Welch, K. 342
Welin, S. 131, 349
Wellman, G. J. 356
Wenger, T. L. 154, 358
Westwood, H. 161, 359
Wetherby, A. M. 348, 355
Wharton, T. 350

Whelan, S. 351
White, C. 349
White, R. 356
White, S. 350
Whitehouse, A. J. 342
Whitehouse, A. J. O. 345
Wieckowski, A. T. 277, 359
Wiersema, J. R. 346
Wiggins, L. 353
Wiggins, L. D. 134, 359
Wilcock, A. A. 308, 359
Wiley, R. E. 352
Williams, D. 359
Williams, G. L. 344
Williams, K. 352
Williams, L. N. 359
Wilson, P. 343
Wing, L. 37, 38, 39. 359
Winter, A. S. 347
Wise, S. J. 359
Wodka, E. L. 135, 359
Wolff, N. 350
Wong, G. T. L. 357
Wong, S. W. 352
Wood, E. 344
Wood, R. 46, 58, 296, 297, 298, 305, 347, 259
Woods, R. 235, 347
Woods, S. E. O. 223, 235, 347, 359
Woolf, S. H. 213, 359
World Federation of Occupational
    Therapists 308, 359
Wozniak, J. 350
Wray, C. 354
Wray, J. 342
Wu, I. C. 157, 359
Wu, L. 351
Wu, S. 159, 359

Xavier, A. 357
Xie, M. 345

Yao, G. L. 358
Yergeau, M. 121, 354, 359
Yilmaz-Yenioglu, B. 157, 359
Young, G. S. 354
Youngstrom, E. A. 347
Yu, B. 222, 359
Yu, Y. 231, 259
Yuen, T. 228, 359

Zadurian, N. 312, 313, 354
Zhang, C. 345

Zhang, X. 358
Zhang, Y. 359
Zhao, J. 359
Zhu, Q. 349
Zhu, X. 153, 359
Ziermans, T. 346

Zisk, A. H. 32, 96, 346, 359
Zou, M. 351
Zubizarreta, S. C. P. 346
Zubler, J. 359
Zwaigenbaum, L. 354